Innovative Endocrinology of Cancer

ADVANCES IN EXPERIMENTAL MEDICINE AND BIOLOGY

A Continuation Order Plan is available for this series. A continuation order will bring delivery of each new volume immediately upon publication. Volumes are billed only upon actual shipment. For further information please contact the publisher.

Innovative Endocrinology of Cancer

Edited by

Lev M. Berstein, MD, PhD, DMS

*Laboratory of Oncoendocrinology, Professor N.N. Petrov Research Institute
of Oncology, St. Petersburg, Russia*

Richard J. Santen, MD

*Division of Endocrinology and Metabolism, University of Virginia Health
Sciences Center, Charlottesville, Virginia, USA*

Springer Science+Business Media, LLC
Landes Bioscience

Springer Science+Business Media, LLC
Landes Bioscience

Printed in the U.S.A.

Springer Science+Business Media, LLC, 233 Spring Street, New York, New York 10013, USA
http://www.springer.com

Please address all inquiries to the publishers:
Landes Bioscience, 1002 West Avenue, 2nd Floor, Austin, Texas 78701, USA
Phone: 512/ 637 5060; FAX: 512/ 637 6079
http://www.landesbioscience.com

Innovative Endocrinology of Cancer, edited by Lev M. Berstein and Richard J. Santen,
Landes Bioscience / Springer Science+Business Media, LLC dual imprint / Springer series: Advances
in Experimental Medicine and Biology

ISBN: 978-0-387-78817-3

While the authors, editors and publisher believe that drug selection and dosage and the specifications and
usage of equipment and devices, as set forth in this book, are in accord with current recommendations
and practice at the time of publication, they make no warranty, expressed or implied, with respect to
material described in this book. In view of the ongoing research, equipment development, changes in
governmental regulations and the rapid accumulation of information relating to the biomedical sciences,
the reader is urged to carefully review and evaluate the information provided herein.

Library of Congress Cataloging-in-Publication Data

Innovative endocrinology of cancer / edited by Lev M. Berstein, Richard J. Santen.
   p. ; cm. -- (Advances in experimental medicine and biology ; v. 630)
Includes bibliographical references and index.
ISBN 978-0-387-78817-3
1. Cancer--Endocrine aspects. I. Berstein, Lev M. II. Santen, Richard J. III. Series.
[DNLM: 1. Breast Neoplasms--physiopathology. 2. Breast Neoplasms--drug therapy. 3. Estrogen
Receptor Modulators--pharmacology. 4. Receptors, Estrogen--physiology. 5. Receptors, Progester-
one--physiology. W1 AD559 v.630 2008 / WP 870 I565 2008]
RC268.2.I56 2008
616.99'4071--dc22
                           2008006861

PREFACE

At the beginning of the 21th century, hormone-associated tumors made up not less than 30-40% of all human cancers.[1] Thus, the importance of the problem—both medical and social—was the first reason for the creation of this volume. Accordingly, the first goal of the book was to review different aspects of the extensive field of research in the area covered by the notion 'hormones and cancer'.

First, however does not necessarily mean main. Most of us know that science is about asking questions and finding credible ways to answer them and that it works best in a culture that welcomes challenges to prevailing dogmas.[2] Thus, the principal aim of this volume is to describe these new and attractive ideas and methods which have animated oncoendocrinolgy in recent years. To fulfill this task, the co-editors of the book were guided by a desire to describe the rich innovation in this field.

As a result, the volume is devoted to the new developments in such topics as mechanisms of hormonal carcinogenesis (contributions of J. Chen et al; J. Russo and I. Russo; L. Berstein), epidemiology and risk factors (contributions of S. Ukraintseva et al; A. Hjartåker et al; A.H. Eliassen and S. Hankinson), hormone production by tumor tissue (contribution of S. Bulun and E. Simpson) and hormonal sensitivity of the latter (contribution of C. Lange et al), genesis, dichotomy and endocrinology of cancer in females (contribution of C. Gründker et al), pharmacogenomics and proteomics in oncoendocrinology (contributions of D. Tyson and D. Ornstein; R. Weinshilboum), biological core of hormonal and antihormonal therapy of cancer (contributions of R. Santen et al; A. Butt et al; S. Sengupta and V. C. Jordan) and its prevention (T. Powles' contribution).

As once was said by prominent writer: 'Novelists are either "large-audience" or "small-audience"'.[3] We are hoping that readership of the book (which testifies that endocrinology of cancer has gone a long and fruitful way) will increase gradually and receive further stimulus needed for subsequent achievements in this interesting area.

Lev M. Berstein, MD, PhD, DMS
Richard J. Santen, MD

1. Parkin DM, Fernandez LM. Use of statistics to assess the global burden of breast cancer. Breast J 2006; 12(Suppl 1):S70-80.
2. Omenn GS. Grand challenges and great opportunities in science, technology, and public policy. Science 2006; 314:1696-704.
3. Bellow S. Something to Remember Me By: Three Tales. New York: Viking, 1991.

ABOUT THE EDITORS...

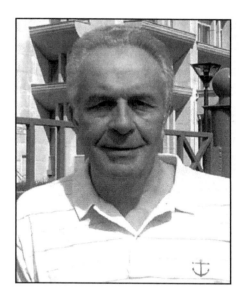

DR. LEV M. BERSTEIN is Chief of Laboratory of Oncoendocrinology at Petrov Research Institute of Oncology, St. Petersburg, Russia. His main scientific interests include mechanisms of hormonal carcinogenesis, risk factors of hormone-associated neoplasms and new approaches to prevention and treatment of the latter. He received several international distinctions (including INTAS grant and UICC Translational Cancer Research Fellowship), and serves as a Member of Council of Russian Endocrine Association, on the editorial boards of two national journals and as a reviewer for *Future Oncology, Journal of Cancer Research and Clinical Oncology, Molecular and Cellular Endocrinology, Cancer Epidemiology, Biomarkers and Prevention* and others. In his bibliography are 7 monographs, 16 chapters and more than 100 papers in peer-reviewed journals. He graduated as MD from Tartu University in Estonia and received his PhD and DMS degrees in Cancer Endocrinology at the Petrov Institute in St. Petersburg.

ABOUT THE EDITORS...

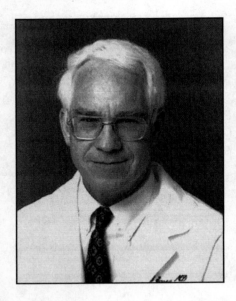

DR. RICHARD SANTEN is Professor of Medicine in the Division of Endocrinology at the University of Virginia Health Sciences Center. He graduated from the University of Michigan Medical School and trained in Internal Medicine at the Cornell/New York Hospital Medical Center and at the University of Michigan. He received fellowship training at the University of Washington School of Medicine. After completion of fellowship, he joined the faculty of the Pennsylvania State University School of Medicine where he rose through the academic ranks to become Evan Pugh Professor of Medicine, Chief of the Division of Endocrinology, Diabetes, and Metabolism, and Vice Chair of the Department of Medicine. Dr. Santen moved to Detroit, Michigan, in 1993 to become Chair of the Department of Medicine at the Wayne State University School of Medicine. He then joined the faculty of the University of Virginia where he presently works. Dr. Santen has contributed to the development of various endocrine treatments of breast cancer and particularly the development of aromatase inhibitors. For that work, he was awarded the Brinker International Award of the Susan Komen Foundation. He currently investigates the basic mechanisms whereby estrogens cause breast tumor growth and is developing tools with which to evaluate the need for estrogen treatment in menopausal women. He is the author of more than 250 scientific publications and 75 chapters and has written three medically related books.

PARTICIPANTS

Hany Abdel-Hafiz
Departments of Medicine, Pathology,
    and Obstetrics and Gynecology
University of Colorado
Health Sciences Center
Aurora, Colorado
USA

Konstantin G. Arbeev
Center for Population Health
    and Aging
Duke University
Durham, North Carolina
USA

Lev M. Berstein
Laboratory of Oncoendocrinology
Professor N.N. Petrov
    Research Institute of Oncology
St. Petersburg
Russia

Terry R. Brown
Department of Biochemistry
    and Molecular Biology
Johns Hopkins Bloomberg
    School of Public Health
Baltimore, Maryland
USA

Serdar E. Bulun
Robert H. Lurie Comprehensive
    Cancer Center
and
Department of Obstetrics
    and Gynecology
Northwestern University
Chicago, Illinois
USA

Alison J. Butt
Cancer Research Program
Garvan Institute of Medical Research
Darlinghurst, New South Wales
Australia

C. Elizabeth Caldon
Cancer Research Program
Garvan Institute of Medical Research
Darlinghurst, New South Wales
Australia

Jin-Qiang Chen
Department of Medicine
University of Virginia
    School of Medicine
Charlottesville, Virginia
USA

Hidtek Eguchi
Department of Molecular
    Epidemiology
Hiroshima University Graduate School
    of Biomedical Sciences
and
Department of Radiobiology
    and Molecular Epidemiology
Radiation Effects Research
    Foundation
Hiroshima
Japan

A. Heather Eliassen
Channing Laboratory
Brigham and Women's Hospital
Boston, Massachusetts
USA

Günter Emons
Department of Gynecology
  and Obstetrics
Georg-August-University
Göttingen
Germany

Ping Fan
Division of Endocrinology
  and Metabolism
University of Virginia Health
  Sciences Center
Charlottesville, Virginia
USA

Carsten Gründker
Department of Gynecology
  and Obstetrics
Georg-August-University
Göttingen
Germany

Andreas R. Günthert
Department of Gynecology
  and Obstetrics
Georg-August-University
Göttingen
Germany

Susan E. Hankinson
Department of Epidemiology
Harvard School of Public Health
Boston, Massachusetts
USA

Shin-ichi Hayashi
Department of Medical Technology
Tohoku University School of Medicine
Hiroshima
Japan

Anette Hjartåker
Department of Etiological Research
Cancer Registry of Norway
Oslo
Norway

Kathryn B. Horwitz
Departments of Medicine, Pathology,
  and Obstetrics and Gynecology
University of Colorado
Health Sciences Center
Aurora, Colorado
USA

Britta M. Jacobsen
Departments of Medicine, Pathology,
  and Obstetrics and Gynecology
University of Colorado
Health Sciences Center
Aurora, Colorado
USA

V. Craig Jordan
Fox Chase Cancer Center
Philadelphia, Pennsylvania
USA

Carol A. Lange
University of Minnesota Cancer Center
Division of Hematology
Departments of Medicine,
Pharmacology, Oncology
  and Transplants
Minneapolis, Minnesota
USA

Hilde Langseth
Department of Etiological Research
Cancer Registry of Norway
Oslo
Norway

Shigeru Masamura
Department of Surgery
Tokyo Dental College
  Ichikawa General Hospital
Sugano, Ichikawa
Japan

Catriona M. McNeil
Cancer Research Program
Garvan Institute of Medical Research
Darlinghurst, New South Wales
Australia

Elizabeth A. Musgrove
Cancer Research Program
Garvan Institute of Medical Research
Darlinghurst, New South Wales
Australia

Kei Nakachi
Department of Molecular
   Epidemiology
Hiroshima University Graduate School
   of Biomedical Sciences
and
Department of Radiobiology
   and Molecular Epidemiology
Radiation Effects Research
   Foundation
Hiroshima
Japan

David K. Ornstein
Department of Urology
University of California Irvine
   Medical Center
Orange, California
USA

Trevor J. Powles
Parkside Oncology Clinic
London
UK

Irma H. Russo
Breast Cancer Research Laboratory
Fox Chase Cancer Center
Philadelphia, Pennsylvania
USA

Jose Russo
Breast Cancer Research Laboratory
Fox Chase Cancer Center
Philadelphia, Pennslyvania
USA

Richard J. Santen
Division of Endocrinology
   and Metabolism
University of Virginia
   Health Sciences Center
Charlottesville, Virginia
USA

Carol A. Sartorius
Departments of Medicine, Pathology,
   and Obstetrics and Gynecology
University of Colorado
Health Sciences Center
Aurora, Colorado
USA

Surojeet Sengupta
Fox Chase Cancer Center
Philadelphia, Pennsylvania
USA

Evan R. Simpson
Prince Henry's Institute of Medical
   Research
Clayton, Victoria
Australia

Tetsuya Sogon
Department of Molecular
   Epidemiology
Hiroshima University Graduate School
   of Biomedical Sciences
and
Department of Radiobiology
   and Molecular Epidemiology
Radiation Effects Research
   Foundation
Hiroshima
Japan

Robert X. Song
Division of Endocrinology
   and Metabolism
University of Virginia
   Health Sciences Center
Charlottesville, Virginia
USA

Monique A. Spillman
Departments of Medicine, Pathology,
   and Obstetrics and Gynecology
University of Colorado
Health Sciences Center
Aurora, Colorado
USA

Robert L. Sutherland
Cancer Research Program
Garvan Institute of Medical Research
Darlinghurst, New South Wales
and
Department of Medicine
St. Vincent's Clinical School
University of New South Wales
Randwick, New South Wales
Australia

Alexander Swarbrick
Cancer Research Program
Garvan Institute of Medical Research
Darlinghurst, New South Wales
Australia

Darren R. Tyson
Departments of Urology, Physiology
    and Biophysics
University of California Irvine
    Medical Center
Orange, California
USA

Svetlana V. Ukraintseva
Center for Population Health
    and Aging
Duke University
Durham, North Carolina
USA

Elisabete Weiderpass
Department of Etiological Research
Cancer Registry of Norway
Oslo
Norway
and
Department of Medical Epidemiology
    and Biostatistics
Karolinska Institutet
Stockholm
Sweden
and
Department of Genetics Epidemiology
Folkhalsan Research Center
Helsinki
Finland

Richard Weinshilboum
Mayo Clinic College of Medicine
Mayo Clinic – Mayo Foundation
Rochester, Minnesota
USA

James D. Yager
Department of Environmental
    Health Sciences
Johns Hopkins Bloomberg School
    of Public Health
Baltimore, Maryland
USA

Anatoly I. Yashin
Center for Population Health
    and Aging
Duke University
Durham, North Carolina
USA

Wei Yue
Division of Endocrinology
    and Metabolism
University of Virginia
    Health Sciences Center
Charlottesville, Virginia,
USA

CONTENTS

8. AROMATASE EXPRESSION IN WOMEN'S CANCERS 112

Serdar E. Bulun and Evan R. Simpson

9. PROTEOMICS OF CANCER OF HORMONE-DEPENDENT
    TISSUES 133

Darren R. Tyson and David K. Ornstein

10. ENDOGENOUS HORMONE LEVELS AND RISK OF BREAST,
     ENDOMETRIAL AND OVARIAN CANCERS:
     PROSPECTIVE STUDIES 148

A. Heather Eliassen and Susan E. Hankinson

11. HORMONAL HETEROGENEITY OF ENDOMETRIAL CANCER 166

Carsten Gründker, Andreas R. Günthert and Günter Emons

12. CELL CYCLE MACHINERY: LINKS WITH GENESIS AND TREATMENT OF BREAST CANCER 189

Alison J. Butt, C. Elizabeth Caldon, Catriona M. McNeil, Alexander Swarbrick, Elizabeth A. Musgrove and Robert L. Sutherland

13. SELECTIVE ESTROGEN MODULATORS AS AN ANTICANCER TOOL: MECHANISMS OF EFFICIENCY AND RESISTANCE 206

Surojeet Sengupta and V. Craig Jordan

ACKNOWLEDGEMENTS

The editors of this book are grateful to all authors of chapters for their innovative input and to the Landes Bioscience staff for their friendly atmosphere and cooperation during preparation of the book.

CHAPTER 1

Mechanisms of Hormone Carcinogenesis:
Evolution of Views, Role of Mitochondria

Jin-Qiang Chen,* Terry R. Brown and James D. Yager

Abstract

Cumulative and excessive exposure to estrogens is associated with increased breast cancer risk. The traditional mechanism explaining this association is that estrogens affect the rate of cell division and apoptosis and thus manifest their effect on the risk of breast cancer by affecting the growth of breast epithelial tissues. Highly proliferative cells are susceptible to genetic errors during DNA replication. The action of estrogen metabolites offers a complementary genotoxic pathway mediated by the generation of reactive estrogen quinone metabolites that can form adducts with DNA and generate reactive oxygen species through redox cycling. In this chapter, we discussed a novel mitochondrial pathway mediated by estrogens and their cognate estrogen receptors (ERs) and its potential implications in estrogen-dependent carcinogenesis. Several lines of evidence are presented to show: (1) mitochondrial localization of ERs in human breast cancer cells and other cell types; (2) a functional role for the mitochondrial ERs in regulation of the mitochondrial respiratory chain (MRC) proteins and (3) potential implications of the mitochondrial ER-mediated pathway in stimulation of cell proliferation, inhibition of apoptosis and oxidative damage to mitochondrial DNA. The possible involvement of estrogens and ERs in deregulation of mitochondrial bioenergetics, an important hallmark of cancer cells, is also described. An evolutionary view is presented to suggest that persistent stimulation by estrogens through ER signaling pathways of MRC proteins and energy metabolic pathways leads to the alterations in mitochondrial bioenergetics and contributes to the development of estrogen-related cancers.

Introduction

Cumulative and excessive exposure to endogenous and exogenous estrogens is an important determinant of breast cancer risk in postmenopausal women.[1-3] The traditional mechanism to explain this association is that estrogens affect the rate of cell division and thus manifest their effect by stimulating the proliferation of breast epithelial cells. Proliferating cells are susceptible to genetic errors during DNA replication which, if uncorrected, can ultimately lead to a malignant phenotype.[4] This paradigm has recently been expanded by a complementary genotoxic pathway mediated by the generation of reactive estrogen quinone metabolites that can form adducts in DNA and generate reactive oxygen species through redox cycling. Evidence supporting a role for estrogen metabolites in animal and human breast carcinogenesis has been reviewed (Fig. 1).[1,4] While both the traditional paradigm and the genotoxic pathway are plausible, the precise role of

*Corresponding Author: Jin-Qiang Chen—Division of Pulmonary and Critical Care, Department of Medicine, University of Virginia School of Medicine, Charlottesville, VA 22908-0546 USA. Email: jinqiang.chen@virginia.edu

Innovative Endocrinology of Cancer, edited by Lev M. Berstein and Richard J. Santen. ©2008 Landes Bioscience and Springer Science+Business Media.

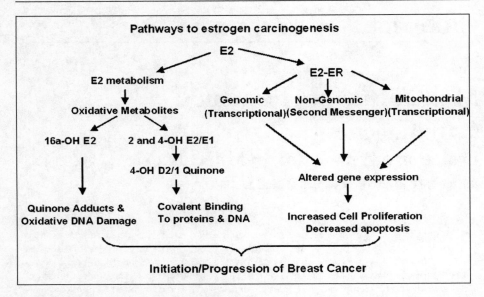

Figure 1. Pathways for estrogen carcinogenesis This figure was taken from Yager JD, Davidson NE. N Engl J Med 2006; 354(3):270-282 with permission granted by New England Journal of Medicine © 2006 Massachusettes Medical Society. All rights reserved.[1]

17-β estradiol (E_2) in breast cancer development is not fully understood, pointing to the involvement of other pathways.

Estrogen receptors (ERs) are ligand-activated transcription factors that mediate the biological activities of estrogens in target tissues. These receptors usually reside in the cytosol where they bind to their ligands and translocate to the nucleus. Like other steroid hormone receptors, the nuclear ERs typically bind as dimers to consensus cis-acting regulatory target DNA sequences termed estrogen responsive elements (EREs) and directly regulate gene transcription. Alternatively, ERs can also interact with other chromatin-bound transcription factors such as AP-1 or Sp1 to enhance or repress gene transcription.[5,6] These have been referred to as the genomic or nuclear-initiated estrogen responses. Alternatively, several rapid, nongenomic pathways mediated by membrane localized ERs also affect cell proliferation and apoptosis.[7,8] Even more intriguing are the recent findings that ERs localize within mitochondria and regulate mitochondrial gene transcription and the intrinsic mitochondrial apoptotic pathways.[9-12] In this chapter, we will discuss novel estrogen activities that are mediated by the ER-dependent mitochondrial pathway and the potential implications of this pathway in estrogen carcinogenesis.

A Novel Paradigm: Estrogen/Estrogen Receptor-Mediated Mitochondrial Pathway

Mitochondria as Important Targets for the Action of Steroid and Thyroid Hormones and Their Respective Receptors

Mitochondria are cellular organelles with a double membrane. Although the outer membrane is relatively smooth, the inner membrane is highly convoluted, forming folds termed cristae. It is on these cristae that metabolic substrates are combined with oxygen to produce ATP (Fig. 2). Mitochondria traditionally participate in multiple cellular functions including: generation of more than 90% of the cell's energy requirements through oxidative phosphorylation; regulation of intracellular calcium homeostasis; control of various ion channels and transporters and participation

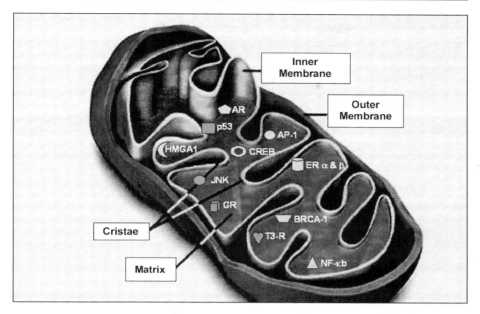

Figure 2. Structural features of mitochondria and the presence of steroid and thyroid hormone receptors and nuclear transcriptional factors within mitochondria. AR: androgen receptor; AP-1: Activation protein-1; BRCA1: protien coded by breast cancer-1 gene; CREB: cyclic AMP response element binding protein; ERα and β: Estrogen receptor α and β; GR: glucocorticoid receptor; JNK: Jun N-terminal kinase; HMGA-1: high mobility group protein A-1; NF-κB: nuclear factor κB; T3R: Thyroid hormone receptor.

in heme and steroid biosynthesis. In addition, mitochondria have a role in regulation of cellular proliferation and apoptosis.[13,14] Each human cell contains hundreds to several thousand copies of the 16.5 kb mitochondrial genome (mtDNA).[15] The coding sequences for 2 rRNAs, 22 tRNAs and 13 proteins are contiguous and without introns. A single major noncoding region, referred to as the displacement loop (D-loop), contains the primary regulatory sequences for transcription and initiation of replication. MtDNA is first transcribed to a larger mitochondrial transcript precursor, from which the 13 mRNAs, 22 tRNAs and 2 rRNAs are derived.

The transcription and translation of the mRNAs into thirteen proteins within mitochondria[16,17] are under the regulation of various molecules.[18] Among these molecules are hormones and other factors, including cortisol,[19,20] androgen,[21] glucocorticoids,[22-27] 1, 25α-dihydroxyvitamin D$_3$,[28] thyroid hormone,[29-31] estrogens,[32] and peroxisome proliferators,[33] that have profound effects on mitochondrial respiratory chain (MRC) activities. Support for the regulatory effects of these hormones on mitochondrial gene transcription, specifically on genes involved in oxidative phosphorylation comes from several types of studies. First, the receptors for glucocorticoids,[18,24,26,34] thyroid hormone,[26,29,35,36] estrogens,[11,12,32,37,38] (see below for details) and androgens,[39] have been detected in mitochondria (Fig. 2); Second, specific steroid hormone responsive elements for glucocorticoids,[40-45] thyroid hormone,[30,46-48] and estrogen,[9,49] are found in the nucleotide sequence of the human mtDNA regulatory region; Third, the ligand-activated glucocorticoid receptor,[18,25] a variant form of the thyroid hormone receptor[30,46-48] and a 45 kDa protein related to peroxisome proliferator-activated receptor γ2[33] have each been shown to mediate stimulatory effects on mitochondrial gene expression; and Fourth, these hormones and their receptors control a number of cellular processes including apoptosis and cell proliferation.[50,51] It is likely that hormonal regulation of mitochondrial gene transcription occurs through mechanisms similar to those that control nuclear gene transcription. These insights extend our understanding of hormone action at the cellular level.

In addition to steroid hormone receptors, other nuclear transcription factors (e.g., NF-κB, AP-1 and p53) have been detected in mitochondria (Fig. 2). The cis-acting regulatory binding sites for these and other transcription factors have been identified in the mtDNA (for review see ref. 18) and their ability to modulate mitochondrial gene expression and affect energy regulation has been observed.

The mitochondria store a host of critical apoptotic activators and inhibitors in their intermembrane space. The release of such factors could represent another mode of action for these hormone receptors and transcription factors within mitochondria.

Collectively, these observations suggest that the mitochondrial genome is an important target for the direct actions of steroid and thyroid hormones and their cognate receptors. The effects of glucocorticoid and thyroid hormones and their receptors on mitochondrial function have been reviewed.[18,26,52,53] Here, we focus on the role of estrogens and ERs in the regulation of mitochondrial function.

Mitochondrial Localization of Estrogen Receptors

During the past decade, a number of studies detected both ERα and ERβ in the cytoplasm of many types of cells and tissues (see ref. 11 for review), although it was unclear whether these receptors were free within the cytoplasm or resided within specific organelles. Monje and colleagues were the first to report the presence of ERα and ERβ in the mitochondria of rat ovarian and uterine tissues.[38,54] More recent studies have definitively demonstrated the presence of ERα and ERβ in mitochondria. For example, Chen et al used confocal microscopy and immunogold electron microscopy to show the predominant localization of ERβ, but also ERα in mitochondria of MCF-7 cells.[11,55] These observations were independently confirmed by Pedram et al.[56] ERβ has also been detected in mitochondria of other cells, including human liver tumor-derived cancer HepG2 cells;[10,57] osteosarcoma SaOS-2 cells,[57] sperm,[39] lens epithelial cells,[58,59] cardiomyocytes[37] and periodontal ligament cells;[60] rat primary neurons and cardiomyocytes[37] and murine hippocampal cells.[37,61] ERα was localized in mitochondria of rat cerebral blood vessels.[62] Interestingly, these cell types exhibit a common requirement for high levels of energy derived from mitochondria to maintain their normal physiological activities.

Stimulation of Mitochondrial Respiratory Chain Gene Expression and Function by Estrogen and ERs

The presence of ERα and ERβ in mitochondria suggests that they may play a key role in the regulation of MRC function by estrogens. As mentioned above, mtDNA encodes 13 proteins that participate in the processes of oxidative phosphorylation. Mounting evidence supports a role for estrogens in mitochondrial gene transcription. For instance, a 16-fold increase in the levels of cytochrome oxidase II(COII) mRNA was observed in GH4C1 rat pituitary tumor cells treated with 0.5 nM E_2 for 6 days.[63] Treatment of ovariectomized female rats with E_2 induced transcript levels of COIII in the hippocampus following treatment for 3 hours.[64] Several mtDNA gene transcripts, including COI, COII, COIII, NADH dehydrogenase subunit 1 (ND1) and ATP synthase subunits 6 and 8, were increased in HepG2 cells and rat hepatocytes treated with ethinyl estradiol (EE).[65-67] In human beast cancer MCF-7 cells, E_2 treatment enhanced the transcript levels of COI, COII and ND1 and these effects were blocked by the ER antagonist, ICI182780, suggesting the involvement of ERs.[10,11] Hsieh et al[68] observed up-regulation of MRC complex IV by the ERβ-selective ligand, diarylpropionitrile (DPN), in rat cardiomyocytes. Jonsson et al[60] observed that E_2-induced attenuation of COI expression in human periodontal ligament cells involved ERβ. Stirone et al[69] reported that in vivo treatment of ovariectomized female rats with E_2 increased the levels of nuclear- and mtDNA-encoded MCR proteins in cerebrovascular mitochondria and increased the energy-producing capacity of these cells.

Whereas the mechanisms of estrogen-induced mitochondrial gene transcription are not fully understood, several lines of evidence support a role for the binding of ERs to EREs in the mtDNA in response to E_2. First, nucleotide sequences with homology to the EREs found in estrogen-responsive nuclear genes have been detected in the D-loop of mouse and human mtDNA.[49,70] Second, using electrophoretic mobility shift assays and surface plasmon resonance analysis, recombinant human ER (rhERα), rhERβ and ERβ present in mitochondrial protein extracts were shown to bind specifically to these mtDNA EREs and this binding was enhanced by E_2 in a time- and dose-dependent manner (Fig. 3).[9,10] The presence of these putative mtDNA EREs and the binding of ERα and ERβ to them lend support for a novel ER signal transduction pathway. These lines of evidence suggest that ERs mediate mtDNA transcription in the same manner as the glucocorticoid receptor which is translocated into the mitochondria and binds to glucocorticoid response elements after treatment with glucocorticoids.[22,25]

The majority of MRC proteins and a number of other proteins involved in the assembly of MRC complexes, the replication and transcription of mtDNA and translation of mtRNAs, are encoded by nuclear DNA, synthesized in the cytosol and subsequently imported into mitochondria. However, proper MRC biogenesis and functions depend on the coordinate expression and correct assembly of both nuclear- and mtDNA-encoded proteins, a complex process that requires a variety of well orchestrated regulatory mechanisms between the physically separate nuclear and mitochondrial compartments.[71,72]

Numerous observations now support a role for estrogens in induction of nuclear-encoded MRC proteins and stimulation of mitochondrial respiration. Treatment of ovariectomized rats with estrogens substantially increased respiratory rate, glycolytic activities and glucose utilization in their uterus in concert with uterine growth.[73] In the liver of EE-treated rats and in E_2-treated HepG2 cells, transcript levels for nuclear genes, e.g., mitochondrial ATP synthase subunit E, were increased along with the enhanced mRNA levels for several mtDNA genes.[65,66] Moreover, these effects were accompanied by increased MRC activity.[66,74] Among the estrogen responsive genes identified in MCF-7 cells was the nDNA-encoded COVII whose promoter region contained a consensus ERE that exhibited E_2-dependent enhancer activity.[75] Several nuclear-encoded MRC genes

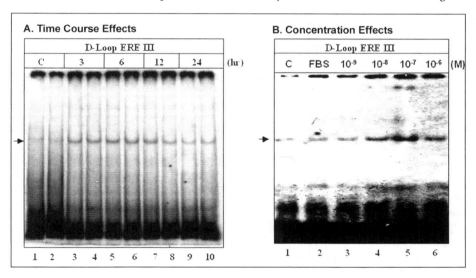

Figure 3. Time- and concentration-dependent effects of E2 on the binding on MCF-7 mitochondrial protein extracts to D-loop ERE III MCF-7 cells cultured in media containing 5% charcoal-striped fetal bovine serum (FBS) for five days were treated with E2 (100 nM) for the indicated time points (A) or with E2 (B) at the indicated concentrations. Mitochondrial protein extracts were prepared and EMSA were performed as described.[9] This figure was taken from Chen et al[9] with permission granted by the *Journal of Cellular Biochemistry*.

(e.g., COVa; and mitochondrial ATP synthase subunits β and F) were up-regulated in dysplastic prostates of Noble rats following administration of testosterone and E2.[76] The nuclear-encoded subunit C isoform of the F0 complex of mitochondrial ATP synthase (F1/F0) and mitochondrial ribosomal protein 3 were up-regulated by estrogens in ERα-positive breast cancer cells.[77] O'Lone et al[78] performed gene expression profiling in aorta of ERα knock out (ERα KO) and ERβKO mice to identify comprehensive gene sets whose levels of expression were regulated by long-term (one week) estrogen treatment. They noted that ERα was essential for the stimulation of a majority of the estrogen-induced genes in the aorta whereas ERβ primarily mediated estrogen-dependent decreases in gene expression. Among the estrogen-regulated genes were those involved in electron transport and the control of reactive oxygen species. Of particular note, the estrogen/ERβ pathway mediated down-regulation of mRNAs for nuclear-encoded subunits in each of the MRC complexes. The estrogen receptor related receptor α, an orphan receptor that is identified as a regulator of cellular energy metabolism, together with its co-activator, proliferator-activator receptor γ 1, played an important role in the regulation of several genes encoding MRC proteins.[79,80]

Morphological observations of abnormal mitochondrial cristae in cardiomyocytes of ERαKO mice[81] and gender differences in mitochondrial morphology and functionality[82,83] suggest that E_2 and ERs are integrally involved in the coordinate expression of mtDNA-and nuclear-encoded subunits. Moreover, nDNA-encoded regulatory/accessory factors are required for mtDNA replication, transcription, translation and assembly.

The effects of E_2/ERs on MRC protein expression are associated with their effects on MRC activities, as reflected by increased superoxide production, O_2 uptake,[66] and intracellular ATP levels.[67,84] The E_2-mediated mitochondrial effects can be inhibited by the pure ER antagonist, ICI182780.[11,74] Estrogen induced higher levels of glutathione (GSH) in mitochondria and nuclei and decreased apoptosis.[67,85] Consistent with these observations is the finding that liver mitochondria from female rats have greater capacity for oxidative phosphorylation than liver mitochondria from male rats.[86] Doan et al observed that prenatal blockade of E_2 synthesis impaired respiratory and metabolic responses to hypoxia in newborn and adult rats.[87]

Taken together, these observations provide significant insights into the molecular mechanism by which E_2 and ERs contribute to the preservation and regulation of mitochondrial function. ERs are present in mitochondria and E_2 enhances mtDNA transcription. Through induction of MRC protein synthesis, E_2 and ERs may regulate mitochondrial structure and function and thus other energy-dependent physiological processes. We proposed (Fig. 4) that once inside the cells, binding of E_2 to ERα and/or ERβ enhances their translocation to the nucleus where they stimulate the expression of nuclear-encoded MRC proteins and protein factors for mtDNA transcription such as mitochondrial transcription factor A (mtTFA) and other accessory factors for assembly of MRC complexes. These proteins are synthesized in the cytosol and imported into mitochondria. On the other hand, binding of E_2 to cytosolic ERβ (or ERα) leads to their import into mitochondria and stimulation of mtDNA transcription and MRC protein synthesis. Assembly of MRC complexes enhances MRC activity, leading to increased ATP and ROS, which could be involved in the control of cellular processes, as described below.

Potential Role of E_2/ER-Mediated Mitochondrial Pathway in Estrogen Carcinogenesis

Estrogens control biogenesis and maintenance of mitochondria through the cross-talk between nuclear and mitochondrial genomes, which appears to control estrogen-induced signaling pathways involved in the cell proliferation, apoptosis and differentiation of both normal and malignant cells.

Potential Role in Cell Proliferation

Estrogens are essential for growth and differentiation of normal, premalignant and malignant cell types including breast epithelial cells, through interaction with ERα and ERβ. The majority of cellular ATP is generated via the MRC.[88] Under physiological conditions, about 2% of electrons leak

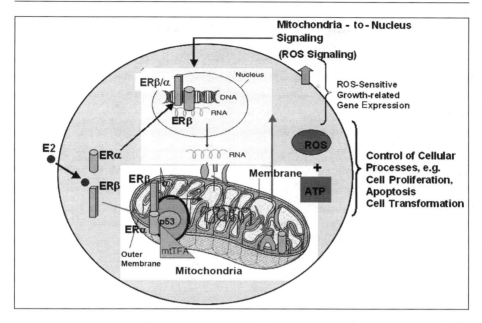

Figure 4. Proposed model for E$_2$/ER-mediated mitochondrial pathway.

from the MRC, which reduce oxygen to superoxide anion and trigger the formation of a cascade of free radicals that are collectively termed reactive oxygen species (ROS).[89] The MRC-generated ATP and ROS are essential for the viability of cells. E$_2$-induced MRC protein synthesis and, perhaps, energy metabolism are physiologically important in E$_2$-target cells and tissues, which have high demand for energy. Therefore, a relative deficiency or overabundance of MRC activities may lead to pathological consequences, depending on the types and ages of the target cells where the energy demand, the availability of E$_2$ and ERs and the duration of their actions vary. Overabundance of E$_2$/ER-mediated MRC protein synthesis and energy metabolism may exist in human breast cells as they are likely exposed to relatively high E$_2$ levels due to the active in situ synthesis of E2.[90-93]

Cell survival, growth and proliferation require large amounts of ATP. For example, cell cycle progression, biosynthetic pathways, kinase-mediated signaling pathways and a wide variety of cross-membrane transporters and channels all require ATP for their proper function. Thus, without sufficient ATP supply, cells are not viable. However, with an excess of ATP, cell proliferation may be enhanced. For example, in rapidly proliferating cells, rates of cell proliferation were closely correlated with enhanced mitochondrial gene expression and MRC activities.[94,95] The E$_2$/ER-mediated mitochondrial pathway may stimulate cell proliferation by overproduction of ATP.

The importance of ATP for regulation of cell proliferation was demonstrated in several studies. Vascular smooth muscle cells respond to ATP by increasing their intracellular calcium concentrations and rate of proliferation. In many cells the extracellular signal-regulated kinase (ERK) cascade plays an important role in cell proliferation. Wilden et al[96] observed that the binding of ATP to an UTP-sensitive P2Y nucleotide receptor activated ERK1/ERK2 in coronary artery smooth muscle cells (CASMC). ATP-induced activation of ERK1/ERK2 is dependent on mitogen-activated protein kinase (MAPK)/ERK kinase. Shen et al[97,98] reported in cultured CASMC that adenosine stimulated phosphorylation of ERK, Jun N-terminal kinase (JNK) and AKT. Moreover, adenosine-induced phosphorylation of these kinases was inhibited by the inhibitors of respective kinase pathways, which, in turn, was associated with abolishment or diminution of adenosine-induced increases in DNA/protein synthesis and cell number. These observations suggest that both ERK1/ERK2and PI3K activities are required for CASMC proliferation. ATP also stimulated the proliferation of several cell types.[99-102]

Recent studies[103-106] have suggested that estrogen-mediated mitochondrial ROS act as signaling molecules to regulate the expression of growth-related proteins. Several proteins involved in redox-regulated signaling pathways, including A-Raf, Akt, protein kinase C(PKC), ERK, MAPK/ERK kinase (MEK) and transcription factors AP-1, nuclear factor κB (NF-κB) and cAMP response element-binding protein (CREB), are targets of both estrogen and ROS. Felty et al[103,104] observed that these same redox sensor kinases and transcription factors were responsible for cell cycle progression in response to estrogen-induced stimulation of mitochondrial ROS. In another study, Felty et al[106] reported that E_2-induction of mitochondrial ROS promoted cell motility through increases of cdc42, activation of Pyk2 and increased phosphorylation of *c-jun* and CREB. These observations suggest that induction of mitochondrial ROS by E_2 acts as a signal to control cell growth and proliferation.

Potential Role of E_2/ER-Mediated ROS to Oxidative Damage and Mutations on mtDNA

Persistent E_2/ER-mediated mitochondrial ROS production may cause mutations in mtDNA and damage to mitochondrial proteins. As mentioned above, in rat hepatocytes and human HepG2 cells treated with E_2 or EE, mitochondrial superoxide levels were enhanced by several fold and inhibited by ICI182780, indicating that these effects were mediated via ERs.[67,74] Under normal conditions, MRC-generated superoxide is detoxified by mitochondrial antioxidant systems that include manganese superoxide dismutase (Mn-SOD), catalase and glutathione. Since estrogens also induce MnSOD expression and activity, the increased superoxide is likely detoxified by MnSOD. However, if the antioxidant system is impaired, superoxide will accumulate within mitochondria. On the other hand, estrogens are known to stimulate the expression of inducible nitric oxide synthase within mitochondria,[107] which catalyzes the generation of nitric oxide (NO^-). Superoxide can combine with nitric oxide to form a highly toxic peroxynitrite species ($OONO^-$). Increased levels of superoxide itself and/or of $OONO^-$ in response to estrogens could lead to oxidative damage to mtDNA and to the redox, heme-containing proteins located in the inner mitochondrial membrane (Fig. 5).

Unlike nuclear DNA, mtDNA is considered by some authors to be highly susceptible to oxidative damage because it is not associated with protective histones and is continually exposed to high levels of ROS generated by MRC. Furthermore, since mitochondria have less-efficient repair mechanisms than the nuclear systems,[108,109] damaged mtDNA may not be efficiently repaired. A high frequency of somatic mtDNA mutations that affect the energetic capability have been described

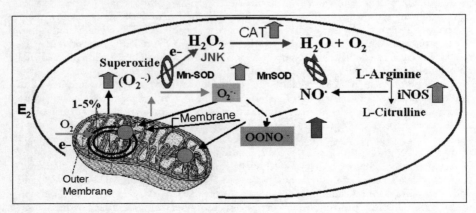

Figure 5. Proposed model for generation, degradation and accumulation of superoxide within mitochondria.

in breast cells.[110,111] In addition, the mtDNA polymorphism, G10398A, results in a nonconservative amino acid substitution of threonine (encoded by the A allele) for alanine (encoded by the G allele) in NADH dehydrogenase subunit 3 (ND3). Canter et al[112] reported that African-American women carrying this variant allele are 60 percent more likely to develop invasive breast cancer than African-American women without this genetic marker. Increased risk of prostate cancer was also observed in African American men who carry this allele.[113] Mutations in nuclear-encoded MRC genes [e.g., succinate dehydrogenase B and C, MRC complex II genes) predispose to two different types of inherited neoplasia syndromes.[114-116] Pathogenic mtDNA mutations that impinge on mitochondrial energy transduction do play a relevant role in the etiology of cancer by any one and/or combination of the following mechanisms: excessive ROS signaling,[117] diminished cellular apoptotic potential[118] or mitochondrial signaling that triggers invasive phenotypes.[119]

ROS-induced mitochondrial dysfunction can also lead to activation of nuclear genes and signaling pathways involved in tumor initiation and progression. For example, ROS can induce stress response pathways that increase the expression of hypoxia induced factor 1α, which, in turn, can activate genes involved in angiogenesis and tumor metastasis.[120] In addition, ROS-mediated disruption of mitochondrial functions has been shown to activate the calcium-dependent PKC pathway, which activates cathepsin L and other downstream genes involved in tumor invasiveness.[119] Whereas only a few nuclear genes are known to be targets of mitochondrial dysfunction in cancer, the effects of mitochondria on nuclear stress signaling in tumor progression may provide clues to the identification of subtypes of tumors that respond to the targeted disruption of specific pathways as effective therapies.

Potential Role in Inhibition of Apoptosis

Apoptosis is a fundamental cellular activity to protect against neoplastic development by eliminating genetically damaged cells or those cells that have been improperly induced to divide by a mitotic stimulus. Inhibition of spontaneous and/or metabolically-induced apoptosis could be one of the mechanisms underlying carcinogenesis.

Estrogens normally inhibit apoptosis in human breast cancer and other types of cells.[121-124] While several membrane ER-mediated pathways mediate E_2-dependent inhibition of apoptosis,[8,125] the E_2/ER-mediated mitochondrial pathway may play a role in the control of apoptosis as well. Mitochondria serve to integrate cellular apoptotic signals and to amplify apoptotic responses.[126] Enhanced MRC gene expression is associated with decreased apoptosis[67,127,128] whereas reduced MRC gene expression and MRC function has been associated with increased apoptosis.[129-132] By regulating E_2-mediated mtDNA gene expression and energy metabolism, mitochondrial ERs may contribute to inhibition of apoptosis.

The role of the mitochondrial ERα in E_2-mediated inhibition of apoptosis was demonstrated by Pedram et al[12] who used several approaches to separate the contributions of the mitochondrial ER from the nuclear and membrane ER signaling pathways in investigating how E2 inhibits UV-induced apoptosis. ER negative HCC-1569 breast cancer and CHO cells were transfected with the ligand binding E domain of ERα targeted to the nucleus, membrane or mitochondria. Anti-apoptotic effects were not seen with the nuclear-targeted E domain ER construct, whereas both the membrane and mitochondria targeted E domain ER constructs inhibited UV-induced apoptosis. To address the mechanism of this protective effect by E2, Pedram et al[12] examined the effects of E_2 treatment on the activity of MnSOD in intact cells and isolated mitochondria. E_2 increased MnSOD activity in both untreated and UV-irradiated intact cells. While others have shown that MnSOD transcription is enhanced by E2, Pedram et al[12] showed that E2 stimulated MnSOD activity just in isolated mitochondria. The E_2-enhanced MnSOD activity was inhibited by ICI182780 in both intact cells and isolated mitochondria. This appears to represent the first report indicating that E_2 can increase MnSOD activity through a process mediated by the E domain of the ER. Additional studies are needed to uncover the mechanism involved and specifically to determine whether it results from a direct interaction between the E domain of ER and MnSOD protein, or as an indirect effect.[133] On the other hand, up-regulation of mtDNA encoded respiratory chain complex IV expression by DPN, an ERβ-selective ligand, was critical for inhibiting mitochondrial apoptotic signaling in rat cardiomyocytes.[134] This finding together with that of Pedram et al[12] suggest that there may be several mechanisms by which the ERs may mediate inhibition of apoptosis following E2 treatment.

It is likely that the E_2/ER-mediated enhancement of cell proliferation and inhibition of apoptosis contribute, at least in part, to estrogen carcinogenesis. Consistent with this notion, MRC gene expression is significantly enhanced in immortalized and transformed cells.[135]

Potential Role in Anti-Cancer Drug Resistance

Tamoxifen (TAM) is an antiestrogen used for treatment of ER-positive human breast cancer. While TAM therapy is initially successful, most tumors become TAM resistant (TAM-R) and the disease ultimately progresses.[136] To date, the majority of studies on TAM-R have focused on the actions of TAM-mediated nuclear- and plasma membrane-ERs, but primary mechanisms leading to TAM-R have yet to be identified. There is evidence that mitochondria are an important target for the action of TAM.[137-142] Proteomic analysis using human breast cancer xenografts identified several MRC proteins whose expression was up-regulated in TAM-R cells.[143] Altered mitochondrial proteome and MRC functions have been observed in adriamycin resistant MCF-7 cells.[144] A role for ERβ in TAM-R is suggested by several observations: a) ERβ expression is up-regulated in TAM-R tumor cells[145] and low levels of ERβ protein predict TAM-R in breast cancer.[146] TAM did not abrogate E_2-induced cell proliferation and transformation of MCF-10F cells,[2,147] in which ERβ is predominantly localized in mitochondria and is involved in E_2-induced expression of MRC proteins. Together, these observations suggest that the E_2/ERβ-mediated mitochondrial pathway could be an important target for TAM and other anti-cancer drugs and that alterations in the E_2/ERβ-mediated mitochondrial function via differential subcellular localization of ERs may contribute to TAM-R and resistance to other anticancer drugs. On the other hand, the mitochondrial localization of ERs can result in fundamental changes in the way cells respond to anti-estrogens. Consistent with this notion, it was reported[148] that long-term treatment of MCF-7 cells with TAM facilitated the translocation of ERα out of the nuclei and enhanced its interaction with epidermal growth factor receptor in the cytoplasm. This change in ERα subcellular localization was thought to be responsible for the acquired TAM-R.

Deregulation of Mitochondrial Bioenergetics in Cancer Cells and Involvement of Estrogens and ERs

Epidemiological studies[149-155] suggest an association of energy imbalance with increased risk of breast, prostate, colon, ovarian, lung and other cancers. While the biological and pathological relevance of these observations remains to be determined, they suggest that altered energy metabolism and utilization is an emerging paradigm in cancer development. It is possible that an imbalance of energy metabolism and utilization could be caused by prolonged exposure to estrogens, which may contribute to estrogen carcinogenesis in the breast, ovary and prostate.

It has long been known that the bioenergetics of cancer cells substantially differ from those of normal cells in that cancer cells need an unusual amount of energy to survive and grow. Cancer cells typically depend more on glycolysis than on oxidative respiration (Warburg effect) in contrast to most normal cells that predominantly rely on oxidative phosphorylation for energy production.[156,157] For example, glycolysis was up-regulated upon malignant transformation in breast cancer tissue.[158] Increasing evidence from recently reviewed studies on bioenergetics of cancer cells indicate that deregulation of bioenergetics is an important hallmark of cancers, including breast cancer[159,160] and plays a crucial role in cancer development. Alterations in energy metabolism pathways including glycolysis, the tricarboxylic acid (TCA) cycle and MRC in cancer cells have been recognized. E_2 and ERs are likely involved in causing these alterations.

Glycolysis is a biochemical pathway catalyzed by enzymes that break hexose sugars into three-carbon molecules, e.g., pyruvate, with generation of two molecules of NADH and ATP. Altered expression of proteins involved in glycolysis has been seen in human colorectal, breast, ovarian and prostate cancers.[160-163] Hexose kinase (HK) catalyzes the first step in glycolysis. Drugs that dissociate HK from the mitochondrial membrane caused apoptosis and interfered with growth pathways.[164] The activity and expression of pyruvate kinase, which catalyzes the last step of glycolysis, was substantially elevated in liver, colon and breast cancer tissues.[158,160,161] E_2 stimulated and TAM inhibited glycolysis in human breast MCF-7 cells.[165] During growth of orthotopic MCF-7 breast cancer xenografts in vivo, the rate of glucose metabolism through glycolysis was increased by E_2 whereas TAM induced growth arrest and a concomitant decrease in glycolytic rate. In congruence, glucose transporter-1 expression was stimulated by E_2 up to 3-fold relative to that found in the presence of TAM, suggesting that E_2-induced changes in glycolysis appeared to be mediated via regulation of glucose transport.[166]

As a biochemical pathway, the TCA cycle, together with electron transport and oxidative phosphorylation, plays a pivotal role in cellular respiration. Altered expression and activity of proteins of the TCA cycle have been seen in breast,[163] prostate[167] and colorectal[162] cancers. Citrate synthase, the enzyme that initiates the TCA cycle, is enhanced in rat cerebral blood vessels following estrogen treatment.[62] Aconitase and isocitrate dehydrogenase (ICDH) catalyze the second and third steps in the TCA cycle. Inhibition of aconitase activity reduced cell proliferation in human prostate carcinoma cells.[168,169] Aconitase and ICDH activities were enhanced by estrogens.[170]

Several lines of evidence indicate that the deregulation of MRC bioenergetics in cancer cells may contribute to cancer development: (i) As mentioned above, many types of mutations in mtDNA and altered expression of MRC proteins and function have been seen in a number of cancer cells including breast and prostate cancer cells.[171-176] A recent proteomic study on breast cancer brain metastases[163] revealed an increased expression of proteins involved in glycolysis, TCA cycle, oxidative phosphorylation and pentose phosphate pathways. This protein profile is consistent with either a selection of predisposed cells or bioenergetics adaptation of the tumor cells to the unique energy metabolism in brain; (ii) As was underlined above, forcing cancer cells into mitochondrial respiration efficiently suppressed cancer growth. Impaired mitochondrial respiration may have a role in metastatic processes;[177] and (iii) Mutations in nuclear-encoded MRC genes [e.g., succinate dehydroganse B and D (SDHB) and SDHC], MRC complex II genes) involved in MRC bioenergetics have been shown to predispose to two different types of inherited neoplasia syndromes.[114-116]

Concluding Remarks, Evolutionary View and Future Directions

The evidence presented supports: (1) mitochondrial localization of ERs in human breast cancer cells and other cell types; (2) a functional role for the mitochondrial ERs in the regulation of MRC energy metabolism; (3) potential implications of the mitochondrial ER-mediated pathway in stimulation of cell proliferation, inhibition of apoptosis and oxidative damage to mitochondrial DNA and (4) deregulation of mitochondrial bioenergetics in cancer cells and involvement of estrogens and ERs in this dysregulation. The regulation of mitochondrial gene transcription and energy metabolism pathways by estrogens and ERs opens a new paradigm to better understand estrogen action at the cellular levels and a potential role for this new pathway in estrogen carcinogenesis.

These data provide a basis for the evolutionary view that persistent stimulation by estrogens and ERs of the expression and activities of proteins involved in the bioenergetics pathways including glycolysis, TCA cycle and MRC may lead to alterations in mitochondrial function, which in turn contributes, at least in part, to initiation and development of hormone-related cancers.

The molecular mechanisms underlying this E_2/ER-mediated pathway and its precise role in estrogen carcinogenesis are still far from being understood. Several important questions need to be addressed: (1) How are ERs imported into mitochondria? (2) Are both or either ERα and ERβ directly involved in E_2-induced MRC protein synthesis? (3) Do ERs mediate the E_2-induced MRC protein synthesis and activity via their interactions with transcription factors within mitochondria? and Finally and importantly, (4) What are the physiological and pathological implications of the overabundance of E_2/ER-mediated mitochondrial effects in cancer cells? New studies should be directed toward answers to these questions. In-depth investigations of these regulatory mechanisms are relevant to the development of novel drugs for the treatment of estrogen-dependent disease, notably cancers.

References

1. Yager JD, Davidson NE. Estrogen carcinogenesis in breast cancer. N Engl J Med 2006; 354(3):270-82.
2. Russo J, Hasan Lareef M, Balogh G et al. Estrogen and its metabolites are carcinogenic agents in human breast epithelial cells. J Steroid Biochem Mol Biol 2003; 87(1):1-25.
3. Feigelson HS, Henderson BE. Estrogens and breast cancer. Carcinogenesis 1996; 17(11):2279-84.
4. Okobia MN, Bunker CH. Estrogen metabolism and breast cancer risk—a review. Afr J Reprod Health 2006; 10(1):13-25.
5. Tsai MJ, O'Malley BW. Molecular mechanisms of action of steroid/thyroid receptor superfamily members. Annu Rev Biochem 1994; 63451-86.
6. Pettersson K, Delaunay F, Gustafsson JA. Estrogen receptor beta acts as a dominant regulator of estrogen signaling. Oncogene 2000; 19(43):4970-78.
7. Song RX, Barnes CJ, Zhang Z et al. The role of Shc and insulin-like growth factor 1 receptor in mediating the translocation of estrogen receptor alpha to the plasma membrane. Proc Natl Acad Sci USA 2004; 101(7): 2076-81.
8. Levin ER. Integration of the extranuclear and nuclear actions of estrogen. Mol Endocrinol 2005; 19(8):1951-59.
9. Chen JQ, Eshete M, Alworth WL et al. Binding of MCF-7 cell mitochondrial proteins and recombinant human estrogen receptors alpha and beta to human mitochondrial DNA estrogen response elements. J Cell Biochem 2004; 93(2):358-73.
10. Chen JQ, Yager JD. Estrogen's effects on mitochondrial gene expression: mechanisms and potential contributions to estrogen carcinogenesis. Ann N Y Acad Sci 2004; 1028258-72.
11. Chen JQ, Delannoy M, Cooke C et al. Mitochondrial localization of ERalpha and ERbeta in human MCF7 cells. Am J Physiol Endocrinol Metab 2004; 286(6):E1011-22.
12. Pedram A, Razandi M, Wallace DC et al. Functional estrogen receptors in the mitochondria of breast cancer cells. Mol Biol Cell 2006; 17(5):2125-37.
13. Green DR, Reed JC, Mitochondria and apoptosis. Science 1998; 281(5381):1309-312.
14. Bossy-Wetzel E, Green DR, Apoptosis: checkpoint at the mitochondrial frontier. Mutat Res 1999; 434(3):243-51.
15. Kelly DP, Scarpulla RC. Transcriptional regulatory circuits controlling mitochondrial biogenesis and function. Genes Dev 2004; 18(4):357-68.
16. Clayton DA. Transcription and replication of mitochondrial DNA. Hum Reprod 2000; 15 Suppl 211-17.
17. Clayton DA. Replication and transcription of vertebrate mitochondrial DNA. Annu Rev Cell Biol 1991; 7453-478.
18. Psarra AM, Solakidi S, Sekeris CE. The mitochondrion as a primary site of action of steroid and thyroid hormones: presence and action of steroid and thyroid hormone receptors in mitochondria of animal cells. Mol Cell Endocrinol 2006; 246(1-2):21-33.
19. Mansour AM, Nass S. In vivo cortisol action on RNA synthesis in rat liver nuclei and mitochondria. Nature 1970; 228(272):665-67.
20. Yu FL, Feigelson P. A comparative study of RNA synthesis in rat hepatic nuclei and mitochondria under the influence of cortisone. Biochim Biophys Acta 1970; 213(1):134-141.
21. Cornwall GA, Orgebin-Crist MC, Hann SR. Differential expression of the mouse mitochondrial genes and the mitochondrial RNA-processing endoribonuclease RNA by androgens. Mol Endocrinol 1992; 6(7):1032-42.
22. Demonacos CV, Karayanni N, Hatzoglou E et al. Mitochondrial genes as sites of primary action of steroid hormones. Steroids 1996; 61(4):226-32.
23. Demonacos C, Djordjevic-Markovic R, Tsawdaroglou N et al. The mitochondrion as a primary site of action of glucocorticoids: the interaction of the glucocorticoid receptor with mitochondrial DNA sequences showing partial similarity to the nuclear glucocorticoid responsive elements. J Steroid Biochem Mol Biol 1995; 55(1):43-55.
24. Scheller K, Sekeris CE, Krohne G et al. Localization of glucocorticoid hormone receptors in mitochondria of human cells. Eur J Cell Biol 2000; 79(5):299-307.
25. Scheller K, Sekeris CE. The effects of steroid hormones on the transcription of genes encoding enzymes of oxidative phosphorylation. Exp Physiol 2003; 88(1):129-40.
26. Scheller K, Seibel P, Sekeris CE. Glucocorticoid and thyroid hormone receptors in mitochondria of animal cells. Int Rev Cytol 2003; 2221-61.

27. Moutsatsou P, Psarra AM, Tsiapara A et al. Localization of the glucocorticoid receptor in rat brain mitochondria. Arch Biochem Biophys 2001; 386(1):69-78.
28. Kessler MA, Lamm L, Jarnagin K et al. 1,25-Dihydroxyvitamin D3-stimulated mRNAs in rat small intestine. Arch Biochem Biophys 1986; 251(2):403-12.
29. Casas F, Rochard P, Rodier A et al. A variant form of the nuclear triiodothyronine receptor c-ErbAalpha1 plays a direct role in regulation of mitochondrial RNA synthesis. Mol Cell Biol 1999; 19(12):7913-24.
30. Wrutniak-Cabello C, Casas F, Cabello G. Thyroid hormone action in mitochondria. J Mol Endocrinol 2001; 26(1):67-77.
31. Enriquez JA, Fernandez-Silva P, Garrido-Perez N et al. Direct regulation of mitochondrial RNA synthesis by thyroid hormone. Mol Cell Biol 1999;19(1):657-70.
32. Chen JQ, Yager JD, Russo J. Regulation of mitochondrial respiratory chain structure and function by estrogens/estrogen receptors and potential physiological/pathophysiological implications. Biochim Biophys Acta 2005; 1746(1):1-17.
33. Casas F, Domenjoud L, Rochard P et al. A 45 kDa protein related to PPARgamma2, induced by peroxisome proliferators, is located in the mitochondrial matrix. FEBS Lett 2000; 478(1-2):4-8.
34. Psarra AM, Bochaton-Piallat ML, Gabbiani G et al. Mitochondrial localization of glucocortocoid receptor in glial (Muller) cells in the salamander retina. Glia 2003; 41(1):38-49.
35. Morrish F, Buroker NE, Ge M et al. Thyroid hormone receptor isoforms localize to cardiac mitochondrial matrix with potential for binding to receptor elements on mtDNA. Mitochondrion 2006; 6(3):143-48.
36. Wrutniak C, Cassar-Malek I, Marchal S et al. A 43-kDa protein related to c-Erb A alpha 1 is located in the mitochondrial matrix of rat liver. J Biol Chem 1995; 270(27):16347-54.
37. Yang SH, Liu R, Perez EJ et al. Mitochondrial localization of estrogen receptor beta. Proc Natl Acad Sci USA 2004; 101(12):4130-35.
38. Monje P, Boland R. Subcellular distribution of native estrogen receptor alpha and beta isoforms in rabbit uterus and ovary. J Cell Biochem 2001; 82(3):467-79.
39. Solakidi S, Psarra AM, Nikolaropoulos S et al. Estrogen receptors {alpha} and {beta} (ER{alpha} and ER{beta}) and androgen receptor (AR) in human sperm: localization of ER{beta} and AR in mitochondria of the midpiece. Hum Reprod 2005; 20(12):3481-87.
40. Ioannou IM, Tsawdaroglou N, Sekeris CE. Presence of glucocorticoid responsive elements in the mitochondrial genome. Anticancer Res 1988; 8(6):1405-09.
41. Demonacos C, Djordjevic-Markovic R, Tsawdaroglou N et al. The mitochondrion as a primary site of action of glucocorticoids: the interaction of the glucocorticoid receptor with mitochondrial DNA sequences showing partial similarity to the nuclear glucocorticoid responsive elements. J Steroid Biochem Mol Biol 1995; 55(1):43-55.
42. Demonacos C, Tsawdaroglou NC, Djordjevic-Markovic R et al. Import of the glucocorticoid receptor into rat liver mitochondria in vivo and in vitro. J Steroid Biochem Mol Biol 1993; 46(3):401-43.
43. Demonacos CV, Karayanni N, Hatzoglou E et al. Mitochondrial genes as sites of primary action of steroid hormones. Steroids 1996; 61(4):226-32.
44. Tsiriyotis C, Spandidos DA, Sekeris CE. The mitochondrion as a primary site of action of glucocorticoids: mitochondrial nucleotide sequences, showing similarity to hormone response elements, confer dexamethasone inducibility to chimaeric genes transfected in LATK- cells. Biochem Biophys Res Commun 1997; 235(2):349-54.
45. Sekeris CE. The mitochondrial genome: a possible primary site of action of steroid hormones. In vivo 1990; 4(5):317-20.
46. Casas F, Rochard P, Rodier A et al. A variant form of the nuclear triiodothyronine receptor c-ErbAalpha1 plays a direct role in regulation of mitochondrial RNA synthesis. Mol Cell Biol 1999; 19(12):7913-24.
47. Enriquez JA, Fernandez-Silva P, Garrido-Perez N et al. Direct regulation of mitochondrial RNA synthesis by thyroid hormone. Mol Cell Biol 1999; 19(1):657-70.
48. Wrutniak C, Cassar-Malek I, Marchal S et al. A 43-kDa protein related to c-Erb A alpha 1 is located in the mitochondrial matrix of rat liver. J Biol Chem 1995; 270(27):16347-54.
49. Sekeris CE. The mitochondrial genome: a possible primary site of action of steroid hormones. In vivo 1990; 4(5):317-20.
50. Sionov RV, Kfir S, Zafrir E et al. Glucocorticoid-induced apoptosis revisited: a novel role for glucocorticoid receptor translocation to the mitochondria. Cell Cycle 2006; 5(10):1017-26.
51. Sionov RV, Cohen O, Kfir S et al. Role of mitochondrial glucocorticoid receptor in glucocorticoid-induced apoptosis. J Exp Med 2006; 203(1):189-201.
52. Bassett JH, Harvey CB, Williams GR. Mechanisms of thyroid hormone receptor-specific nuclear and extra nuclear actions. Mol Cell Endocrinol 2003; 213(1):1-11.

53. Psarra AM, Solakidi S, Sekeris CE. The mitochondrion as a primary site of action of regulatory agents involved in neuroimmunomodulation. Ann N Y Acad Sci 2006; 1088:12-22.

54. Monje P, Zanello S, Holick M et al. Differential cellular localization of estrogen receptor alpha in uterine and mammary cells. Mol Cell Endocrinol 2001; 181(1-2):117-29.

55. Chen JQ, Eshete M, Alworth WL et al. Binding of MCF-7 cell mitochondrial proteins and recombinant human estrogen receptors alpha and beta to human mitochondrial dna estrogen response elements. J Cell Biochem 2004; 93(2):358.

56. Pedram A, Razandi M, Wallace DC et al. Functional Estrogen Receptors in the Mitochondria of Breast Cancer Cells. Mol Biol Cell 2006; 17(5):2125-37.

57. Solakidi S, Psarra AM, Sekeris CE. Differential subcellular distribution of estrogen receptor isoforms: localization of ERalpha in the nucleoli and ERbeta in the mitochondria of human osteosarcoma SaOS-2 and hepatocarcinoma HepG2 cell lines. Biochim Biophys Acta 2005; 1745(3):382-92.

58. Cammarata PR, Chu S, Moor A et al. Subcellular distribution of native estrogen receptor alpha and beta subtypes in cultured human lens epithelial cells. Exp Eye Res 2004; 78(4):861-71.

59. Cammarata PR, Flynn J, Gottipati S et al. Differential expression and comparative subcellular localization of estrogen receptor beta isoforms in virally transformed and normal cultured human lens epithelial cells. Exp Eye Res 2005; 81(2):165-75.

60. Jonsson D, Nilsson J, Odenlund M et al. Demonstration of mitochondrial oestrogen receptor beta and oestrogen-induced attenuation of cytochrome c oxidase subunit I expression in human periodontal ligament cells. Arch Oral Biol 2007; 52(7):669-76.

61. Milner TA, Ayoola K, Drake CT et al. Ultrastructural localization of estrogen receptor beta immunoreactivity in the rat hippocampal formation. J Comp Neurol 2005; 491(2):81-95.

62. Stirone C, Duckles SP, Krause DN et al. Estrogen increases mitochondrial efficiency and reduces oxidative stress in cerebral blood vessels. Mol Pharmacol 2005; 68(4):959-65.

63. Van Itallie CM, Dannies PS. Estrogen induces accumulation of the mitochondrial ribonucleic acid for subunit II of cytochrome oxidase in pituitary tumor cells. Mol Endocrinol 1988; 2(4):332-37.

64. Bettini E, Maggi A. Estrogen induction of cytochrome c oxidase subunit III in rat hippocampus. J Neurochem 1992; 58(5):1923-29.

65. Chen J, Schwartz DA, Young TA et al. Identification of genes whose expression is altered during mitosuppression in livers of ethinyl estradiol-treated female rats. Carcinogenesis 1996; 17(12):2783-86.

66. Chen J, Gokhale M, Li Y et al. Enhanced levels of several mitochondrial mRNA transcripts and mitochondrial superoxide production during ethinyl estradiol-induced hepatocarcinogenesis and after estrogen treatment of HepG2 cells. Carcinogenesis 1998; 19(12):2187-93.

67. Chen J, Delannoy M, Odwin S et al. Enhanced mitochondrial gene transcript, ATP, bcl-2 protein levels and altered glutathione distribution in ethinyl estradiol-treated cultured female rat hepatocytes. Toxicol Sci 2003; 75(2):271-78.

68. Hsieh YC, Yu HP, Suzuki T et al. Upregulation of mitochondrial respiratory complex IV by estrogen receptor-beta is critical for inhibiting mitochondrial apoptotic signaling and restoring cardiac functions following trauma-hemorrhage. J Mol Cell Cardiol 2006; 41(3):511-21.

69. Stirone C, Duckles SP, Krause DN et al. Estrogen increases mitochondrial efficiency and reduces oxidative stress in cerebral blood vessels. Mol Pharmacol 2005; 68(4):959-65.

70. Hatzoglou E, Sekeris CE. The detection of nucleotide sequences with strong similarity to hormone responsive elements in the genome of eubacteria and archaebacteria and their possible relation to similar sequences present in the mitochondrial genome. J Theor Biol 1997; 184(3):339-44.

71. Grivell LA. Nucleo-mitochondrial interactions in mitochondrial gene expression. Crit Rev Biochem Mol Biol 1995; 30(2):121-64.

72. Garesse R, Vallejo CG. Animal mitochondrial biogenesis and function: a regulatory cross-talk between two genomes. Gene 2001; 263(1-2):1-16.

73. Roberts, Szego CM. The influence of steroids on uterine respiration and glycolysis. J Biol Chem 1953; 201(1):21-30.

74. Chen J, Li Y, Lavigne JA et al. Increased mitochondrial superoxide production in rat liver mitochondria, rat hepatocytes and HepG2 cells following ethinyl estradiol treatment. Toxicol Sci 1999; 51(2):224-35.

75. Watanabe T, Inoue S, Hiroi H et al. Isolation of estrogen-responsive genes with a CpG island library. Mol Cell Biol 1998; 18(1):442-49.

76. Thompson CJ, Tam NN, Joyce JM et al. Gene expression profiling of testosterone and estradiol-17 beta-induced prostatic dysplasia in Noble rats and response to the antiestrogen ICI 182,780. Endocrinology 2002; 143(6):2093-105.

77. Weisz A, Basile W, Scafoglio C et al. Molecular identification of ERalpha-positive breast cancer cells by the expression profile of an intrinsic set of estrogen regulated genes. J Cell Physiol 2004; 200(3):440-50.

78. O'Lone R, Knorr K, Jaffe IZ et al. Estrogen Receptors {alpha} and {beta} Mediate Distinct Pathways of Vascular Gene Expression, Including Genes Involved in Mitochondrial Electron Transport and Generation of Reactive Oxygen Species. Mol Endocrinol 2007 [Epub ahead of print].

79. Huss JM, Torra IP, Staels B et al. Estrogen-related receptor alpha directs peroxisome proliferator-activated receptor alpha signaling in the transcriptional control of energy metabolism in cardiac and skeletal muscle. Mol Cell Biol 2004; 24(20):9079-91.

80. Huss JM, Kelly DP. Nuclear receptor signaling and cardiac energetics. Circ Res 2004; 95(6):568-78.

81. Zhai P, Eurell TE, Cooke PS et al. Myocardial ischemia-reperfusion injury in estrogen receptor-alpha knockout and wild-type mice. Am J Physiol Heart Circ Physiol 2000; 278(5): H1640-47.

82. Rodriguez-Cuenca S, Pujol E, Justo R et al. Sex-dependent thermogenesis, differences in mitochondrial morphology and function and adrenergic response in brown adipose tissue. J Biol Chem 2002; 277(45):42958-63.

83. Justo R, Frontera M, Pujol E et al. Gender-related differences in morphology and thermogenic capacity of brown adipose tissue mitochondrial subpopulations. Life Sci 2005; 76(10):1147-58.

84. Degani H, Shaer A, Victor TA et al. Estrogen-induced changes in high-energy phosphate metabolism in rat uterus: 31P NMR studies. Biochemistry 1984; 23(12):2572-77.

85. Chen J, Gokhale M, Schofield B et al. Inhibition of TGF-beta-induced apoptosis by ethinyl estradiol in cultured, precision cut rat liver slices and hepatocytes. Carcinogenesis 2000; 21(6):1205-11.

86. Justo R, Boada J, Frontera M et al. Gender dimorphism in rat liver mitochondrial oxidative metabolism and biogenesis. Am J Physiol Cell Physiol 2005; 289(2): C372-78.

87. Doan VD, Gagnon S, Joseph V. Prenatal blockade of estradiol synthesis impairs respiratory and metabolic responses to hypoxia in newborn and adult rats. Am J Physiol Regul Integr Comp Physiol 2004; 287(3): R612-18.

88. Papa S. Mitochondrial oxidative phosphorylation changes in the life span. Molecular aspects and physiopathological implications. Biochim Biophys Acta 1996; 1276(2):87-105.

89. Boyer PD. The ATP synthase—a splendid molecular machine. Annu Rev Biochem 1997; 66717-49.

90. Brodie A, Lu Q, Nakamura J. Aromatase in the normal breast and breast cancer. J Steroid Biochem Mol Biol 1997; 61(3-6):281-86.

91. Santner RJ, Santner SJ, Pauley RJ et al. Estrogen production via the aromatase enzyme in breast carcinoma: which cell type is responsible? J Steroid Biochem Mol Biol 1997; 61(3-6):267-71.

92. Chen S, Itoh T, Wu K. et al. Transcriptional regulation of aromatase expression in human breast tissue. J Steroid Biochem Mol Biol 2002; 83(1-5):93-99.

93. Yue W, Santen RJ, Wang JP et al. Aromatase within the breast. Endocr Relat Cancer 1999; 6(2):157-64.

94. Kim H, You S, Kim IJ et al. Increased mitochondrial-encoded gene transcription in immortal DF-1 cells. Exp Cell Res 2001; 265(2):339-47.

95. Dong X, Ghoshal K, Majumder S et al. Mitochondrial transcription factor A and its downstream targets are up-regulated in a rat hepatoma. J Biol Chem 2002; 277(45):43309-18.

96. Wilden PA, Agazie YM, Kaufman R et al. ATP-stimulated smooth muscle cell proliferation requires independent ERK and PI3K signaling pathways. Am J Physiol 1998; 275(4 Pt 2): H1209-15.

97. Shen J, Halenda SP, Sturek M et al. Cell-signaling evidence for adenosine stimulation of coronary smooth muscle proliferation via the A1 adenosine receptor. Circ Res 2005; 97(6):574-82.

98. Shen J, Halenda SP, Sturek M et al. Novel mitogenic effect of adenosine on coronary artery smooth muscle cells: role for the A1 adenosine receptor. Circ Res 2005; 96(9):982-90.

99. Heo JS, Han HJ. ATP stimulates mouse embryonic stem cell proliferation via protein kinase C, phosphatidylinositol 3-kinase/Akt and mitogen-activated protein kinase signaling pathways. Stem Cells 2006; 24(12):2637-48.

100. Yu SM, Chen SF, Lau YT et al. Mechanism of extracellular ATP-induced proliferation of vascular smooth muscle cells. Mol Pharmacol 1996; 50(4):1000-09.

101. Wagstaff SC, Bowler WB, Gallagher JA et al. Extracellular ATP activates multiple signalling pathways and potentiates growth factor-induced c-fos gene expression in MCF-7 breast cancer cells. Carcinogenesis 2000; 21(12):2175-81.

102. Schafer R, Sedehizade F, Welte T et al. ATP- and UTP-activated P2Y receptors differently regulate proliferation of human lung epithelial tumor cells. Am J Physiol Lung Cell Mol Physiol 2003; 285(2): L376-85.

103. Felty Q, Roy D. Mitochondrial signals to nucleus regulate estrogen-induced cell growth. Med Hypotheses 2005; 64(1):133-41.

104. Felty Q, Roy D. Estrogen, mitochondria and growth of cancer and noncancer cells. J Carcinog 2005; 4(1):1.

105. Felty Q, Xiong WC, Sun D et al. Estrogen-induced mitochondrial reactive oxygen species as signal-transducing messengers. Biochemistry 2005; 44(18):6900-09.

106. Felty Q, Singh KP, Roy D. Estrogen-induced G(1)/S transition of G(0)-arrested estrogen-dependent breast cancer cells is regulated by mitochondrial oxidant signaling. Oncogene 2005; 24(31):4883-93.

107. Karpuzoglu E, Fenaux JB, Phillips RA et al. Estrogen up-regulates inducible nitric oxide synthase, nitric oxide and cyclooxygenase-2 in splenocytes activated with T-cell stimulants: role of interferon-gamma. Endocrinology 2006; 147(2):662-71.

108. Richard SM, Bailliet G, Paez GL et al. Nuclear and mitochondrial genome instability in human breast cancer. Cancer Res 2000; 60(15):4231-37.

109. Bianchi NO, Bianchi MS, Richard SM. Mitochondrial genome instability in human cancers. Mutat Res 2001; 488(1):9-23.

110. Parrella P, Xiao Y, Fliss M et al. Detection of mitochondrial DNA mutations in primary breast cancer and fine-needle aspirates. Cancer Res 2001; 61(20):7623-26.

111. Tan DJ, Bai RK, Wong LJ. Comprehensive scanning of somatic mitochondrial DNA mutations in breast cancer. Cancer Res 2002; 62(4):972-76.

112. Canter JA, Kallianpur AR, Parl FF et al. Mitochondrial DNA G10398A polymorphism and invasive breast cancer in African-American women. Cancer Res 2005; 65(17):8028-33.

113. Mims MP, Hayes TG, Zheng S et al. Mitochondrial DNA G10398A polymorphism and invasive breast cancer in African-American women. Cancer Res 2006; 66(3):1880; author reply 1880-81.

114. Habano W, Sugai T, Nakamura S et al. Reduced expression and loss of heterozygosity of the SDHD gene in colorectal and gastric cancer. Oncol Rep 2003; 10(5):1375-80.

115. Neumann HP, Pawlu C, Peczkowska M et al. Distinct clinical features of paraganglioma syndromes associated with SDHB and SDHD gene mutations. Jama 2004; 292(8):943-51.

116. Baysal BE, Ferrell RE, Willett-Brozick JE et al. Mutations in SDHD, a mitochondrial complex II gene, in hereditary paraganglioma. Science 2000; 287(5454):848-51.

117. Petros JA, Baumann AK, Ruiz-Pesini E et al. mtDNA mutations increase tumorigenicity in prostate cancer. Proc Natl Acad Sci USA 2005; 102(3):719-24.

118. Shidara Y, Yamagata K, Kanamori T et al. Positive contribution of pathogenic mutations in the mitochondrial genome to the promotion of cancer by prevention from apoptosis. Cancer Res 2005; 65(5):1655-63.

119. Amuthan G, Biswas G, Zhang SY et al. Mitochondria-to-nucleus stress signaling induces phenotypic changes, tumor progression and cell invasion. EMBO J 2001; 20(8):1910-20.

120. Gao N, Ding M, Zheng JZ et al. Vanadate-induced expression of hypoxia-inducible factor 1 alpha and vascular endothelial growth factor through phosphatidylinositol 3-kinase/Akt pathway and reactive oxygen species. J Biol Chem 2002; 277(35):31963-71.

121. Perillo B, Sasso A, Abbondanza C et al. 17beta-estradiol inhibits apoptosis in MCF-7 cells, inducing bcl-2 expression via two estrogen-responsive elements present in the coding sequence. Mol Cell Biol 2000; 20(8):2890-901.

122. Kim JK, Pedram A, Razandi M et al. Estrogen Prevents Cardiomyocyte Apoptosis through Inhibition of Reactive Oxygen Species and Differential Regulation of p38 Kinase Isoforms. J Biol Chem 2006; 281(10):6760-67.

123. Patten RD, Pourati I, Aronovitz MJ et al. 17beta-estradiol reduces cardiomyocyte apoptosis in vivo and in vitro via activation of phospho-inositide-3 kinase/Akt signaling. Circ Res 2004; 95(7):692-99.

124. Mattson MP, Robinson N, Guo Q. Estrogens stabilize mitochondrial function and protect neural cells against the pro-apoptotic action of mutant presenilin-1. Neuroreport 1997; 8(17):3817-21.

125. Song RX, Santen RJ. Membrane initiated estrogen signaling in breast cancer. Biol Reprod 2006; 75(1):9-16.

126. Kroemer G, Reed JC. Mitochondrial control of cell death. Nat Med 2000; 6(5):513-19.

127. Ikeuchi M, Matsusaka H, Kang D et al. Overexpression of mitochondrial transcription factor a ameliorates mitochondrial deficiencies and cardiac failure after myocardial infarction. Circulation 2005; 112(5):683-90.

128. Matsuyama S, Xu Q, Velours J et al. The Mitochondrial F0F1-ATPase proton pump is required for function of the proapoptotic protein Bax in yeast and mammalian cells. Mol Cell 1998; 1(3):327-36.

129. Comelli M, Di Pancrazio F, Mavelli I. Apoptosis is induced by decline of mitochondrial ATP synthesis in erythroleukemia cells. Free Radic Biol Med 2003; 34(9):1190-99.

130. Mills KI, Woodgate LJ, Gilkes AF et al. Inhibition of mitochondrial function in HL60 cells is associated with an increased apoptosis and expression of CD14. Biochem Biophys Res Commun 1999; 263(2):294-300.

131. Wang J, Silva JP, Gustafsson CM et al. Increased in vivo apoptosis in cells lacking mitochondrial DNA gene expression. Proc Natl Acad Sci USA 2001; 98(7):4038-43.

132. Wolvetang EJ, Johnson KL, Krauer K et al. Mitochondrial respiratory chain inhibitors induce apoptosis. FEBS Lett 1994; 339(1-2):40-44.

133. Yager JD, Chen JQ. Mitochondrial estrogen receptors—new insights into specific functions. Trends Endocrinol Metab 2007; 18(3):89-91.
134. yHsieh YC, Yu HP, Suzuki T et al. Upregulation of mitochondrial respiratory complex IV by estrogen receptor-beta is critical for inhibiting mitochondrial apoptotic signaling and restoring cardiac functions following trauma-hemorrhage. J Mol Cell Cardiol 2006; 41(3):511-21.
135. Torroni A, Stepien G, Hodge JA et al. Neoplastic transformation is associated with coordinate induction of nuclear and cytoplasmic oxidative phosphorylation genes. J Biol Chem 1990; 265(33):20589-93.
136. Muss HB. Endocrine therapy for advanced breast cancer: a review. Breast Cancer Res Treat 1992; 21(1):15-26.
137. Cardoso CM, Custodio JB, Almeida LM et al. Mechanisms of the deleterious effects of tamoxifen on mitochondrial respiration rate and phosphorylation efficiency. Toxicol Appl Pharmacol 2001; 176(3):145-52.
138. Cardoso CM, Moreno AJ, Almeida LM et al. 4-Hydroxytamoxifen induces slight uncoupling of mitochondrial oxidative phosphorylation system in relation to the deleterious effects of tamoxifen. Toxicology 2002; 179(3):221-32.
139. Cardoso CM, Moreno AJ, Almeida LM et al. Comparison of the changes in adenine nucleotides of rat liver mitochondria induced by tamoxifen and 4-hydroxytamoxifen. Toxicol In vitro 2003; 17(5-6):663-70.
140. Tuquet C, Dupont J, Mesneau A et al. Effects of tamoxifen on the electron transport chain of isolated rat liver mitochondria. Cell Biol Toxicol 2000; 16(4):207-19.
141. Kallio A, Zheng A, Dahllund J et al. Role of mitochondria in tamoxifen-induced rapid death of MCF-7 breast cancer cells. Apoptosis 2005; 10(6):1395-410.
142. Zhao Y, Wang LM, Chaiswing L et al. Tamoxifen protects against acute tumor necrosis factor alpha-induced cardiac injury via improving mitochondrial functions. Free Radic Biol Med 2006; 40(7):1234-41.
143. Besada V, Diaz M, Becker M et al. Proteomics of xenografted human breast cancer indicates novel targets related to tamoxifen resistance. Proteomics 2006; 6(3):1038-48.
144. Strong R, Nakanishi T, Ross D et al. Alterations in the mitochondrial proteome of adriamycin resistant MCF-7 breast cancer cells. J Proteome Res 2006; 5(9):2389-95.
145. Speirs V, Malone C, Walton DS et al. Increased expression of estrogen receptor beta mRNA in tamoxifen-resistant breast cancer patients. Cancer Res 1999; 59(21):5421-24.
146. Hopp TA, Weiss HL, Parra IS et al. Low levels of estrogen receptor beta protein predict resistance to tamoxifen therapy in breast cancer. Clin Cancer Res 2004; 10(22):7490-99.
147. Lareef MH, Garber J, Russo PA et al. The estrogen antagonist ICI-182-780 does not inhibit the transformation phenotypes induced by 17-beta-estradiol and 4-OH estradiol in human breast epithelial cells. Int J Oncol 2005; 26(2):423-29.
148. Fan P, Wang J, Santen RJ et al. Long-term Treatment with Tamoxifen Facilitates Translocation of Estrogen Receptor {alpha} out of the Nucleus and Enhances its Interaction with EGFR in MCF-7 Breast Cancer Cells. Cancer Res 2007; 67(3):1352-60.
149. Jasienska G, Thune I, Ellison PT. Energetic factors, ovarian steroids and the risk of breast cancer. Eur J Cancer Prev 2000; 9(4):231-39.
150. Simopoulos AP. Energy imbalance and cancer of the breast, colon and prostate. Med Oncol Tumor Pharmacother 1990; 7(2-3):109-20.
151. Malin A, Matthews CE, Shu XO et al. Energy balance and breast cancer risk. Cancer Epidemiol Biomarkers Prev 2005; 14(6):1496-501.
152. Silvera SA, Jain M, Howe GR et al. Energy balance and breast cancer risk: a prospective cohort study. Breast Cancer Res Treat 2005; 1-10.
153. Silvera SA, Jain M, Howe GR et al. Energy balance and breast cancer risk: a prospective cohort study. Breast Cancer Res Treat 2006; 97(1):97-106.
154. Chang SC, Ziegler RG, Dunn B et al. Association of energy intake and energy balance with postmenopausal breast cancer in the prostate, lung, colorectal and ovarian cancer screening trial. Cancer Epidemiol Biomarkers Prev 2006; 15(2):334-41.
155. Suzuki S, Platz EA, Kawachi I et al. Intakes of energy and macronutrients and the risk of benign prostatic hyperplasia. Am J Clin Nutr 2002; 75(4):689-97.
156. Warburg O. On the origin of cancer cells. Science 1956; 123(3191):309-14.
157. Warburg O. On respiratory impairment in cancer cells. Science 1956; 124(3215):269-70.
158. Balinsky D, Platz CE, Lewis JW. Enzyme activities in normal, dysplastic and cancerous human breast tissues. J Natl Cancer Inst 1984; 72(2):217-24.
159. Garber K. Energy deregulation: licensing tumors to grow. Science 2006; 312(5777):1158-59.
160. Isidoro A, Martinez M, Fernandez PL et al. Alteration of the bioenergetic phenotype of mitochondria is a hallmark of breast, gastric, lung and oesophageal cancer. Biochem J 2004; 378(Pt 1):17-20.

161. Isidoro A, Casado E, Redondo A et al. Breast carcinomas fulfill the Warburg hypothesis and provide metabolic markers of cancer prognosis. Carcinogenesis 2005; 26(12):2095-104.
162. Bi X, Lin Q, Foo TW et al. Proteomics analysis of colorectal cancer reveals alterations in metabolic pathways-mechanism of tumorigenesis. Mol Cell Proteomics 2006; 5(6):1119-30.
163. Chen EI, Hewel J, Krueger JS et al. Adaptation of energy metabolism in breast cancer brain metastases. Cancer Res 2007; 67(4):1472-86.
164. Pedersen PL, Mathupala S, Rempel A et al. Mitochondrial bound type II hexokinase: a key player in the growth and survival of many cancers and an ideal prospect for therapeutic intervention. Biochim Biophys Acta 2002; 1555(1-3):14-20.
165. Neeman M, Degani H. Metabolic studies of estrogen- and tamoxifen-treated human breast cancer cells by nuclear magnetic resonance spectroscopy. Cancer Res 1989; 49(3):589-94.
166. Rivenzon-Segal D, Boldin-Adamsky S, Seger D et al. Glycolysis and glucose transporter 1 as markers of response to hormonal therapy in breast cancer. Int J Cancer 2003; 107(2):177-82.
167. Dakubo GD, Parr RL, Costello LC et al. Altered metabolism and mitochondrial genome in prostate cancer. J Clin Pathol 2006; 59(1):10-16.
168. Juang HH. Modulation of iron on mitochondrial aconitase expression in human prostatic carcinoma cells. Mol Cell Biochem 2004; 265(1-2):185-94.
169. Juang HH. Modulation of mitochondrial aconitase on the bioenergy of human prostate carcinoma cells. Mol Genet Metab 2004; 81(3):244-52.
170. Yadav RN. Isocitrate dehydrogenase activity and its regulation by estradiol in tissues of rats of various ages. Cell Biochem Funct 1988; 6(3):197-202.
171. Copeland WC, Wachsman JT, Johnson FM et al. Mitochondrial DNA alterations in cancer. Cancer Invest 2002; 20(4):557-69.
172. Chatterjee A, Mambo E, Sidransky D. Mitochondrial DNA mutations in human cancer. Oncogene 2006; 25(34):4663-74.
173. Brandon M, Baldi P, Wallace DC. Mitochondrial mutations in cancer. Oncogene 2006; 25(34):4647-62.
174. Krieg RC, Knuechel R, Schiffmann E et al. Mitochondrial proteome: cancer-altered metabolism associated with cytochrome c oxidase subunit level variation. Proteomics 2004; 4(9):2789-95.
175. Capuano F, Varone D, D'Eri N et al. Oxidative phosphorylation and F(O)F(1) ATP synthase activity of human hepatocellular carcinoma. Biochem Mol Biol Int 1996; 38(5):1013-22.
176. Haugen DR, Fluge O, Reigstad LJ et al. Increased expression of genes encoding mitochondrial proteins in papillary thyroid carcinomas. Thyroid 2003; 13(7):613-20.
177. Schulz TJ, Thierbach R, Voigt A et al. Induction of oxidative metabolism by mitochondrial frataxin inhibits cancer growth: Otto Warburg revisited. J Biol Chem 2006; 281(2):977-81.

CHAPTER 2

Adaptation to Estradiol Deprivation Causes Up-Regulation of Growth Factor Pathways and Hypersensitivity to Estradiol in Breast Cancer Cells

Richard J. Santen,* Robert X. Song, Shigeru Masamura, Wei Yue, Ping Fan, Tetsuya Sogon, Shin-ichi Hayashi, Kei Nakachi and Hidtek Eguchi

Abstract

Deprivation of estrogen causes breast tumors in women to adapt and develop enhanced sensitivity to this steroid. Accordingly, women relapsing after treatment with oophorectomy, which substantially lowers estradiol for a prolonged period, respond secondarily to aromatase inhibitors with tumor regression. We have utilized in vitro and in vivo model systems to examine the biologic processes whereby Long Term Estradiol Deprivation (LTED) causes cells to adapt and develop hypersensitivity to estradiol. Several mechanisms are associated with this response including up-regulation of ERα and the MAP kinase, PI-3-kinase and mTOR growth factor pathways. ERα is 4-10 fold up-regulated as a result of demethylation of its C promoter, This nuclear receptor then co-opts a classical growth factor pathway using SHC, Grb-2 and Sos. This induces rapid nongenomic effects which are enhanced in LTED cells.

The molecules involved in the nongenomic signaling process have been identified. Estradiol binds to cell membrane-associated ERα which physically associates with the adaptor protein SHC and induces its phosphorylation. In turn, SHC binds Grb-2 and Sos which results in the rapid activation of MAP kinase. These nongenomic effects of estradiol produce biologic effects as evidenced by Elk-1 activation and by morphologic changes in cell membranes. Additional effects include activation of the PI-3-kinase and mTOR pathways through estradiol-induced binding of ERα to the IGF-1 and EGF receptors.

A major question is how ERα locates in the plasma membrane since it does not contain an inherent membrane localization signal. We have provided evidence that the IGF-1 receptor serves as an anchor for ERα in the plasma membrane. Estradiol causes phosphorylation of the adaptor protein, SHC and the IGF-1 receptor itself. SHC, after binding to ERα, serves as the "glue" which tethers ERα to SHC binding sites on the activated IFG-1 receptors. Use of siRNA methodology to knock down SHC allows the conclusion that SHC is needed for ERα to localize in the plasma membrane.

In order to abrogate growth factor induced hypersensitivity, we have utilized a drug, farnesylthiosalicylic acid, which blocks the binding of GTP-Ras to its membrane acceptor protein, galectin 1 and reduces the activation of MAP kinase. We have shown that this drug is a potent

*Corresponding Author: Richard J. Santen—Division of Endocrinology and Metabolism, University of Virginia Health Sciences Center, Charlottesville, Virginia, USA. Email: rjs5y@virginia.edu

Innovative Endocrinology of Cancer, edited by Lev M. Berstein and Richard J. Santen. ©2008 Landes Bioscience and Springer Science+Business Media.

inhibitor of mTOR and this provides the major means for inhibition of cell proliferation. The concept of "adaptive hypersensitivity" and the mechanisms responsible for this phenomenon have important clinical implications. The efficacy of aromatase inhibitors in patients relapsing on tamoxifen could be explained by this mechanism and inhibitors of growth factor pathways should reverse the hypersensitivity phenomenon and result in prolongation of the efficacy of hormonal therapy for breast cancer.

Introduction

Cancer cells adapt in response to the pressure exerted upon them by various hormonal treatments. Ultimately, this process of adaptation renders them insensitive to hormonal therapy. In patients, clinical observations suggest that long term deprivation of estradiol causes breast cancer cells to develop enhanced sensitivity to the proliferative effects of estrogen. Premenopausal women with advanced hormone dependent breast cancer experience objective tumor regressions in response to surgical oophorectomy which lowers estradiol levels from mean levels of approximately 200 pg/ml to 10 pg/ml.[1] After 12-18 months on average, tumors begin to regrow even though estradiol levels remain at 10 pg/ml. Notably tumors again regress upon secondary therapy with aromatase inhibitors which lower estradiol levels to 1-2 pg/ml. These observations suggest that tumors develop hypersensitivity to estradiol as demonstrated by the fact that untreated tumors require 200 pg/ml of estradiol to grow whereas tumors regrowing after oophorectomy require only 10 pg/ml. We have shown in prior studies that up-regulation of growth factor pathways contributes to the phenomenon of hypersensitivity.[2-10] Ultimately these tumors adapt further and grow exclusively in response to growth factor pathways and do not require estrogens for growth.

In order to provide direct proof that hypersensitivity does develop and to study the mechanisms involved, we have utilized cell culture and xenograft models of breast cancer as experimental tools.[5,8,9,11-13]

Phenomenon of Hypersensitivity: Mechanisms and Pathways

To induce hypersensitivity, wild type MCF-7 cells require culturing over a 6-24 month period in estrogen-free media to mimic the effects of ablative endocrine therapy such as induced by surgical oophorectomy or aromatase inhibitors.[11,12] This process involves Long Term Estradiol Deprivation and the adapted cells are called by the acronym, LTED cells. As evidence of hypersensitivity, a three log lower concentration of estradiol can stimulate proliferation of LTED cells compared to wild type MCF-7 cells (Fig. 1A).[7] We reasoned that the development of hypersensitivity could involve modulation of the genomic effects of estradiol acting on transcription, nongenomic actions involving plasma membrane related receptors, cross talk between growth factor and steroid hormone stimulated pathways, or interactions among these various effects.[5,7-9,11-13]

We initially postulated that enhanced receptor mediated transcription of genes related to cell proliferation might be involved. Indeed, the levels of ERα increased 4-10 fold during long term estradiol deprivation.[11] The up-regulation of ER alpha results from demethylation of promoter A and C of the estrogen receptor (Fig. 1B and 1C). The transcripts stimulated by this promoter increase by 149 fold and the DNA of this segment exhibits a marked increase in demethylation. [13a]We initially reasoned that the up-regulation of ERα would directly result in hypersensitivity to estradiol (E_2). Accordingly, to directly examine whether enhanced sensitivity to E_2 in LTED cells occurred at the level of ER mediated transcription, we quantitated the effects of estradiol on transcription in LTED and in wild type MCF-7 cells. As transcriptional readouts, we measured the effect of E_2 on progesterone receptor (PgR) and pS2 protein concentrations and on ERE-CAT reporter activity (Fig. 2A-F).[9,13] We observed no shift to the left in estradiol dose response curves (the end point utilized to detect hypersensitivity) for any of these responses (i.e., PgR, pS2, CAT activity) when comparing LTED with wild type MCF-7 cells. On the other hand, basal levels (i.e., no estrogen added) of transcription of three ER/ERE related reporter genes were greater in LTED than in wild type MCF-7 cells (Fig. 2D-F).[13]

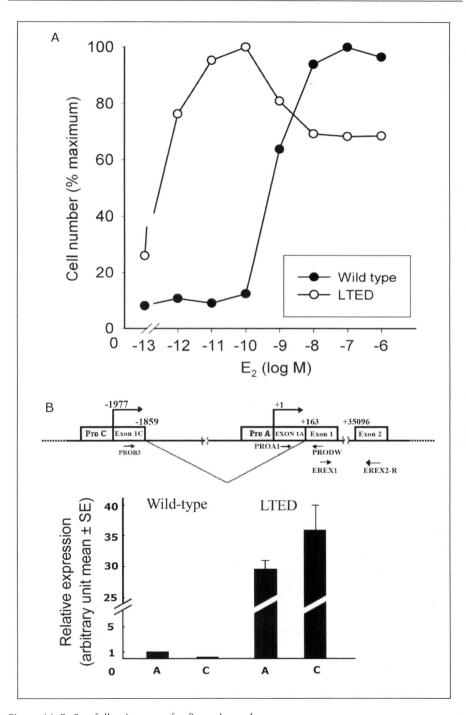

Figure 1A-B. See following page for figure legend.

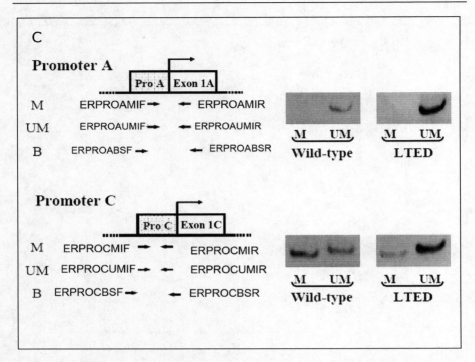

Figure 1. A, viewed on previous page) E_2-induced cell proliferation. Wild type MCF-7 and LTED cells were plated in 6 well plates at a density of 60,000 cells/well. After 2 days the cells were refed with phenol-red and serum free IMEM (improved modified Eagles medium) and cultured in this medium for another 2 days before treatment with various concentrations of E_2 in the presence of ICI 182,780 (fulvestrant) at a 1 nmol concentration to abrogate the effects of any residual estradiol in the medium. Cell number was counted 5 days after treatment.[7,9] From: Yue W et al. Endocrinology 2002; 143(9):3221-9;[9] with permission of The Endocrine Society. B, viewed on previous page) Schematic representation of a part of ER alpha gene organization is shown. The transcription start site of Promoter A is defined as +1. Relative expression of ER alpha mRNA from promoters A and C in wild type and LTED cells is shown. Expression levels of ER alpha mRNA from promoters A and C were quantified by RT-PCR. C) COBRA assay for gene promoter C of ER α in wild type and LTED cells: an image of the polyacrilamide gel showing the methylated (M) and unmethylated (UM) products. B,C) From: Sogon T et al. J Steroid Biochem Mol Biol 2007; 105(1-5):106-14;[13a] with permission of Elsevier.

To interpret these data, we used the classic definition for hypersensitivity, namely a significant shift to the left in the dose causing 50% of maximal stimulation. Accordingly, these data suggest that hypersensitivity of LTED cells to the proliferative effects of estradiol does not occur primarily at the level of ER-mediated gene transcription (Fig. 2A-C) but may be influenced by the higher rates of maximal transcription (Fig. 2D-F).

We next considered that adaptation might involve dynamic interactions between pathways utilizing steroid hormones and those involving MAP kinase and PI-3-kinase for growth factor signaling (Fig. 3A).[5,7-9,11-16] Our initial approach demonstrated that basal levels of MAP kinase were elevated in LTED cells in vitro (Fig. 2B, top panel) and in xenografts (data not shown) and were inhibited by the pure antiestrogen, fulvestrant.[8,11]

We further demonstrated that activated MAP kinase is implicated in the enhanced growth of LTED cells since inhibitors of MAP kinase such as PD98059 or U-0126 block the incorpora-

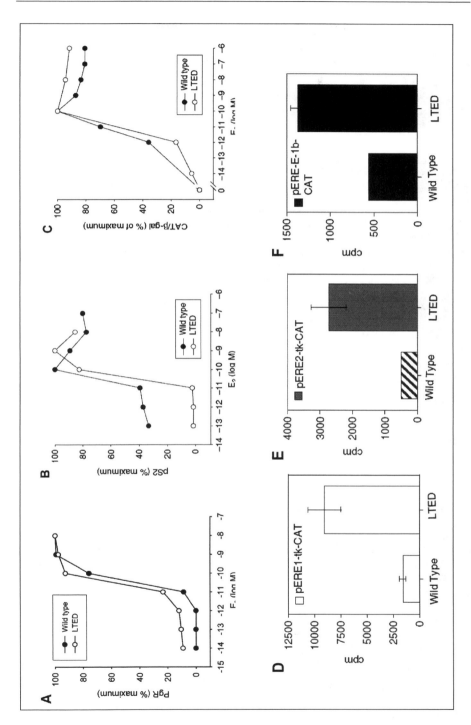

Figure 2. See following page for figure legend.

Figure 2, viewed on previous page. A-C) Wild–type MCF-7 and LTED cells, deprived of E_2, were treated with different concentrations of E_2. Cytosols were measured for PgR (A), pS2 protein (B) and ERE-TK-CAT activity (C) 48 h after E_2 treatment. A-C) From: Yue W et al. Endocrinology 2002; 143(9):3221-9;[9] with permission of The Endocrine Society. D-F) ER trans-activation function in wild-type MCF-7 and LTED cells under basal conditions. Wild type and LTED cells were deprived of estrogen and transfected with ERE-TK-CAT (D), pERE-2-TK-CAT E) or pERE-E1b-CAT (F) reporter plasmids in conjunction with pCMV-beta Gal plasmid as internal control. Two days later, cell cytosols were collected and assayed for CAT activities using the same amount of beta-galactosidase units.[9,11,13] D-F) From: Jeng MH et al. Endocrinology 1998; 139(10):4164-74;[13] with permission of The Endocrine Society.

tion of tritiated thymidine into DNA.[7] To demonstrate proof of the principle of MAP kinase participation, we stimulated activation of MAP kinase in wild type MCF-7 cells by administering TGFα (data not shown). Administration of TGFα caused a two log shift to the left in the ability of estradiol to stimulate the growth of wild type MCF-7 cells. To demonstrate that this effect was related specifically to MAP kinase and not to a nonMAP kinase mediated effect of TGF alpha, we co-administered PD 98059. Under these circumstances, the two log left shift in estradiol dose response, returned back to the baseline dose response curve.[7] As further evidence of the role of MAP kinase, we administered U-0126 to LTED cells and examined its effect on level of sensitivity to estradiol. This agent partially shifted dose response curves to the right by approximately one-half log (data not shown).

While an important component, MAP kinase did not appear to be solely responsible for hypersensitivity to estradiol. Blockade of this enzyme did not completely abrogate hypersensitivity. Accordingly, we examined the PI-3-kinase pathway to determine if it was up-regulated in LTED cells as well (Fig. 3B) and examined several signaling molecules downstream from this regulatory kinase.[16] We determined that LTED cells exhibit an enhanced activation of AKT (Fig. 3B, second panel), P70 S6 kinase (Fig. 3B, third panel) and PHAS-1/4E BP-1 (Fig. 3B, fourth panel; see also below).[16] Dual inhibition of PI-3- kinase with Ly 294002 (specific PI-3-kinase inhibitor) and MAP kinase with U-0126 shifted the level of sensitivity to estradiol more dramatically: more than two logs to the right (Fig. 3C).[7]

One possible mechanism to explain the activation of MAP kinase would be through nongenomic effects of estrogen acting via ERα located in or near the cell membrane.[17-19] We postulated that membrane associated ERα might utilize a classical growth factor pathway to transduce its effects in LTED cells. The adaptor protein SHC represents a key modulator of tyrosine kinase activated peptide hormone receptors.[14-15,20] Upon receptor activation and auto-phosphorylation, SHC binds rapidly to specific phosphotyrosine residues of receptors through its PTB or SH2 domain and becomes phosphorylated itself on tyrosine residues of the CH domain.[14,15] The phosphorylated tyrosine residues on the CH domain provide the docking sites for the binding of the SH2 domain of Grb2 and hence recruit SOS, a guanine nucleotide exchange protein. Formation of this adapter complex allows Ras activation via SOS, leading to the activation of the MAPK pathway.[20]

We postulated that estrogen deprivation might trigger activation of a nongenomic, estrogen-regulated, MAP kinase pathway which utilizes SHC.[14-15,20-22] We employed MAP kinase activation as an endpoint with which to demonstrate rapid nongenomic effects of estradiol (Fig. 4A). The addition of E_2 stimulated MAP kinase phosphorylation in LTED cells within minutes. The increased MAP kinase phosphorylation by E_2 was time and dose-dependent, being greatly stimulated at 15 min and remaining elevated for at least 30 min. Maximal stimulation of MAP kinase phosphorylation was at 10^{-10} M of E_2.

We then examined the role of peptides known to be involved in growth factor signaling pathways that activate MAP kinase. SHC proteins are known to couple tyrosine kinase receptors to the MAPK pathway and activation of SHC involves the phosphorylation of SHC itself.[20-22] To investigate if the SHC pathway was involved in the rapid action of estradiol in LTED cells, we immunoprecipitated tyrosine phosphorylated proteins and tested for the presence of SHC under

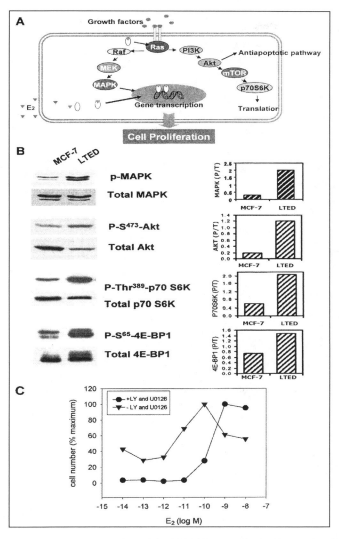

Figure 3. A) Diagrammatic representation of the MAP kinase and PI-3-kinase signaling pathways activated when growth factors bind to their trans-membrane receptors. After auto-phosphorylation of the receptor, a series of events occurs which results in the activation of Ras. Downstream from Ras is the activation of the MAP kinase pathway with its components Raf and Mek and the activation of the PI-3-kinase pathway with its downstream components Akt, mTOR and p70S6K. At the same time, estradiol binds to the estrogen receptor and initiates transcription in the nucleus. B, top) Comparison of total and activated MAP kinase, detected with a phosphospecific antibody directed against activated MAP kinase and an antibody directed against total MAP kinase, in WT (wild-type MCF-7) and LTED cells. The right portion of the panel is a quantitation of the ratio of activated to total MAP kinase in WT and LTED cells.[16] B, second, third and fourth panels) Use of phosphospecific antibodies to quantitate the levels of activated Akt (second panel), p70S6 kinase (third panel) and 4E-BP1 (fourth panel) in wild type MCF-7 and LTEDS cells.[16] C) Treatment of LTED cells with an inhibitor of MAP kinase (U-0126) and PI-3- kinase (LY 292004) to demonstrate a shift to the right of LTED cells to a normal level of sensitivity to estradiol.[7,9] From: Yue W et al. J Steroid Biochem Mol Biol 2003; 86(3-5):265-74;[8] ©2003 with permission from Elsevier.

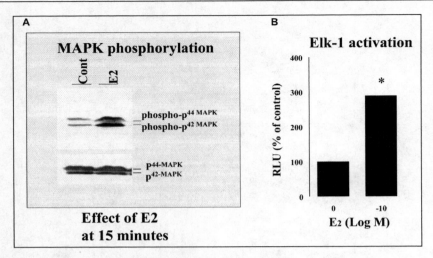

Figure 4. A) Effect of 0.1 nM estradiol on levels of activated and total MAP kinase measured 15 min after addition of steroid. Shown on the top segment is activated MAP kinase as assessed by an antibody specific for activated MAP kinase and on the bottom segment, total MAP kinase. B) Effect of 0.1 nM estradiol on the activation of ELK-1.

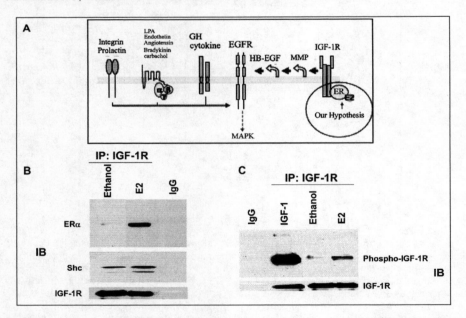

Figure 5. A) Diagrammatic representation of a model in which estradiol binds to ER⬚ which then binds to the adaptor protein, SHC. At the same time estradiol causes phosphorylation of the IGF-1-R, which provides a binding site for SHC. In this model, estradiol signals through the IGF-1-R and activates MAP kinase which then acts through Elk-1 to initiate gene transcription. B) Estradiol-induced protein complex formation among ERα, SHC and IGF-1-R. MCF-7 cells were treated with vehicle, 1 ng/ml IGF-1, or E2 at 0.1 nM for the times indicated. Lysates were immunoprecipitated with IGF-1-R antibody. The nonspecific monoclonal antibody (IgG) served as a negative control.28 C) Estradiol increases the phosphorylation of the IGF-1-R.

E_2 treatment. E_2 rapidly stimulated SHC tyrosine phosphorylation in a dose and time dependent fashion with a peak at 3 minutes.[20] The pure estrogen receptor antagonist, fulvestrant, blocked E_2-induced SHC and MAPK phosphorylation at 3 min and 15 min respectively. To demonstrate that the classical ER alpha mediated this response, we transfected a siRNA against ER alpha and showed down-regulation of this receptor and also abrogated the effect of estradiol to rapidly enhance MAP kinase activation. The time frame suggests that SHC is an upstream component in E_2-induced MAPK activation.

We reasoned that the adapter protein SHC may directly or indirectly associate with ERα in LTED cells and thereby mediate E_2-induced activation of MAP kinase. We considered this likely in light of recent evidence regarding ERα membrane localization.[23-25] To test this hypothesis, we immunoprecipitated SHC from nonstimulated and E_2-stimulated LTED cells and then probed immunoblots with anti-ERα antibodies. Our data showed that the ERα/SHC complex pre-existed before E_2 treatment and E_2 time-dependently increased this association.[20] In parallel with SHC phosphorylation, we observed a maximally induced association between ERα and SHC at 3 min (data not shown). MAP kinase pathway activation by SHC requires SHC association with the adapter protein Grb2 and then further association with SOS. By immunoprecipitation of Grb2 and detection of both SHC and SOS, we demonstrated that the SHC-Grb2-SOS complex constitutively existed at relatively low levels in LTED cells, but was greatly increased by treatment of cells with 10^{-10} M E_2 for 3 min.[20]

After the demonstration of protein-protein interactions, we wished to provide evidence that these biochemical steps resulted in biologic effects. Accordingly, we evaluated the role of estrogen activated MAP kinase on the function of the transcription factor, Elk-1. When activated, Elk-1 serves as a down stream mediator of cell proliferation. The phosphorylation of Elk1 by MAPK can up-regulate its transcriptional activity through phosphorylation. By cotransfection of LTED cells with both GAL4-Elk and its reporter gene GAL4-luc,[26,27] we were able to show that E_2 dose-dependently increased Elk-1 activation at 6 hours as shown by luciferase assay (Fig. 4B).[20]

We also wished to demonstrate biologic effects on cell morphology. To examine E_2 effects on reorganization of the actin cytoskeleton, we visualized the distribution of F-actin by phalloidin staining and also redistribution of the ERα localization in LTED and MCF-7 cells (data not shown).[20] Untreated MCF-7 cells expressed low actin polymerization and a few focal adhesion points. After E_2 stimulation, in contrast, the cytoskeleton underwent remodeling associated with formation of cellular ruffles, lamellipodia and leading edges, alterations of cell shape and loss of mature focal adhesion points. A sub-cellular redistribution of ERα to these dynamic membranes upon E_2 stimulation represented another important feature. The ER antagonist ICI 182 780 at 10^{-9} M blocked E_2-induced ruffle formation as well as redistribution of ERα to the membrane with little effect by itself. Therefore, these studies further demonstrated the rapid action of E2 with respect to dynamic membrane alterations in LTED cells.

A key unanswered question was how the ER could localize in the plasma membrane when it does not contain membrane localization motifs. We postulated that the IGF-1-receptor and SHC might be involved in this process (Fig. 5A).[28] A series of studies by other investigators suggested that ERα and the IGF-1 receptor might interact.[28] We tested the model that estradiol caused binding of SHC to ERα but also caused phosphorylation of the IGF-1 receptor. In this way, SHC would serve as the "glue" which would tether ER alpha to the plasma membrane where it would bind to the SHC acceptor site. To assess this possibility, we immunoprecipitated IGF-1 receptors before and after addition of estradiol. This caused SHC to bind to the IFG-1 receptor (Fig. 5C) and caused the IGF-1 receptor to become phosphorylated (Fig. 5B,C). In order to prove a causal effect for this role of SHC, we utilized an siRNA methodology to knock down SHC and showed that this prevented ERα from binding to the IGF-1 receptor.[28] As further evidence, we conducted confocal microscopy experiments to show that knockdown of SHC prevented ERα from localizing in the plasma membrane (data not shown).[29]

Ellis Levin and colleagues recently showed that ER alpha must be palmitylated before it can localize in the plasma membrane.[29A] Although speculative, we postulate that ER alpha requires palmitylation to travel to the plasma membrane but activated SHC serves to tether it to the membrane via IGF-1-R. In contrast to our previous concept that SHC serves as the "bus" to carry ER alpha to the membrane, we now postulate that SHC is the "glue" that tethers ER alpha there after binding to the IGF-1-R. Further studies will be necessary to dissect out each component of these interactions and their biologic relevance.

From the data reviewed, we conclude that membrane related ERα plays a role in cell proliferation and in activation of MAP kinase. It appeared likely then that LTED cells might exhibit enhanced functionality of the membrane ERα system. As evidence of this, we examined the ability of estradiol to cause the phosphorylation of SHC in wild type and MCF-7 cells and also to cause association of SHC with the membrane ERα. We demonstrated a marked enhancement of both of these processes in LTED as opposed to wild type cells. Considering all of these data together, it is still not clear at the present time what is responsible for enhancement of the nongenomic ERα mediated process.

If adaptive hypersensitivity results from the up-regulation of growth factor pathways, an inhibitor of MAP kinase and downstream PI-3-kinase pathways could be important in abolishing hypersensitivity and in inhibiting cell proliferation. We had been studying the effects of a MAP kinase inhibitor, farnesylthiosalicylic acid (FTS), which has been shown to block proliferation of LTED cells. This agent interferes with the binding of GTP-Ras to its acceptor site in the plasma membrane, a protein called galectin 1.[30] While examining its downstream effects, we have shown that this agent is also a potent inhibitor of phosphoinositol-3-kinase (PI-3-kinase). We postulated that an agent which blocks not only the MAP kinase pathway but also downstream actions of the PI-3-kinase pathway might be ideal to inhibit hypersensitivity. Accordingly, we have intensively studied the effects of FTS on mTOR.

The mammalian target of rapamycin, mTOR, is a Ser/Thr protein kinase involved in the control of cell growth and proliferation.[31] One of the best characterized substrates of mTOR is PHAS-1 (also called 4E-BP1).[32,33] PHAS-I/4E-BP1 binds to eIF4E and represses cap-dependent translation by preventing eIF4E from binding to eIF4G.[32,33] When phosphorylated by mTOR, PHAS-I/4E-BP1 dissociates from eIF4E, allowing eIF4E to engage eIF4G, thus increasing the formation of the eIF4F complex needed for the proper positioning of the 40S ribosomal subunit and for efficient scanning of the 5'-UTR.[31] In cells, mTOR is found in mTORC1, a complex also containing raptor, a newly discovered protein of 150kDa. It has been proposed that raptor functions in TORC1 as a substrate-binding subunit which presents PHAS-I/4E-BP1 to mTOR for phosphorylation.[31,32] Our results suggest that FTS inhibits phosphorylation of the mTOR effectors, PHAS-I/4E-BP1 and S6K1, in response to estrogen stimulation of breast cancer cells.[2]

To investigate the effects of FTS on mTOR function, we utilized 293T cells and monitored changes in the phosphorylation of PHAS-I/4E-BP1.[2] Incubating cells with increasing concentrations of FTS decreased the phosphorylation of PHAS-I/4E-BP1, as evidenced by a decrease in the electrophoretic mobility. To determine whether FTS also promoted dephosphorylation of Thr36 and Thr45, the preferred sites for phosphorylation by mTOR[31], an immunoblot was prepared with PThr36/45 antibodies. Increasing FTS markedly decreased the reactivity of PHAS-I/4E-BP1 with the phosphospecific antibodies (Fig. 6A,B).

To investigate further the inhibitory effects of FTS on mTOR signaling, we determined the effect of the drug on the association of mTOR, raptor and mLST8 (Fig. 6A,B). AU1-mTOR and HA-tagged forms of raptor and mLST8 were overexpressed in 293T-cells, which were then incubated with increasing concentrations of FTS before AU1-mTOR was immunoprecipitated with anti-AU1 antibodies. Immunoblots were prepared with anti-HA antibodies to assess the relative amounts of HA-raptor and HA-mLST8 that co-immunoprecipitated with AU1-mTOR. Both HA-tagged proteins were readily detectable in immune complexes from cells incubated in the absence of FTS, indicating that mTOR, raptor and mLST8 form a complex in 293T cells. FTS did not change the amount AU1-mTOR that immunoprecipitated; however, increasing concentrations of FTS produced a progressive decrease in the amount of HA-raptor that co-immunoprecipitated. The half maximal effect on raptor dissociation from mTOR was observed at approximately 30 μM

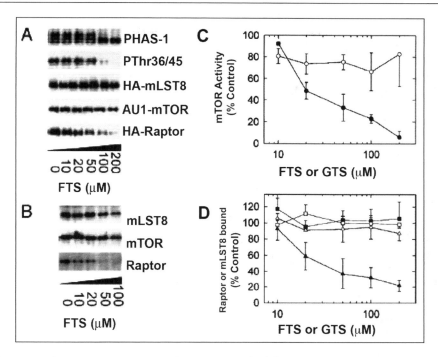

Figure 6. Left) FTS promotes raptor dissociation and inhibits mTOR activity in cell extracts. A) 293T cells were transfected with pcDNA3 alone (vector) or with a combination of pcDNA3-AU-1-mTOR, pcDNA3-3-HA-raptor and pcDNA3-3HA-mLST8. Extracts of cells were incubated with increasing concentration of FTS for 30 min before AU-1-mTOR was immunoprecipitated. Samples of the immune complexes were incubated with (γ32P)-ATP and recombinant (HIS 6) PHAS-1 and then subjected to SDS-PAGE. A phosphor image of a dried gel was obtained to detect ^{32}P-PHAS1 and an immunoblot was prepared with PThr36/45 antibodies. Other samples of the immune complexes were subjected to SDS-PAGE and immunoblots were prepared with antibodies to the HA epitope or to mTOR.[2] B) Extracts of nontransfected 293T cells were incubated with increasing concentrations of FTS before mTOR was immunoprecipitated with mTab 1. A control immuno-precipitation was conducted using nonimmune IgG(NI). Immune complexes were subjected to SDS-PAGE and immunoblots were prepared with antibodies to mLST8, mTOR and raptor.[2] Right) Relative effects of increasing concentrations of FTS and GTS on mTOR activity and the association of mTOR and raptor. Samples of extracts from 293T cells overexpressing AU1-mTOR, HA-raptor and HA-mLST8 were incubated for 1 hr with increasing concentrations of FTS (•, ♦, ■) or GTS (O,△, □) before immunopreciptations were conducted with anti-AU 1 antibodies.[2] A) mTOR kinase activity (•, O) was determined by measuring^{32}P incorporation into (HIS6) PHAS-1 in immune complex kinase assays performed with (γ32P)-ATP. B) The relative amounts of HA-raptor (♦, △) and HA-mLST8 (■, □) that co-immunoprecipitated with AU-1-mTOR were determined after immunoblotting with anti-HA antibodies. The results (mean values ± SE for five experiments) are expressed as percentages of the mTOR activity (C) or co-immununoprecipitating proteins (D) from samples incubated without FTS or GTS and have been corrected for the amounts of AU-1-mTOR immunopecipitated.[2] From: McMahon LP et al. J Mol Endocrinol 2005; 19(1):175-183;[2] with permission of The Endocrine Society.

FTS (Fig. 6A,B). Results obtained with over-expressed proteins are not necessarily representative of responses of endogenous proteins. Therefore, experiments were conducted to investigate the effect

FTS on the endogenous TORC1 in nontransfected cells. Similar results were found indicating the FTS blocks the association of raptor from mTOR.[2]

Incubating cells with FTS produced a stable decrease in mTOR activity that persisted even when mTOR was immunoprecipitated. The dose response curves for FTS-mediated inhibition of AU1-mTOR activity (Fig. 6C,D) and dissociation of AU1-mTOR and HA-raptor were very similar, with half maximal effects occurring between 20-30 μM. These results indicate that FTS inhibits mTOR in cells by promoting dissociation of raptor from mTORC1.

These studies provide direct evidence that FTS inhibits mTOR activity. The finding that the inhibition of mTOR activity by increasing concentrations of FTS correlated closely with the dissociation of the mTOR-raptor complex, both in cells and in vitro (Fig. 6), supports the conclusion that FTS acts by promoting dissociation of raptor from mTORC1.

Since FTS blocks both MAP kinase and mTOR, it was reasonable to conclude that it could block cell proliferation. For that reason, we conducted extensive studies to demonstrate that FTS blocks the growth of LTED cells. As shown in Figure 7A, B, FTS blocks the growth on LTED cells both in vitro and in vivo.

Our studies to date have predominantly concentrated on long term estradiol deprivation as a mode of development of resistance to aromatase inhbitors. More recently, we have examined the effect of long term tamoxifen treatment (LTTT) on MCF-7 cells. Interestingly, this maneuver also causes enhanced sensitivity to estradiol, both in vitro and in vivo.[34,35] While the up-regulation of MAP kinase is only transitory for a period of 2-3 months, these cells become hypersensitive to EGF-R mediated pathways. At the same time, we have demonstrated increased complex formation between ER alpha and the EGF-R and between ER alpha and cSRC. These studies also demonstrate that the tamoxifen resistant cells become hypersensitive to the inhibitory properties of the EGF-R tyrosine kinase inhibitor, AG 1478.

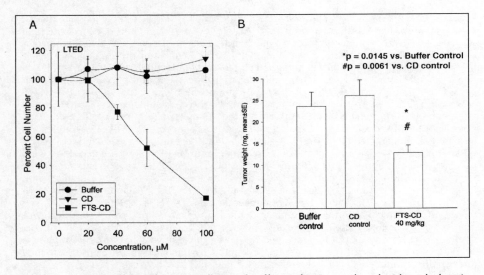

Figure 7. A) In vitro effects of FTS on cell growth. Effects of FTS complexed with cyclodextrin (CD) for solubility were compared with buffer or cyclodextrin (CD) alone on the number of LTED cells expressed as a percent of maximum number. The ordinate shows the concentration of FTS used. B) In vivo effects of FTS on cell growth. LTED cells were implanted into castrate nude mice to form xenografts. Silastic implants delivering estradiol at amounts sufficient to provide plasma levels of estradiol of 5 pg/ml were implanted. One group received buffer alone, the second cyclodextrin alone and the third FTS 40 mg/kg complexed to cyclodextrin. The effects of FTS-CD compared to CD control were statistically significant at p = 0.0061.

Significance of Our Findings to Development of Further Therapies

Our data suggest that cells adapt to hormonal therapy by up-regulation of growth factor pathways and ultimately become resistant to that therapy. Blockade of the pathways involved might then allow enhancement of the duration of responsiveness to various hormonal agents. Studies by Osborne and Schiff et al[36,37] and by Nicholson and his group[38,39] have demonstrated this phenomenon both in vitro and in vivo. For example, Schiff and Osborne have treated HER-2/neu transfected MCF-7 cells with a cocktail of three kinase inhibitors: pertuzmab, gefitamab and traztuzmab as well as tamoxifen.[40] Each sequential growth factor inhibitor caused a further delay in development of resistance. Only 2/20 tumors began to regrow as a reflection of resistance when the four agents were used in combination (i.e., tamoxifen, pertuzmab, gefitimab and traztuzmab).

There are multiple agents currently in development to block growth factor pathways. Agents are available to block HER-1, 2, 3 and 4; EGF-R, IGF-R, mTOR, MAP kinase, Raf and MEK. Each of these agents might potentially be used in combination with an endocrine therapy. At the present time, this strategy is being used in several studies. A recent presentation demonstrated proof of the principle of this concept. Women with metastatic breast cancer selected to be ERα and HER-2 positive were treated either with an aromatase inhibitor alone or in combination with Herceptin. The percent of patients achieving clinical benefit (i.e., complete objective tumor regression, partial regression or stable disease for >6 months) was 27.9% percent in the aromatase inhibitor alone group and 42.9% in the combined group, a statistically significant ($p = 0.026$) finding.[41] Further studies will be necessary to determine the optimal combinations of growth factor and aromatase inhibitors in the future. However, based upon the Tandem study (examining the efficacy of aromatase inhibitor plus Herceptin), this approach appears to be promising.

Synthesis of Our Current Thinking

Our current working model to explain adaptive hypersensitivity can be summarized as follows. Long term estradiol deprivation causes a four to ten fold up-regulation of the amount of ERα present in cell extracts and an increase in basal level of transcription of several estradiol stimulated genes. The up-regulation of the ER results from demethylation of promoter C of the ER. The lack of shift to the left in the dose response curves of these transcriptional endpoints suggested that hypersensitivity is not mediated primarily at the transcriptional level (Fig. 1 and 2). On the other hand, rapid, nongenomic effects of estradiol such as the phosphorylation of SHC and binding of SHC to ERα are easily demonstrable and appear enhanced in the LTED cells. Taken together, these observations suggest that adaptive hypersensitivity is associated with an increased utilization of nongenomic, plasma membrane mediated pathways. This results in an increased level of activation of the MAP kinase as well as the PI-3-kinase and mTOR pathways. All of these signals converge on downstream effectors which are directly involved in cell cycle functionality and which probably exert synergistic effects at that level. As a reflection of this synergy, E2F1, an integrator of cell cycle stimulatory and inhibitory events, is hypersensitive to the effects of estradiol in LTED cells.[7] Thus, our working hypothesis at present is that hypersensitivity reflects upstream nongenomic ERα events as well as downstream synergistic interactions of several pathways converging at the level of the cell cycle.

It is clear that primary endocrine therapies can exert pressure on breast cancer cells that causes them to adapt as a reflection of their inherent plasticity. Based upon this concept, we postulate that certain patients may become resistant to tamoxifen as a result of developing hypersensitivity to the estrogenic properties of tamoxifen. Up-regulation of growth factor pathways involving erb-B-2, IGF-1 receptor and the EGF receptor are associated with this process.[2] The estrogen agonistic properties of tamoxifen under these circumstances might explain the superiority of clinical responses in patients receiving aromatase inhibitors as opposed to tamoxifen. It is possible to counteract the effects of the adaptive processes leading to growth factor up-regulation. If breast cancer cells are exceedingly sensitive to small amounts of estradiol or to the estrogenic properties of tamoxifen, one therefore needs highly potent aromatase inhibitors to block estrogen synthesis or pure antiestrogens such as fulvestrant. Blockade of the downstream effects of the IGF-1-R,

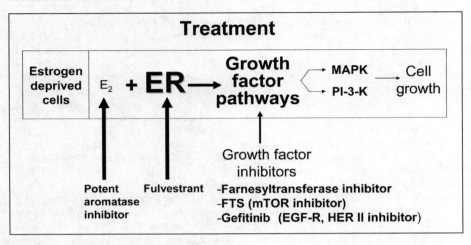

Figure 8. Practical implications of the effects of up-regulation of growth factor pathways and development of hypersensitivity to estradiol. Potent aromatase inhibitors are useful to counteract the enhanced sensitivity to estradiol resulting from adaptation to prolonged estradiol deprivation. A pure antiestrogen such as fulvestrant can counteract the up-regulation of the ER that occurs. Growth factor inhibitors such as FTS, farnesyl-transferase inhibitors and growth factor inhibitors such as Iressa and others can be used to block up-regulation of growth factor pathways.

EGF-R and erb-B-2 pathways would also be beneficial and allow continuing responsiveness to aromatase inhibitors or tamoxifen.

Disruption of each of several key steps could reduce the level of sensitivity to estradiol and block cell growth. Figure 8 illustrates the potential sites for disruption of adaptive hypersensitivity. An agent that blocks the nodal points through which several growth factor pathways must pass might be a more suitable therapy than combination of several growth factor blocking agents. Our preliminary data suggest that FTS blocks two nodal points, the functionality of Ras and the activity of mTOR. FTS also effectively inhibits the proliferation of MCF-7 breast cancer cells in culture. Since this agent blocks MAP kinase as well as mTOR, it may be ideal for the prevention of adaptive hypersensitivity and prolongation of the effects of hormonal therapy in breast cancer. We are currently conducting further studies in xenograft models to demonstrate its efficacy. We envision the possibility that women with breast cancer will receive a combination of aromatase inhibitors plus FTS. In this way, the beneficial effects of the aromatase inhibitor may be prolonged and relapses due to growth factor over-expression might be prevented or retarded.

Acknowledgments
These studies have been supported by NIH RO-1 grants Ca 65622 and Ca 84456 and Department of Defense Centers of Excellence Grant DAMD17-03-1-0229.

References
1. Santen RJ, Manni A, Harvey H et al. Endocrine treatment of breast cancer in women. Endocr Rev 1990; 11(2):221-265.
2. McMahon LP, Yue W, Santen RJ et al. Farnesylthiosalicylic acid inhibits mammalian target of rapamycin (mTOR) activity both in cells and in vitro by promoting dissociation of the mTOR-raptor complex. J Mol Endocrinol 2005; 19(1):175-183.
3. Santen RJ, Song RX, Zhang Z et al. Long-term estradiol deprivation in breast cancer cells up-regulates growth factor signaling and enhances estrogen sensitivity. Endocr Relat Cancer 2005; 12(Suppl.1): S61-73.

4. Shim WS, DiRenzo J, DeCaprio JA et al. Segregation of steroid receptor coactivator-1 from steroid receptors in mammary epithelium. Proc Natl Acad Sci USA 1999; 96(1):208-13.
5. Shim WS, Conaway M, Masamura S et al. Estradiol hypersensitivity and mitogen-activated protein kinase expression in long-term estrogen deprived human breast cancer cells in vivo. Endocrinology 2000; 141(1):396-405.
6. Yue W, Wang J, Li Y et al. Farnesylthiosalicylic acid blocks mammalian target of rapamycin signaling in breast cancer cells. Int J Cancer 2005; 117(5):746-754.
7. Yue W, Wang JP, Conaway M et al. Activation of the MAPK pathway enhances sensitivity of MCF-7 breast cancer cells to the mitogenic effect of estradiol. Endocrinology 2002; 143(9):3221-3229.
8. Yue W, Wang JP, Conaway MR et al. Adaptive hypersensitivity following long-term estrogen deprivation: involvement of multiple signal pathways. Journal of Steroid Biochemistry & Molecular Biology 2003; 86(3-5):265-74.
9. Song RX. Membrane-initiated steroid signaling action of estrogen and breast cancer. Seminars in Reproductive Medicine 2007; 25(3):187-197.
10. Song RX, Fan P, Yue W, Chen Y, Santen RJ. Role of receptor complexes in the extranuclear actions of estrogen receptor alpha in breast cancer. Endocrine-Related Cancer 2006; 13 (Suppl 1):S3-S13.
11. Jeng MH, Yue W, Eischeid A et al. Role of MAP kinase in the enhanced cell proliferation of long term estrogen deprived human breast cancer cells. Breast Cancer Res Treat 2000; 62(3):167-175.
12. Masamura S, Santner SJ, Heitjan DF et al. Estrogen deprivation causes estradiol hypersensitivity in human breast cancer cells. J Clin Endocrinol Metab 1995; 80(10):2918-2925.
13. Jeng MH, Shupnik MA, Bender TP et al. Estrogen receptor expression and function in long-term estrogen-deprived human breast cancer cells. Endocrinology 1998; 139(10):4164-74.
13a. Sogon T, Masamura S, Hayashi S-I et al. J Steroid Biochem Mol Biol 2007; 105(1-3):106-14.
14. Pelicci G, Lanfrancone L, Salcini AE et al. Constitutive phosphorylation of SHC proteins in human tumors. Oncogene 1995; 11(5):899-907.
15. Pelicci G, Dente L, De Giuseppe A et al. A family of SHC related proteins with conserved PTB, CH1 and SH2 regions. Oncogene 1996; 13(3):633-641.
16. Yue W, Wang JP, Li Y et al. Farnesylthiosalicylic acid blocks mammalian target of rapamycin signaling in breast cancer cells. Int J Cancer 2005; 117(5):746-54.
17. Migliaccio A, Di Domenico M, Castoria G et al. Tyrosine kinase/p21ras/MAP-kinase pathway activation by estradiol-receptor complex in MCF-7 cells. EMBO J 1996; 15(6):1292-1300.
18. Kelly MJ, Lagrange AH, Wagner EJ et al. Rapid effects of estrogen to modulate G protein-coupled receptors via activation of protein kinase A and protein kinase C pathways. Steroids 1999; 64(1-2):64-75.
19. Valverde MA, Rojas P, Amigo J et al. Acute activation of Maxi-K channels (hSlo) by estradiol binding to the beta subunit [see comments]. Science 1999; 285(5435):1929-1931.
20. Song RX, McPherson RA, Adam L et al. Linkage of rapid estrogen action to MAPK activation by ERalpha-SHC association and SHC pathway activation. J Mol Endocrinol 2002; 16(1):116-127.
21. Dikic I, Batzer AG, Blaikie P et al. SHC binding to nerve growth factor receptor is mediated by the phosphotyrosine interaction domain. J Biol Chem 1995; 270(25):15125-15129.
22. Boney CM, Gruppuso PA, Faris RA et al. The critical role of SHC in insulin-like growth factor-I-mediated mitogenesis and differentiation in 3T3-L1 preadipocytes. J Mol Endocrinol 2000; 14(6):805-813.
23. Collins P, Webb C. Estrogen hits the surface. [see comments]. Nature Medicine 1999; 5(10):1130-1131.
24. Watson CS, Campbell CH, Gametchu B. Membrane oestrogen receptors on rat pituitary tumour cells: immuno-identification and responses to oestradiol and xenoestrogens. [Review] [45 refs]. Exp Physiol 1999; 84(6):1013-1022.
25. Watson CS, Norfleet AM, Pappas TC et al. Rapid actions of estrogens in GH3/B6 pituitary tumor cells via a plasma membrane version of estrogen receptor-alpha. Steroids 1999; 64(1-2):5-13.
26. Duan R, Xie W, Burghardt RC et al. Estrogen receptor-mediated activation of the serum response element in MCF-7 cells through MAPK-dependent phosphorylation of Elk-1. J Biol Chem 2001; 276(15):11590-11598.
27. Roberson MS, Misra-Press A, Laurance ME et al. A role for mitogen-activated protein kinase in mediating activation of the glycoprotein hormone alpha-subunit promoter by gonadotropin-releasing hormone. Mol Cell Biol 1995; 15(7):3531-3539.
28. Song RX, Barnes CJ, Zhang Z et al. The role of SHC and insulin-like growth factor 1 receptor in mediating the translocation of estrogen receptor alpha to the plasma membrane. Proc Natl Acad Sci USA 2004; 101(7):2076-81.
29. Song RX, Santen RJ. Role of IFG-1R in mediating nongenomic effects of estrogen receptor alpha. Paper presented at: The Endocrine Society's 85th Annual Meeting (USA). Philadelphia, 2003.
29a. Pedram A, Razandi M, Sainson RC et al. A conserved mechanism for steroid receptor translocation to the plasma membrane. J Biol Chem. 2007; 282(31):22278-88.

30. Haklai R, Weisz MG, Elad G et al. Dislodgment and accelerated degradation of Ras. Biochemistry 1998; 37(5):1306-14.
31. Harris TE, Lawrence JC Jr. TOR signaling. [Review] [221 refs]. Science's Stke [Electronic Resource]: Sci STKE 2003; (212):ref 15.
32. Lawrence JC Jr, Brunn GJ. Insulin signaling and the control of PHAS-I phosphorylation. [Review] [102 refs]. Prog Mol Subcell Biol 2001; 26:1-31.
33. Brunn GJ, Hudson CC, Sekulic A et al. Phosphorylation of the translational repressor PHAS-I by the mammalian target of rapamycin. Science 1997; 277(5322):99-101.
34. Berstein L, Zheng H, Yue W et al. New approaches to the understanding of tamoxifen action and resistance. Endocr Relat Cancer. 2003; 10(2):267-77.
35. Fan P, Wang J, Santen RJ et al. Long-term treatment with tamoxifen facilitates translocation of estrogen receptor alpha out of the nucleus and enhances its interaction with EGFR in MCF-7 breast cancer cells. Cancer Res 2007; 67(3):1352-1360.
36. Osborne CK, Hamilton B, Titus G et al. Epidermal growth factor stimulation of human breast cancer cells in culture. Cancer Res 1980; 40(7):2361-2366.
37. Osborne CK, Fuqua SA. Mechanisms of Tamoxifen Resistance. Breast Cancer Res Treat 1994; 32:49-55.
38. Hiscox S, Morgan L, Green TP et al. Elevated Src activity promotes cellular invasion and motility in tamoxifen resistant breast cancer cells. Breast Cancer Res Treat 2006; 97(3):263-274.
39. Hiscox S, Morgan L, Barrow D et al. Tamoxifen resistance in breast cancer cells is accompanied by an enhanced motile and invasive phenotype: inhibition by gefitinib ('Iressa', ZD1839). Clin Exp Metastasis 2004; 21(3):201-212.
40. Schiff R, Massarweh SA, Shou J et al. Advanced concepts in estrogen receptor biology and breast cancer endocrine resistance: implicated role of growth factor signaling and estrogen receptor coregulators. [Review] [97 refs]. Cancer Chemother Pharmacol 2005; 56(Suppl 1):10-20.
41. Mackey JR, Kaufman B, Clemens M et al. Trastuzumab prolongs progression-free survival in hormone dependent and HER2-positive metastatic breast cancer. Breast Cancer Res Treat 2006: 100:(Suppl 1): S5, Ab 3.

Chapter 3

Role of Endocrine-Genotoxic Switchings in Cancer and Other Human Diseases:
Basic Triad

Lev M. Berstein*

Abstract

Cancer is one of the leading causes of human death and belongs to the group of main chronic noncommunicable diseases (NCD). Certain specific features of NCD have raised the concept of 'normal' and 'successful' aging. The apparent paradox of simultaneous increase with aging of the diseases connected with estrogen deficiency as well as with estrogenic excess can be explained by the existence of the phenomenon of the switching of estrogen effects. An isolated or combined with the weakening of hormonal effect increase in genotoxic action of estrogens can modify the course of age-associated pathology. In particular, such changes in estrogen effect may alter the biology of tumors to make them less favorable/more aggressive. Two other endocrine-genotoxic switchings (EGS) involving phenomena of Janus (dual) function of glucose and adipogenotoxicosis may produce similar influences on tumor and other NCD biology. These three phenomena form a 'basic triad' and can act independently of each other or in concert. EGS and their inductors may serve as targets for prevention and, probably, treatment of main noncommunicable diseases. The measures to correct components of the 'triad' can be divided into several groups aimed to optimally orchestrate the balance between endocrine and DNA-damaging effects of estrogens, glucose and adipose tissue-related factors.

Introduction

Cancer (including tumors of hormone dependent tissues) is one of the leading causes of human death and belongs to the group of main chronic noncommunicable diseases (NCD).[1,2] In addition to cancer, several NCD such as atherosclerosis, arterial hypertension, diabetes, neurodegenerative pathology, chronic pulmonary disease and osteoporosis increase with advancing age.[2] The burden of these diseases, as is well known, becomes particularly prevalent in the second half of life, after age 50-60. Notwithstanding the quite demonstrative increase in the average age when these diseases are diagnosed, the characteristics of them including clinical course and individual time of onset are highly variable. Under the surface of the same nosological form can be hidden distinctive pathological processes, which result in differences in aggressiveness, alterations in the frequency of their appearance in the population, changes in the rate/velocity of progression and reaction to treatment. In aggregate, these distinctions may lead to different levels of mortality and—as reflection of that—to individually different life span.

*Lev M. Berstein—Laboratory of Oncoendocrinology, Prof. N.N. Petrov Research Institute of Oncology, St. Petersburg, Russia. Email: levmb@endocrin.spb.ru

Innovative Endocrinology of Cancer, edited by Lev M. Berstein and Richard J. Santen.
©2008 Landes Bioscience and Springer Science+Business Media.

In the attempt to explain such widespread and not rarely discussed differences in morbidity and mortality at the later stages of ontogenesis, the concept was proposed that aging could either be normal or successful.[3,4] According to this concept[4] successful aging was characterized by three components: (1) (relatively) high mental and physical function, (2) active engagement with life, including close relationships with others and most importantly (3) (relatively) low risk of disease and disease-related disability. With complete understanding that the term successful aging may itself have the unintended effect of defining a significant part of population as unsuccessful and therefore as failing, the authors hoped that their classification will invite researchers to investigate the heterogeneity among middle-age and older people and to discover its causes—genetic, psychosocial and environmental.[5]

The possible causes of these distinctions are not, of course, limited to those presented above. The key applicable word is "heterogeneity" and this applies to the mechanisms of hormonal carcinogenesis (see in detail the chapters by Chen and Yager and Santen et al in this volume) as well as to the factors predisposing to the two principal types of the latter—promotional or stochastic/mitogenic and genotoxic.[6-9]

During several recent years we have attempted to understand what conditions may advance or be associated with a shift from promotional to less favorable genotoxic type of hormone-induced carcinogenesis and from less to more aggressive variants of several other noncommunicable diseases. Subsequently, we have focused upon three events: phenomenon of switching of estrogen effects (PSEE), Janus, or dual, function of glucose (JFG) and adipogenotoxicosis (AdG).[10-12] This treatise will first provide an introductory background and then, present an analysis of these phenomena (forming so called 'basic triad') as well as the practical implications following from them.

General Principle: Types of Effects

The world rather often is binary. Although transitions from the one state to another sometimes are not possible, in fact, in biology and medicine almost nothing goes according to one scenario. Even in seemingly very strict situations, like cell fate determination involving Notch signaling, all cells in a given population can adopt an alternative fate, but some maintain this new destiny stably, whereas others revert to the default state.[13] In case of the whole organism choices are understandably manifold and variable. Nevertheless, with reference to hormones and some hormone-associated substances their different activities (taking into account possible associations with cancer and other NCD) may be reduced to the two primary: hormonal or endocrine and DNA-damaging or genotoxic.[9,10] Factors inducing or supporting an increase in the ratio of genotoxic/hormonal effects can be considered correspondingly as direct or indirect genotoxicants. Endocrine-genotoxic switchings (transitions which alter function in the direction of DNA-damaging effects) may be not only induced but also spontaneous/constitutive, e.g., in genetically or otherwise predisposed persons. These switchings can be manifested by a) an isolated increase of genotoxic effects without a decrease in hormonal effect (relative predominance) as well as with b) combined trend toward an increase in genotoxic effects and decrease in hormonal effects (absolute predominance), Figure 1. Understandably, it is not enough to admit that the coin has two sides; depending of situation it is essential also to clarify which side and when is more important.[14]

Phenomenon of Switching of Estrogen Effects (PSEE)

Although an idea that estrogen-induced carcinogenesis per se and the modulating action of estrogens on carcinogenesis are different notions was emphasized a rather long time ago,[15] drawing a line between these two events is not very easy. One explanation for such difficulty lies in the absence of complete understanding of whether the modifying effect of hormones involves only epigenetic pathways.[16]

Those who believe in the exclusive role of estrogens as mitogenic and promoting factors proposed that increased hormonal stimulation is an important link in the process of hormone dependent tumor development. The attention of these investigators was attracted first by the observation of enhanced proliferation in target tissues under conditions of excessive estrogenic influence.

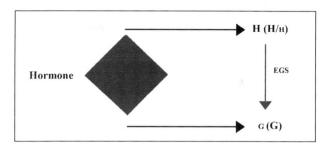

Figure 1. The principle of endocrine-genotoxic switchings applied to hormones, hormone-related substances and changes in target tissues. H—hormonal effect (not changed or decreased); G—genotoxic effect (increased); EGS—spontaneous or induced endocrine-genotoxic switchings.

Thus, in other words, it was concluded that "no increased proliferation—no hormone-induced carcinogenesis".

Later studies stated that though "... proliferation is necessary, it may not be sufficient for neoplastic transformation"[6,17] and suggested several additions to the proffered scheme. This, after passing through critique, discussions and several intermediate concepts,[16] led finally to contemporary point of view which indicates that mitogenic as well as mutagenic effects of estrogens act in concert to initiate and promote the development of cancer.[6,8,18] Initially, rather extensive research has concentrated upon possible procarcinogenic properties of 16α-hydroxylated estrogens, including their genotoxic effects.[19] More recently, 4-hydroxylated metabolites of estradiol and estrone and their further metabolic conversions, in preference to the 2-hydrohylated derivatives, have been the focus of studies in the context of estrogen-induced cancer.[7,20,21] Additionally, recent observations demonstrated the ability of estradiol to activate human CYP1B1 (estrogen-4-hydroxylase) gene via ER-alpha, thereby providing insights into the homeostasis of estrogen metabolism as well the interaction of potential pathways of estrogen-induced carcinogenesis.[22]

The dual role of estrogen in tumor development as both a hormone stimulating cell proliferation and as a procarcinogen that induces genetic damage, indicates that the search of conditions or factors modulating the genotoxic component in total estrogenic (genomic and nongenomic) effect can be essential. Such factors may influence both the hormonal carcinogenesis process and biological properties of the developing hormone-dependent tumors.[9,23]

As we demonstrated previously, in oophorectomized rats, tobacco smoke induces phased changes in uterotrophic action of estrogens, which finally result in attenuation of the hormonal (H) component of their effect (dynamics of uterine weight and proliferation index, etc) and in increase of the rate of genotoxic (G) damage (COMET assay). The phenomenon was referred as switching of estrogen effects (PSEE).[10,24] Interestingly, although it is known that smoking increases 2-hydroxylation of estrogens[25] the same factor may stimulate CYP1B1 in the aerodigestive tract,[26] thus denoting one of the pathways through which estrogenic DNA-damaging activity can be increased.

In a recently performed investigation, the hormonal and genotoxic effects of estradiol (E2) and their possible modification by diluted tobacco smoke condensate (TSC) were studied in breast cancer MCF-7 cell line.[27] TSC decreased effect of E2 on the cell counts and opposed the anti-apoptotic influence of this hormone (Fig. 2A,B). The combination of TSC with E2 promoted progesterone receptor B induction after 5 days of cocultivation (Fig. 2C). However, in long-term (3 mo) studies in vivo the same combination of agents led to a diminution of this hormonal estrogenic effect.[24] In addition, in MCF-7 cells treated with TSC and E2 (in the lesser of two studied concentrations, 10^{-11} M) the immunocytochemical staining of oxidative DNA damage marker, 8-OHdG, revealed higher values than in cells processed with these agents separately (Fig. 2D).[27]

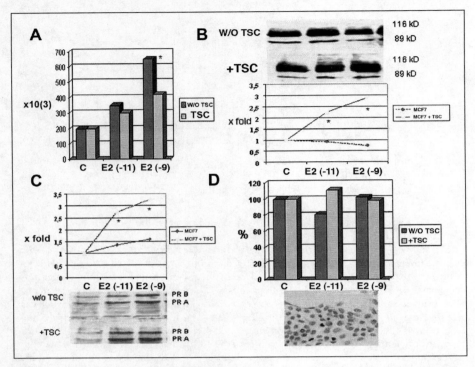

Figure 2. Modification of estradiol (E2) effects by tobacco smoke condensate (TSC) in MCF-7 cells. Diluted TSC was used in final concentration equivalent to 2.5 mcg of cigarette tar/ml medium and E2 as 10^{-11} M and 10^{-9} M. The duration of experiments varied between 2 and 5 days. A) Cell counts. Cell growth was monitored by cell number counting. Briefly, cells growing in 6-well plates were treated with E2 and/or TSC as indicated in figure legend. Cells were rinsed with 0.9% saline, lysed in ZAP buffer and counted with a model Z1 Coulter counter. B) Apoptosis. This parameter was evaluated by the cleavage of poly-ADP ribose polymerase (PARP) and immunoblotting. Cells were washed with ice phosphate-buffered saline and extracted with binding buffer. Equal amounts of protein from cell extracts were analyzed on SDS-polyacrilamide gels and transferred to PVDF membranes. The membranes were probed with rabbit polyclonal antiPARP antibody, 1:1000 (Cell Signaling). The immunoblots were incubated with antirabbit secondary antibodies and further developed using the chemiluminescence detection system (Pierce). Data are presented as 116 kD/89 kD ratios. C) Progesterone receptor (B isoform). In this case PVDF membranes were probed with mouse monoclonal antiprogesterone receptor antibodies, 1:1000 (Cell Signaling). The immunoblots were incubated with antimouse secondary antibodies and developed using the chemiluminescence detection system. Data are presented as PR B ratio in relation to control values. D) 8-hydroxy-2'-deoxyguanosine (8-OH-dG). Cells were fixed with ethanol and acetone and evaluated by immunocytochemical method with mouse monoclonal anti-8-OH-dG antibody 4E9, 1:200 (Trevigen). Data are presented as relative scores.

The latter data are in line with observations demonstrating higher levels of DNA adducts in cervical tissue of young smoking women taking oral estrogen-containing contraceptives in comparison with nonsmokers or contraceptive nonusers.[28] They also correspond with data reporting higher excretion of carcinogenic and genotoxic cathecholestrogens (in particular, 4-hydroxyestrogens) in smoking postmenopausal women treated with estradiol valerate, Proginova (Table 1).[29] It is noteworthy that before the start of estrogen replacement therapy, the excretion of 4-hydroxyestrone and 4-hydroxyestradiol in smokers was not higher than in nonsmokers. This observation suggests that

Table 1. *Urinary excretion of estrogen metabolites as means and standard deviations, nmol/24 h in nonsmoking and smoking postmenopausal women receiving estrogen replacement therapy, ERT*

Urinary Estrogen Fraction	Nonsmokers		Smokers	
	Before ERT	**After ERT**	**Before ERT**	**After ERT**
E1	9.70 ± 8.60	1232.6 ± 295.2	14.46 ± 13.24	951.5 ± 181.2
E2	2.87 ± 2.14	212.6 ± 42.2	3.65 ± 2.60	235.7 ± 40.5
E3	4.38 ± 2.37	178.3 ± 75.2	3.31 ± 2.49	131.2 ± 83.2
4-OHE1	2.29 ± 1.28[a]	28.8 ± 10.6	1.09 ± 0.51[a]	43.7 ± 18.2
4-OHE2	0.07 ± 0.08	23.5 ± 15.6[a]	0.10 ± 0.13	60.8 ± 25.3[a]
2-OHE1	8.88 ± 8.42	226.9 ± 68.3[a]	6.52 ± 3.78	330.9 ± 80.0[a]
2-OHE2	2.19 ± 2.09	36.4 ± 11.7	2.05 ± 0.56	45.8 ± 9.2
2-MOE1	2.49 ± 1.57	53.4 ± 15.1	2.36 ± 0.79	51.3 ± 21.9
2-MOE2	0.37 ± 0.26	3.10 ± 0.80	0.41 ± 0.25	3.20 ± 1.10
16α-OHE1	3.79 ± 3.40	104.8 ± 78.1	2.46 ± 1.40	105.8 ± 66.8

[a]Difference between smokers and nonsmokers is significant (p at least <0.05). E1, estrone; E2, estradiol; E3, estriol; 4-OHE1, 4-hydroxyestrone; 4-OHE2, 4-hydroxyestradiol; 2-OHE1, 2-hydroxyestrone; 2-OHE2, 2-hydroxyestradiol; 2-MOE1, 2-methoxyestrone; 2-MOE2, 2-methoxyestradiol; 16α-OHE1, 16α-hydroxyestrone. Reprinted from Berstein LM, Tsyrlina EV, Kolesnik OS et al. J Steroid Biochem Mol Biol 2000; 72:143-7. With permission from Elsevier.

only the combination of external estrogen and smoking promotes the switch into the direction of increased formation of genotoxic estrogen metabolites.[10,29]

For the subject under consideration and in addition to the named estrogen metabolism features, the sensitivity of target tissues to estrogens is without doubt of importance too. About 30-40% of breast cancers lack steroid receptors (ER and/or PR) at diagnosis, a finding which predicts an unfavorable prognosis and a limited response to usage of hormone therapy.

Opinions differ as to whether receptor negative cancers arise from R(−) compartment within the mammary epithelium or represent evolution from R(+) to R(−) state. Evidence in support of the idea on distinct etiologic pathways rather than different stages in the natural history of breast cancer has been recently growing.[30,31] Receptor-positive and receptor-negative breast cancer subtypes may have associations with distinctive risk factors and heterogeneity by hormone-receptor status related to initial existence of the two separate types of cancer (R+ and R−) is rather possible.[30,32]

The mechanisms leading to the development of receptor-negative breast cancer (BC) warrant further studies. Existing interpretations are not definitive and can be reduced to the role of several genetic (including BRCA1 and BRCA2) and epigenetic factors, interrelations with the presence of EGF and erbB2/HER-2/neu receptors in tumor tissue and certain features of endocrine (reproductive) system which consider the level of estrogen in the blood and intratumoral aromatase/estrogen synthetase activity.[31,33-35]

Taking into account the principal characteristics of the phenomenon of switching of estrogen effects (PSEE) described above, the assumption has been made that weakening of hormonal and strengthening of genotoxic activity of estrogens may be of importance in predisposing to disturbances in estrogen signal transduction and preferential formation of receptor-negative BC.[24] In fact, statistically significant distinction between smoking and nonsmoking BC patients was revealed only in reproductive period and only in regard of ER+ PR− tumors, which were overrepresented in smokers (t = 2.18, p < 0.05; χ^2 = 5.01, p = 0.025).[36] Predominant formation of the tumors with a phenotype presumably reflecting failure of estrogenic signal transduction and insufficient induction of estrogen-dependent proteins including PR[37,38] in smoking females with conserved menstrual cycle, suggests that tobacco smoke promotes PSEE mainly in the case of excessive or at least nondeficient estrogenic stimulation.

A contemporary view links the origin of receptor-positive and receptor-negative breast tumors correspondingly with luminal and basal type of mammary epithelium.[39] Interestingly, the diminished survival observed in BC patients who smoke[40] can be associated with receptor-negative phenotype[36,41] and with switch to a basal/myoepithelial lineage. The same switch was discovered under influence of progestins which partly explains the higher BC risks and poorer prognosis on postmenopausal estrogen-progestin replacement therapy (HRT).[42] Effects of HRT differ depending on women age and are more favorable during a rather short (first 5-7 yrs after menopause) "critical window".[43] Thus it is possible that endocrine predominance in estrogen effect leads to less aggressive luminal subtype of BC, while genotoxic predominance in the action of these hormones, associated in particular with smoking, promotes more clinically tough and mostly receptor-negative mammary carcinoma type. Of note, in receptor-negative endometrial cancer type II, mutations of p53 are found[44] which arrest cellular check-points activation and promote proliferation of cells with signs of DNA damage.[45] Consequently, inefficient DNA repair may tentatively be included into the orbit of events directly or indirectly supporting a PSEE-associated genotoxic switch. Other genetic and epigenetic abnormalities related to DNA-damaging estrogen action may also be involved into this process.

We made an attempt to find additional factors inducing the phenomenon of switching of estrogen effects. The accumulated experimental data suggests that PSEE can be divided into complete switching with a simultaneous increase of genotoxic component and decrease of hormonal component in estrogenic effect and incomplete, with an isolated increase in DNA-damaging capacity only. The inductors of PSEE may be classified in a corresponding manner as complete and incomplete. Summing up results received in oophorectomized rats injected with estradiol, complete PSEE inductors include long-term treatment with tobacco smoke and drinking of 15% ethanol (i.e., in levels equal to chronic alcoholism). The group of incomplete inductors included consumption of alcohol in more moderate, 5%, concentration, single whole-body γ-irradiation in the lesser (0.2 Grays) of two investigated doses and aging.[10,24] Certain xenoestrogens may work in a similar fashion. Fortunately they are distributed in nature in low concentrations. Although their action may be mediated primarily through aryl hydrocarbonic receptors, or AhR,[46] this action may be estrogen-dependent as well. Indeed, dioxins induce DNA adducts formation in liver of intact but not oophorectomized rats[47] and in MCF-10A cells TCDD and estradiol do not provoke oxidative stress separately while induce it in combination.[48]

Thus, it is possible that low-concentrated but widespread progenotoxic "natural agents" combined with estrogenic stimulation might be a dangerous risk factor for cancer and some other chronic noncommunicable diseases. PSEE is manifested in such conditions as an increased genotoxic effect of estrogens, which may be or may be not coupled with retained hormonal, e.g., mitogenic, influence of these hormones.[9] The same rationale should be taken into consideration when analysis goes beyond estrogens.

Janus (Dual) Function of Glucose

Major investigative attention has focused during several recent decades upon the metabolic syndrome. The abnormalities associated with this syndrome, first of all hyperinsulinemia and insulin resistance, may increase the risk of hormone dependent cancer and predispose to simultaneous development of other frequent and, in the end, lethal chronic human illnesses (like cardiovascular disease, stroke, type 2 diabetes, etc.). Typical characteristics of the metabolic syndrome may include also visceral obesity, hypertension, chronic low-level inflammatory state, dyslipidemia and—rather often—impaired carbohydrate tolerance.[49-51]

Together with aging-related events, one of the greatest contribution to the current expansion of noncommunicable pathology is the combined influence of disordered nutrition and impaired physical activity.[1,2] In most parts of the world (understandably, with some exceptions), as food became more available, new insights into the relationship between carbohydrates and chronic diseases became apparent. A high glycemic load is associated with increased risk of these diseases including cancer and a pathogenic role in the process can be played by postprandial hypergly-cemia.[52,53] In concert with hyperinsulinemia and activation of IGF-I and mammalian target of rapamycin (mTOR) systems, glucose along with some other nutrients, creates a metabolic/mitogenic platform for the amplification of cellular proliferation.[54,55] Importantly, according to some observations, intrinsic or nutritionally induced glucose intolerance may increase risk of hormone dependent cancer to a higher degree than does overt diabetes.[56]

In mammalian cells the glucose fate begins with glucose transport and metabolism and ends, among innumerable other functions, with two actions, which can be considered as principal.[10,11,57] The first, which may be designated as an endocrine effect, is realized due to the ability of glucose to be a stimulus for hormonal secretion, particularly, for insulin production in pancreatic β-cells. The gradual β-cell failure, occurring as normal glucose tolerant individuals progress to type 2 diabetes, includes the whole group of different processes and reactions among which sensitivity of these cells to glucose, glucotoxicity and output of insulin are of primary importance.[58,59] The second principal function of glucose may be designated as a genotoxic, or progenotoxic. Oxidative damage to DNA is characteristic of overt diabetes mellitus[60] and hyperglycemia may contribute (under participation of mitochondrial electron transport chain) to the generation of oxidative stress resulting in damage to lipids, proteins and DNA in a variety of cells.[61,62]

Specifically, it has been shown recently that oral glucose challenge stimulates reactive oxygen species, or ROS, generation by blood mononuclear cells.[63] As has been hypothesized by us, the individual (that is on the person-to-person basis) shift in the ratio between hormonal (blood insulin) and genotoxic (ROS generation in mononuclears by luminol-dependent/latex-induced chemiluminescence) effects of glycemic load may reflect a Janus, or dual, role of glucose and probably can be associated with predisposition to the certain type of human pathology.[9,10,57] It was assumed that even among healthy people different reaction to glucose can be apparent. Preferential inclination of the probands to endocrine or genotoxic predominance may occur and this working hypothesis was confirmed by subsequent research.[10,11] Thirty eight healthy subjects (37 females, 1 male, age 19-58 years) without signs of glucose tolerance impairment were included into the study. All participants were given glucose (40 g/1 m² of body surface) after a 12- to 14-hrs overnight fast. Venous blood samples were taken at 0 and 120 min and processed for the preparation of mononuclear cells and for hormonal-biochemical measurements.

The average stimulation of ROS generation in mononuclears (parameter A) by oral glucose was equal at 120 min 1,77 (or + 77%) in the entire studied group. When ROS stimulation (120/0 min) with factor ≥2 had been evaluated it was observed in 9 of 38 subjects (i.e., in 23,7%). This group of people was designated as "GIGT+", or the group with glucose-induced genotoxicity. Correspondingly, the second group of 29 people (in which this stimulation was less than 2 or was not discovered at all) was designated as "GIGT-".[11] When several additional parameters have been compared in these groups, it was revealed that along with relative predominance of glucose-stimulated ROS generation over the level of reactive insulinemia (see parameter A/B), the only other noticeable distinction seen in people who belonged to the group "GIGT+" was lower glucose-induced C-peptide secretion (Table 2). This shows that "GIGT+ individuals" are really characterized by combination of increased glucose-induced ROS production and lower β-cells reaction to glucose (notably, the absence of distinctions in absolute values of insulinemia may reflect not only process of insulin production but also the rate of its biological clearance).[58] No difference between two compared groups was discovered in relation to the age of subjects, their BMI value, or levels of reactive glycemia, basal lipidemia and concentrations of thiobarbiturate-reactive products and carbonylated proteins (Table 2). Yet, a rather clear tendency to higher plasma levels of the TNF-α and lower concentrations of blood leptin (especially at 120 min) was observed in "GIGT+" group of subjects (Fig. 3). Although it is well known that increased TNF serum content may be associated with insulin resistance,[50,51] glucotoxins of different origin including alpha-dicarbonyl methylglyoxal are considered as an inductors of TNF.[64] Therefore, the combination of TNF excess with glucose-induced genotoxicity seems rather possible, perhaps reflecting a link in the chain of further pathological reactions. Additionally, the observed increase in the

Table 2. Comparison of the data in groups with and without glucose-induced genotoxicity, GIGT

Parameter	Group		p
	GIGT–	GIGT+	
Age	38,1 ± 2,3	34,9 ± 3,4	0,50
BMI	26,1 ± 0,8	25,6 ± 2,1	0,81
Glucose, 120/0 min	1,012 ± 0,037	0,922 ± 0,059	0,23
CML, 120/0 min (A)	1,05 ± 0,09	4,09 ± 0,73	0,0002
Insulin, 120/0 min (B)	11,96 ± 5,63	16,51 ± 13,2	0,71
A/B	0,43 ± 0,11	2,78 ± 0,93	0,0004
C-peptide, 120/0 min	3,84 ± 0,72	2,01 ± 0,59	0,19
CHOL, mmol/l	5,78 ± 0,21	5,71 ± 0,43	0,86
TG, mmol/l	1,01 ± 0,07	0,91 ± 0,07	0,48
LPS, cond.units	335,4 ± 20,0	323,2 ± 27,8	0,75
TBRPs, nmol/l	3,37 ± 0,29	3,90 ± 0,70	0,41
CP, cond.units	313,9 ± 24,9	294,3 ± 39,8	0,68

BMI—body mass index; CML, 120/0 (chemiluminescence data in mononuclears, cond. un., on 120 min. after peroral glucose load, to chemiluminescence data in blood mononuclears isolated after fasting); Insulin, 120/0 (ratio of blood insulin level on 120 min. after peroral glucose load, to fasting insulinemia); CHOL—blood cholesterol; TG—triglycerides; LPS—total (β + preβ) lipoproteins; TBRPs—thiobarbiturate-reactive products; CP—carbonylated proteins. Reprinted from Berstein LM, Vasilyev DA, Poroshina TE et al. Hormone Metabol Research 2006; 38:650-5 with permission from Georg Thieme Verlag KG.

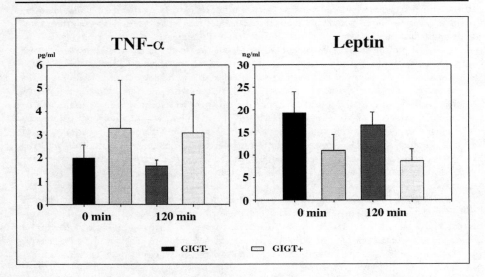

Figure 3. Plasma TNF-α and leptin concentrations after fasting and on 120 min of oral glucose load in subjects without (GIGT–) and with (GIGT+) signs of glucose-induced genotoxicity.

ratio of TNF-α to leptin seems rather characteristic and will be discussed below in the section entitled "Adipogenotoxicosis".

According to the data of S.W. Choi et al[65] the higher was the basal glycemia level in diabetic patients, the higher was rate of DNA damage in their lymphocytes (COMET assay). In our studies, notwithstanding the absence of difference between compared groups in glycemia level (Table 2) and in the comets' tail length in the basal state, a tendency to higher stimulation of comet processing with H_2O_2 was discovered in "GIGT+ subjects". Thus in aggregate, if dual function of glucose is realized in the "genotoxic mode", the phenotype (and probably genotype) of probands may be rather distinctive to that discovered in glucose-induced "endocrine prevalence". As a result, a specific pro-endocrine or promutagenic basis for different chronic diseases or for different features of the same disease can be created.[9-11] Such an assumption, in addition to other evidence, is supported by the data indicating signs of DNA damage only in subgroups of patients with atherosclerosis as well diabetes.[60,66] When searching for the factors which may promote a switch into the direction of glucose-induced genotoxic effect it should be underlined that though aging and obesity are sometimes considered as an inductors of excessive ROS production due to the insulin-related reactions, there are also data which (depending of cellular context) contradict with such notion.[67] Of note, our preliminary data show that tumor presence appears to be more important than the age of subjects in securing of the mentioned switch.[68] Of course, other possible modifiers of dual (Janus) function of glucose should be taken into account too. For instance, smoking can influence glucose tolerance starting from young adulthood[69] and according to our observations the incidence of smokers in "GIGT+" group was higher than in "GIGT–" subjects. Altogether, mechanistic and clinical associations related to presented findings as well as their significance for preventive measures deserve attention and further exploration.

Adipogenotoxicosis

Under conditions of glucose intolerance, free fatty acids acquire functionality as the principal energetic substrates, in accordance with the Randle cycle. Their excessive oxidation together with an age-dependent decrease in mitochondrial function, dysfunction of receptors of peroxisome proliferator-activated receptors (in particular PPARγ), etc., assist in furthering the progression of insulin resistance and the formation of a cluster of other metabolic propathogenic factors.[49,50,70] These observations together with data on the association of obesity with insulin resistance and increased cancer risk[50,71,72] (see also chapter of A. Hjartaker et al. in this volume) quite naturally rekindle interest in the role of adipose tissue. The latter, viewed previously as primarily an energy depository, is actually a functionally active endocrine organ producing steroid hormones (including estrogens) as well as hormone-like peptide molecules known as adipokines or adipocytokines (leptin, resistin, adiponectin, PAI-1, TNFα, visfatin, etc.).[73,74] Peptide hormones of adipose tissue may influence tumor growth directly as well as through the reproductive system and other mechanisms[75] and their problastomogenic effects may differ considerably. For example, leptin (probably via activation of MAP-kinase) increases aromatase activity and the proliferation index in mammary cancer cell lines, while a decrease of blood adiponectin concentration is described as a prospective risk factor for breast and endometrial cancer.[76,77] Accordingly, special attention is directed to mammary fat, since it is essential for the development of mammary epithelium. This occurs by providing signals that mediate ductal morphogenesis, by playing a vital role in defining the level of stromal-epithelial interactions and by contributing significantly to tumor growth starting from its early stages until further distinct clinical progression.[79,80] It is appropriate to re-emphasize here again that mechanisms of hormonal carcinogenesis, besides stimulation of cell proliferation, include formation of DNA adducts and mutagenesis in the target tissue.[6-8]

Importantly, adipose tissue consists not only of adipocytes but also of several other cell types, including macrophages.[73,74] Macrophages as a part on the nonfat compartment of adipose tissue, are increased in obesity and as a result of certain hormonal and nonhormonal signals.[81,82] They are responsible for almost all adipose tissue TNFα expression and for significant amounts of nitric oxide (NO) and IL-6 production.[73,81] These products are often considered as pro-inflammatory mediators and effectors resulting in oxidative stress[83] and, finally, in the genotoxic cellular damage. Since features of oxidative stress were indeed reported recently in human adipose tissue and its cell lines,[84-86] we decided to study properties of mammary fat in breast cancer patients. Our aim was to find factors possibly contributing to the shift of these properties from hormonal to pro-inflammatory/genotoxic. We have coined the term, adipogenotoxicosis to characterize this process.[12]

Samples of mammary fat located 1.5-2.0 cm from the tumor have been taken within 10-15 min after surgery in 95 patients with breast cancer. The tumors were mainly intraductal breast carcinomas, stages $T_{1-2}N_{0-1}M_0$. Twenty five patients (mean age 42.6 ± 1.3) that had menses comprised the premenopausal group. The others 70 patients (mean age 63.2 ± 1.0) were postmenopausal for not less than 1 year. Among the latter, 23 patients showed signs of modest fasting hyperglycemia (6.1-7.5 mmol/l, n = 15) or overt compensated diabetes mellitus (n = 8). With respect to body mass most patients (>70%) were normal (BMI 18.5-24.9) or overweight (BMI 25.0-29.9) but not obese (BMI >30.0). Correspondingly, taking all this into account we compared the ability of mammary fat explants from premenopausal or postmenopausal breast cancer patients to release substances associated with adipocytes (leptin, adiponectin) or non-adipose cells, mainly macrophages (TNFα, IL-6, NO), into culture medium. In addition we studied the release of thiobarbiturate-reactive products (TBRPs), a marker of lipid peroxidation, as well as aromatase activity and estrogen 4-hydroxylase (CYP1B1) expression in mammary fat.[12]

The most demonstrative results are presented in Table 3. Immunohistochemical staining for macrophage marker CD68 did not differ between the two groups. However, the release of NO and, especially, TNFα from adipose tissue showed a tendency to increase in the postmenopausal period (oppositely to the trend demonstrated by leptin and adiponectin). This was manifested also as a quite notable tendency to increase in the TNFα/adiponectin ratio from 4.56 ± 1.32 in the premenopausal group to 8.60 ± 2.06 in the postmenopausal group.

The menopausal status (pre or post) of cancer patients did not affect aromatase activity in their mammary fat samples, contrary to CYP1B1 expression and TBRP release into culture medium, which were higher in the premenopausal group (Table 3). In the latter group, in case of higher CYP1B1 expression and NO and IL-6 release, an increased aromatase activity in adipose tissue was found. In postmenopausal patients with fasting hyperglycemia, IL-6 level and IL-6/adiponectin ratio in incubation medium were notably higher than in the patients with normal blood glucose (Fig. 4). Thus, trends in the ratio TNFα/leptin in "GIGT+" group (see previous section), in mentioned several lines above ratio TNFα/adiponectin in mammary fat of postmenopausal patients and in the ratio IL-6/adiponectin under influence of hyperglycemia (Fig. 4) allow to conclude that just these parameters demonstrate in certain situations the domination of inflammatory/progenotoxic signs with rather high constancy. Notably, no differences were found between breast cancer patients with body mass index above or below the average as concerns the secretion of TNF, IL-6 and NO, as well as adiponectin and leptin by adipose tissue. This demonstrates, that unlike the role of menstrual status and glucose intolerance, obesity was not a factor promoting the shift from hormonal to genotoxic properties of adipose tissue in our studies.[12]

Thus, attributing to the features of progenotoxic switch in mammary fat not only an upsurge of TNFα, IL-6 and NO (related mainly to nonfat cells[73,81]) but increased expression of CYP1B1 as well and taking into account discovered aromatase-related 'associations', it may be concluded that this switch, or adipogenotoxicosis, is present not only in the postmenopausal (elderly) breast cancer patients. Besides, estrogens and their catechol derivatives are likely to be implicated in it to a not lesser extent than the well-known aforementioned pro-inflammatory molecules are. A tendency for the simultaneous decrease in the local release of peptide hormones (primarily, adiponectin) derived from adipocytes suggests that adipogenotoxicosis combines the loss of certain endocrine functions and the gain of progenotoxic effects. The mediating role of free fatty acids as ROS inductors[87] and recent data on TNFα ability to cause DNA damage through the generation of ROS[88] deserve mentioning too.

Future studies of adipogenotoxicosis should be focused on correlations between the hormonal and progenotoxic properties of adipose tissue and the clinical and morphological characteristics of

Table 3. *The release of studied factors to the medium, aromatase activity and expression of CYP1B1 and CD68 in mammary adipose tissue of breast cancer patients*

Group of Patients	Leptin (ng/100 mg of Tissue)	Adiponectin (mcg/100 mg of Tissue)	TNFα (pg/100 mg of Tissue)	NO (ng/100 mg of Tissue)	TBRPs (Extinction Units/100 mg of Tissue)	Aromatase Activity (fM/mg Protein/hr)	CYP1B1 (Conditional Units)	CD68 (Conditional Units)
PreMP	38,0 ± 9,9	8,4 ± 0,4	49,3 ± 9,5	283,6 ± 46,9	3,95 ± 0,63	7,22 ± 1,23	2,73 ± 0,18	2,47 ± 0,27
PostMP	25,5 ± 5,7	7,7 ± 0,2	83,1 ± 10,7	389,9 ± 52,8	2,54 ± 0,23	7,07 ± 0,75	2,25 ± 0,16	2,17 ± 0,17
p	0,24	0,13	0,06	0,27	0,01	0,92	0,08	0,35

PreMP—premenopausal; PostMP—postmenopausal. Methods: leptin, adiponectin, TNFα by ELISA, NO (nitric oxide) by Griess reaction, TBRPs by reaction with thiobarbituric acid, aromatase activity as 3H2O release from 3H-1-β-androstenedione, CYP1B1 and CD68 by semi-quantitative immunohistochemical evaluation. Reprinted from Berstein LM, Kovalevskij AY, Poroshina TE et al. International J Cancer 2007 with permission from John Wiley & Sons Inc.

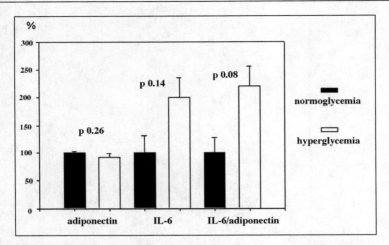

Figure 4. Release of adiponectin and IL-6 by mammary fat explants of patients with normo- and hyperglycemia.

breast cancer in order to check whether genotoxic shift is associated with a less favorable course of the disease. These studies should take into account the comparison of fat located in close proximity to a tumor and distantly from it (with the aim to address "the cause and effect" problem). If the adipogenotoxicosis hypothesis is confirmed, this may lead to development of specific fat-targeted interventions with the intent of preventing and treating cancer and probably some other main chronic diseases.

Basic Triad: Interactions and Implications

Figure 5 provides a brief overview of the issues addressed in this treatise. The triple endocrine-genotoxic switchings in estrogen, glucose and adipose tissue 'systems' composing the so called 'basic triad' can occur independently as well as interact with each other. Examples of such interactions include a trend toward adipogenotoxicosis in subjects with glucose intolerance (Fig. 4) and an association of PPAR-γ and -α and their target gene UDP-glucuronosyltransferase 1A9 simultaneously with glucose utilization, sensitization to insulin, free fatty acids mobilization and inactivation of genotoxic catecholestrogens.[89] Tobacco smoking appears to be a rather universal inducer of the three phenomena (PSEE, Janus/dual function of glucose and adipogenotoxicosis). Of note, prolonged smoking is able to increase the rate of many noncommunicable diseases (NCD). Furthermore, when the incidence does not increase, as in the case of breast and especially endometrial cancer,[90] the course of such diseases in smokers is characterized with poorer clinical outcomes.[40]

Even though human aging does not have a specifically ordered, biologically based program,[55,91] its type is no doubt of importance for the most people. The idea that hormone-related genotoxic shifts are associated with higher NCD aggressiveness and "less successful aging" is supported by several sets of observational data including: the apparently decreased survival in breast cancer patients with higher concentration of certain catecholestrogen fractions in tumor tissue;[92] the more frequent and severe diabetes complications in patients with the signs of oxidative stress and DNA damage;[60,61,93] and the correlation of DNA adducts in cells of thoracic aortas with stage of atherosclerosis.[66,94] Since fetal programming is considered nowadays rather frequently as a starting point for the rise of human pathology characteristic for the second half of life and even as a cause of reduced longevity,[95] attempts were made to find deviations in DNA adducts in young healthy adults born with low birthweight in comparison with age matched normal birthweight controls.[96] Of note, so called 'edge effects' of hormones on the very early and late stages of ontogenesis may involve a DNA-destroying mechanism appearing as a characteristic feature of their procarcinogenic

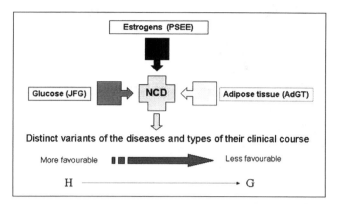

Figure 5. The components of 'basic triad' or triple endocrine-genotoxic switchings: possible association with noncommunicable diseases (NCD). PSEE—phenomenon of switching of estrogen effects; JFG—Janus/dual function of glucose; AdGT—adipogenotoxicosis; H, G—transition from hormonal effects to predominance of genotoxic effects.

influence.[9] Thus, all three mentioned allied or independent events (adipogenotoxicosis, Janus role of glucose and PSEE) should be viewed when discussing mechanisms of the development of major noncommunicable human diseases. The potential existence of two types of aberration with endocrine or genotoxic predominance should be considered and related to measures for their prevention. The aims of prevention should include well-known targets but also try to go beyond them. In this regard an advisable approach might include: correctors of steroid and peptidergic signaling (SERMs, SARMs, modifiers of aromatase, IGF-1, Ras-MAPK-PI3-kinase-system and so on—see chapters of R. Santen et al.; S. Bulun and E. Simpson; S. Sengupta and V.C. Jordan; T. Powles); alleviators of glucose intolerance and insulin resistance (e.g., diet and dietary restriction, biguanides, statins, glitazones, cannabinoid receptor blockers),[49,55,97-100] various antioxidants and antigenotoxicants,[21,101,102] more or less selective mTOR inhibitors,[55,103,104] but also an effort to reach the optimal balance in the ratio of the hormonal and genotoxic effects discussed above.

Acknowledgements

Drs. E. Tsyrlina, D. Vasilyev, A. Kovalevskij, I. Kovalenko, A. Kotov, T. Poroshina, K. Pozharisski, R.J. Santen, W. Yue and J-P. Wang.

Studies were supported by RFBR, INTAS and UICC grants.

References

1. Zimmet P. Globalization, coca-colonization and the chronic disease epidemic: can the Doomsday scenario be averted? J Intern Med 2000; 247(3):301-10.
2. Unwin N, Alberti KG. Chronic noncommunicable diseases. Ann Trop Med Parasitol 2006; 100(5-6):455-64.
3. Baltes PB, Baltes MM. Psychological perspectives on successful aging: The model of selective optimization with compensation. In: Baltes PB, Baltes MM., eds. Successful aging: perspectives from the behavioral sciences. Cambridge, England: Cambridge University Press, 1990:1-34.
4. Rowe JW, Kahn RL. Human aging: usual and successful. Science 1987; 237(4811):143-9.
5. Kahn RL. Guest editorial. On "Successful ageing and well-being: self-rated and compared with Rowe and Kahn". The Gerontologist 2002; 42:725-726.
6. Liehr JG. Dual role of oestrogens as hormones and procarcinogens: tumour initiation by metabolic activation of oestrogens. Eur J Cancer Prevention 1997; 6:3-10.
7. Cavalieri EL, Li KM, Balu N et al. Catechol ortho-quinones: the electrophilic compounds that form depurinating DNA adducts and could initiate cancer and other diseases. Carcinogenesis 2002; 23:1071-7.
8. Santen RJ. Endocrine-responsive cancer. In: Larsen PR. et al. eds. Williams' Textbook of Endocrinology. Philadelphia: W.B.Saunders Comp, 2003:1797-833.

9. Berstein LM. Modern concepts of hormonal carcinogenesis: mechanisms, predisposing factors, consequences. In: Berstein LM, ed. Hormones, age and cancer. St. Peterburg: Nauka, 2005:38-67.

10. Berstein LM, Tsyrlina EV, Vasilyev DA et al. Phenomenon of the switching of estrogen effects and joker function of glucose: similarities, relation to age-associated pathology, approaches to correction. Annals NY Acad Sci 2005; 1057:235-246.

11. Berstein LM, Vasilyev DA, Poroshina TE et al. Glucose-induced effects and joker function of glucose: endocrine or genotoxic prevalence? Hormone Metabol Research 2006; 38:650-5.

12. Berstein LM, Kovalevskij AY, Poroshina TE et al. Signs of proinflammatory/genotoxic switch (adipogenotoxicosis) in mammary fat of breast cancer patients: role of menopausal status, estrogens and hyperglycemia. International J Cancer 2007; 121:514-9..

13. Ehebauer M, Hayward P, Martinez Arias A. Notch, a universal arbiter of cell fate decisions. Science 2006; 314(5804):1414-5.

14. Flexner S, Flexner D. Wise words: the origins, meanings and time-honored wisdom of proverbs. New York: Avon Books 1993.

15. Burrows H, Horning E. Oestrogens and neoplasia. Springfield, Illinois: Ch C Thomas Publ, 1952.

16. Henderson B, Feigelson H. Hormonal carcinogenesis. Carcinogenesis 2000; 21:427-33.

17. Li JJ, Li SA, Oberley TD et al. Carcinogenic activities of various steroidal and nonsteroidal estrogens in the hamster kidney: relation to hormonal activity and cell proliferation. Cancer Res 1995; 55:4347-51.

18. Yue W, Santen RJ, Wang JP et al. Genotoxic metabolites of estradiol in breast: potential mechanism of estradiol induced carcinogenesis. J Steroid Biochem Mol Biol 2003; 86(3-5):477-86.

19. Suto A, Telang NT, Tanino H et al. In vitro and in vivo modulation of growth regulation in the human breast cancer cell line MCF-7 by estradiol metabolites. Breast Cancer 1999; 6:87-92.

20. Jefcoate CR, Liehr JG, Santen RJ et al. Tissue-specific synthesis and oxidative metabolism of estrogens. J Natl Cancer Inst Monograph 2000; 27:95-112.

21. Cavalieri EL, Chakravarti D, Guttenplan J et al. Catechol estrogen quinones as initiators of breast and other human cancers: Implications for biomarkers of susceptibility and cancer prevention. Biochim Biophys Acta 2006; 1766:63-78.

22. Tsuchiya Y, Nakajima M, Kyo S. et al. Human CYP1B1 is regulated by estradiol via estrogen receptor. Cancer Res 2004; 64:3119-25.

23. Berstein LM. Hormonal carcinogenesis. St. Petersburg: Nauka Publ, 2000.

24. Berstein L, Tsyrlina E, Poroshina T et al. Switching (overtargeting) of estrogen effects and its potential role in hormonal carcinogenesis. Neoplasma 2002; 49:21-25.

25. Michnovicz JJ, Herschcopf RJ, Nagamura H. Increased 2-hydroxylation of estradiol as a possible mechanism for the anti-estrogenic effect of cigarette smoking. New Engl J Med 1986; 315:1305-09.

26. Port JL, Yamaguchi K, Du B et al. Tobacco smoke induces CYP1B1 in the aerodigestive tract. Carcinogenesis 2004; 25:2275-81.

27. Berstein LM, Yue W, Wang JP et al. Estrogenic effects and their modification by tobacco smoke in wild type and estrogen deprived breast cancer cell lines. Paper presented at: The Endocrine Society's (USA) 89th Annual Meeting. Canada: Toronto, 2007.

28. King MM, Hollingsworth A, Cuzick J et al. The detection of adducts in human cervix tissue DNA using ^{32}P-postlabelling: a study of the relationship with smoking history and oral contraceptive use. Carcinogenesis 1994; 15:1097-100.

29. Berstein LM, Tsyrlina EV, Kolesnik OS et al. Catecholestrogens excretion in smoking and nonsmoking postmenopausal women receiving estrogen replacement therapy. J Steroid Biochem Mol Biol 2000; 72:143-7.

30. Tarone RE, Chu KC. The greater impact of menopause on ER– than ER+ breast cancer incidence: a possible explanation. Cancer Causes and Control 2002; 13:7-14.

31. Althuis MD, Fergenbaum JH, Garcia-Closas M et al. Etiology of hormone receptor-defined breast cancer: a systematic review of the literature. Cancer Epidemiol Biomarkers Prev 2004; 13:1558-68.

32. Anderson WF, Matsuno R. Breast cancer heterogeneity: a mixture of at least two main types? J Natl Cancer Inst 2006; 98:948-51.

33. Fan S, Ma YX, Wang C et al. Role of direct interaction in BRCA1 inhibition of estrogen receptor activity. Oncogene 2001; 20:77-87.

34. Sorlie T, Tibshirani R, Parker J et al. Repeated observation of breast tumor subtypes in independent gene expression data sets. Proc Natl Acad Sci USA 2003; 100:8418-23.

35. Fazzari A, Catalano MG, Comba A et al. The control of estrogen and progesterone receptor expression in MCF-7 breast cancer cells: effects of estradiol and sex hormone binding globulin. Mol Cell Endocrinol 2001; 172:31-6.

36. Berstein LM, Tsyrlina EV, Poroshina TE et al. Genotoxic factors associated with the development of receptor-negative breast cancer: potential role of the phenomenon of switching of estrogen effects. Experimental Oncology 2006; 28(1):64-9.

37. Fuqua SAW. Estrogen and progesterone receptors and breast cancer. In: Harris JR et al, eds. Diseases of breast. Philadelphia: Lippincott-Raven 1996; 185-200.

38. Osborne CK, Schiff R, Arpino G et al. Endocrine responsiveness: understanding how progesterone receptor can be used to select endocrine therapy. Breast 2005; 14(6):458-65.

39. Abd El-Rehim DM, Pinder SE, Paish CE et al. Expression of luminal and basal cytokeratins in human breast carcinoma. J Pathol 2004; 203:661-71.

40. Fentiman IS, Allen DS, Hamed D. Smoking and prognosis in women with breast cancer. Int J Clin Pract 2005; 59(9):1051-4.

41. Manjer J, Malina J, Berglund G et al. Smoking associated with hormone receptor negative breast cancer. Int J Cancer 2001; 91(4):580-4.

42. Sartorius CA, Harvell DM, Shen T et al. Progestins initiate a luminal to myoepithelial switch in estrogen-dependent human breast tumors without altering growth. Cancer Res 2005; 65:9779-88.

43. Sherwin BB. Estrogen and cognitive functioning in women. Endocr Rev 2003; 24:133-51.

44. Hecht JL, Mutter GL. Molecular and pathologic aspects of endometrial carcinogenesis. J Clin Oncol 2006; 24:4783-91.

45. Schwartz D, Rotter V. p53-dependent cell cycle control: response to genotoxic stress. Semin Cancer Biol 1998; 8(5): 325-36.

46. Safe S, Wormke M, Samudio I. Mechanisms of inhibitory aryl hydrocarbon receptor-estrogen receptor crosstalk in human breast cancer cells. J Mammary Gland Biol Neoplasia 2000; 5:295-306.

47. Tritscher AM, Seacat AM, Yager JD et al. Increased oxidative DNA damage in livers of TCDD treated intact but not ovariectomized rats. Cancer Letters 1996; 98:219-25.

48. Chen ZH, Hurh YJ, Na HK et al. Resveratrol inhibits TCDD-induced expression of CYP1A1 and CYP1B1 and catechol estrogen-mediated oxidative DNA damage in cultured human mammary epithelial cells. Carcinogenesis 2004; 25:2005-13.

49. Dilman VM. Development, ageing and disease. A new rationale for an intervention strategy. Chur (Switzerland): Harwood Acad Publ 1994.

50. Reaven GM. The insulin resistance syndrome. Curr Atheroscler Rep 2003; 5:364-71.

51. Fernandez-Real JM, Ricart W. Insulin resistance and chronic cardiovascular inflammatory syndrome. Endocrine Rev 2003; 24:278-301.

52. Brand-Miller JC. Glycemic load and chronic disease. Nutr Rev 2003; 61(5 Pt 2):S49-S55.

53. Silvera SA, Jain M, Howe GR et al. Dietary carbohydrates and breast cancer risk: A prospective study of the roles of overall glycemic index and glycemic load. Int J Cancer 2005;114:653-8.

54. Kwon G, Marshall CA, Liu H et al. Glucose-stimulated DNA synthesis through mammalian target of rapamycin (mTOR) is regulated by KATP channels: effects on cell cycle progression in rodent islets. J Biol Chem 2006; 281(6):3261-7.

55. Blagosklonny MV. Aging and immortality. Quasi-programmed senescence and its pharmacological inhibition. Cell Cycle 2006; 18:2087-102.

56. Saydah SH, Loria CM, Eberhardt MS et al. Abnormal glucose tolerance and the risk of cancer death in the United States. Amer J Epidemiol 2003; 157:1092-100.

57. Bershtein LM. (The joker function of glucose in the development of main noncommunicable human diseases). Vestn. Russian Acad Med Sci 2005; N2:48-51.

58. Ferrannini E, Gastaldelli A, Miyazaki Y et al. β-cell function in subjects spanning the range from normal glucose tolerance to overt diabetes: a new analysis. J Clin Endocr Metabol 2005; 90:493-500.

59. Rossetti L, Giacarri A, DeFronzo RA. Glucose toxicity. Diabetes Care 1990; 13:610-30.

60. Dandona P, Thusu K, Cook S et al. Oxidative damage to DNA in diabetes mellitus. Lancet 1996; 347:444-5.

61. Ceriello A, Quatraro A, Giugliano D. Diabetes mellitus and hypertension: the possible role of hyperglycaemia through oxidative stress. Diabetologia 1993;36:265-6.

62. Lin Y, Berg AH, Iyengar P et al. The hyperglycemia-induced inflammatory response in adipocytes: the role of reactive oxygen species. J Biol Chem 2005; 280:4617-26.

63. Mohanty P, Hamouda W, Garg R et al. Glucose challenge stimulates reactive oxygen species (ROS) generation by leucocytes. J Clin Endocrinol Metabol 2000; 85:2970-3.

64. Vlassara H, Cai W, Crandall J et al. Inflammatory mediators are induced by dietary glycotoxins, a major risk factor for diabetic angiopathy. Proc Natl Acad Sci USA 2002; 99:15596-601.

65. Choi SW, Benzie IF, Lam CS et al. Inter-relationship between DNA damage, ascorbic acid and glycaemic control in type 2 diabetes mellitus. Diabetic Med 2005; 22:1347-53.

66. Andreassi MG, Botto N. DNA damage as a new emerging risk factor in atherosclerosis. Trends Cardiovasc Med 2003; 13:270-5.

67. Dandona P, Aljada A, Mohanty P et al. Insulin inhibits intranuclear factor kB in mononuclear cells in obese subjects: evidence for an anti-inflammatory effect? J Clin Endocrinol Metabol 2001; 86:3257-65.

68. Vasilyev DA, Poroshina TE, Kovalenko IG et al. . [Carbohydrates-induced endocrine and genotoxic effects as a potential cancer risk factor]. Presented at 2nd Russian Conference on fundamental oncology. St Petersburg 2006.

69. Houston TK, Person SD, Pletcher MJ et al. Active and passive smoking and development of glucose intolerance among young adults in a prospective cohort: CARDIA study. BMJ 2006; 332(7549):1064-9.

70. Smith SR, Wilson PWF. Editorial: free fatty acids and atherosclerosis—guilty or innocent? J Clin Endocrinol Metabol 2006; 91(7):2506-8.

71. Calle EE, Kaaks R. Overweight, obesity and cancer: epidemiological evidence and proposed mechanisms. Nat Rev Cancer 2004; 4:579-91.

72. Berstein LM. Macrosomy, obesity and cancer. New York: Nova Sci Publ 1997.

73. Kershaw EE, Flier JS. Adipose tissue as an endocrine organ. J Clin Endocrinol Metabol 2004; 89:2548-56.

74. Scherer PE. Adipose tissue: from lipid storage compartment to endocrine organ. Diabetes 2006; 55:1537-45.

75. Lorincz AM, Sukumar S. Molecular links between obesity and breast cancer. Endocr Relat Cancer 2006; 13:279-92.

76. Catalano S, Marsico S, Giordano C et al. Leptin enhances, via AP-1, expression of aromatase in the MCF-7 cell line. J Biol Chem 2003; 278:28668-76.

77. Mantzoros C, Petridou E, Dessypris N et al. Adiponectin and breast cancer risk. J Clin Endocrinol Metabol 2004; 89:1102-7.

78. Matsuzawa Y. Adipocytokines, insulin resistance and main noncommunicable diseases. In: Berstein LM, ed. Hormones, age and cancer. St Peterburg: Nauka 2005:159-69.

79. Celis JE, Moreira JM, Cabezon T et al. Identification of Extracellular and Intracellular Signaling Components of the Mammary Adipose Tissue and Its Interstitial Fluid in High Risk Breast Cancer Patients: Toward Dissecting The Molecular Circuitry of Epithelial-Adipocyte Stromal Cell Interactions. Mol Cell Proteomics 2005; 4:492-522.

80. Iyengar P, Espina V, Williams TW et al. Adipocyte-derived collagen VI affects early mammary tumor progression in vivo, demonstrating a critical interaction in the tumor/stroma microenvironment. J Clin Invest 2005; 115:1163-76.

81. Weisberg SP, McCann D, Desai M et al. Obesity is associated with macrophage accumulation in adipose tissue. J Clin Invest 2003; 112:1796-808.

82. Neels JG, Olefsky JM. Inflamed fat: what starts the fire? J Clin Invest 2006; 116:33-5.

83. Trayhurn P, Wood IS. Inflammatory cytokines and the pleiotropic role of white adipose tissue. Br J Nutr 2004; 92:347-55.

84. Furukawa S, Fujita T, Shimabukuro M et al. Increased oxidative stress in obesity and its impact on metabolic syndrome. J Clin Invest 2004; 114:1752-61.

85. Lin Y, Berg AH, Iyengar P et al. The hyperglycemia-induced inflammatory response in adipocytes: the role of reactive oxygen species. J Biol Chem 2005; 280:4617-26.

86. Schaffer A, Muller-Landner U, Scholmerich J et al. Role of adipose tissue as an inflammatory organ in human diseases. Endocr Rev 2006; 27:449-67.

87. Tripathy D, Mohanty P, Dhindsa S et al. Elevation of free fatty acids induces inflammation and impairs vascular reactivity in healthy subjects. Diabetes 2003; 52:2882-7.

88. Yan B, Wang H, Rabbani ZN et al. Tumor necrosis factor-alpha (TNF-alpha) is a potent endogenous mutagen that promotes cellular transformation. Cancer Res 2006; 66:11565-70.

89. Barbier O, Villeneuve L, Bocher V et al. The UDP-glucuronosyltransferase 1A9 enzyme is a peroxisome proliferator-activated receptor α and γ target gene. J Biol Chem 2003; 278:13975-83.

90. Baron JA, Greenberg ER. Cigarette smoking and neoplasms of the female reproductive tract and breast. Seminars in Reproductive Endocrinology 1989; 7:335-43.

91. Kirkwood TBL. Understanding the odd science of aging. Cell 2005; 120:437-47.

92. Castagnetta LA, Granata OM, Traina A et al. Tissue content of hydroxyestrogens in relation to survival of breast cancer patients. Clin Cancer Res 2002; 8:3146-55.

93. Blasiak J, Arabski M, Krupa R. DNA damage and repair in type 2 diabetes mellitus. Mutat Res 2004; 554(1-2):297-304.

94. Binkova B, Smerhovsky Z, Strejc P et al. DNA-adducts and atherosclerosis: a study of accidental and sudden death of males. Mutat Res 2002; 501(1-2):115-28.

95. Ozanne SE, Hales CN. Poor fetal growth followed by rapid postnatal catch-up growth leads to premature death. Mech Ageing Dev 2005; 126:852-4.

96. Hillestrom PR, Weimann A, Jensen CB et al. Consequences of low birthweight on urinary excretion of DNA markers of oxidative stress in young men. Scand J Clin Lab Invest 2006; 66(5):363-70.
97. Alegret M, Silvestre JS. Pleiotropic effects of statins and related experimental approaches. Methods Find Exp Clin Pharmacol 2006; 28(9):627-56.
98. Berstein LM. Clinical usage of hypolipidemic and antidiabetic drugs in the prevention and treatment of cancer. Cancer Lett 2005; 224(2):203-12.
99. Anisimov VN, Berstein LM, Egormin PA et al. Effect of metformin on life span and on the development of spontaneous mammary tumors in HER-20/neu transgenic mice. Exp Gerontol 2005; 40(8-9):449-66.
100. Klebanov S. Can short-term dietary restriction and fasting have a long-term anticarcinogenic effect? Interdiscip. Top Gerontol 2007; 35:176-92.
101. De Flora S, Ferguson LR. Overview of mechanisms of cancer chemopreventive agents. Mutat Res 2005; 591:8-15.
102. Baur JA, Pearson KJ, Price NL et al. Resveratrol improves health and survival of mice on a high-calorie diet. Nature 2006; 444(7117):337-42.
103. Yue W, Wang J, Santen RJ et al. Farnesylthyosalicylic acid blocks mammalian target of rapamycin signaling in breast cancer cells. International J Cancer 2005; 117(5):746-54.
104. Dowling RJ, Zakikhamni M, Fantus IG et al. Metformin inhibits mammalian target of rapamycin-dependent translation initiation in breast cancer cells. Cancer Res. 2007; 67:10804-12.

CHAPTER 4

Breast Development, Hormones and Cancer

Jose Russo* and Irma H. Russo

Abstract

Breast cancer originates in undifferentiated terminal structures of the mammary gland. The terminal ducts of the Lob 1 of the human female breast, which are the sites of origin of ductal carcinomas, are at their peak of cell replication during early adulthood, a period during which the breast is more susceptible to carcinogenesis. The susceptibility of Lob 1 to undergo neoplastic transformation has been confirmed by in vitro studies, which have shown that this structure has the highest proliferative activity, estrogen receptor content and rate of carcinogen binding to the DNA. The higher incidence of breast cancer observed in nulliparous women supports this concept, whereas the protection afforded by early full-term pregnancy in women could be explained by the higher degree of differentiation of the mammary gland at the time in which an etiologic agent or agents act.

Introduction

The Lobule type 1 of the human breast or terminal ductal lobular unit (TDLU) had been identified as the site of origin of the most common breast malignancy, the ductal carcinoma and corresponds to a specific stage of development of the mammary parenchyma.[1-5] The finding that the lobules type 1 that are undifferentiated structures originate the most undifferentiated and aggressive neoplasm acquires relevance to the light that these structures are more numerous in the breast of nulliparous women, who are, in turn, at a higher risk of developing breast cancer. The Lobule 1 found in the breast of nulliparous women never went through the process of differentiation, whereas the same structures, when found in the breast of postmenopausal parous women did.[4]

Defining the Cell of Origin of Breast Cancer

The relationship of lobular differentiation, cell proliferation and hormone responsiveness of the mammary epithelium is just beginning to be unraveled. Of interest is the fact that the content of estrogen receptor (ERα) and progesterone receptor (PgR) in the lobular structures of the breast is directly proportional to the rate of cell proliferation. These three parameters are maximal in the undifferentiated Lob 1, decreasing progressively in Lob 2, Lob 3 and Lob 4 (Fig. 1). The determination of the rate of cell proliferation, expressed as the percentage of cells that stain positively with Ki-67 antibody, has revealed that proliferating cells are predominantly found in the epithelium lining ducts and lobules and less frequently in the myoepithelium and in the intralobular and interlobular stroma. Ki-67 positive cells are most frequently found in Lob 1. The percentage of positive cells is reduced by three-fold in Lob 2 and by more than ten-fold in Lob 3.[6,7] ERα and PgR positive cells are found exclusively in the epithelium; the myoepithelium and the stroma are

*Corresponding Author: Jose Russo—Breast Cancer Research Laboratory, Fox Chase Cancer Center, 333 Cottman Avenue, Philadelphia, PA 19111, USA. Email: j_russo@fccc.edu

Innovative Endocrinology of Cancer, edited by Lev M. Berstein and Richard J. Santen. ©2008 Landes Bioscience and Springer Science+Business Media.

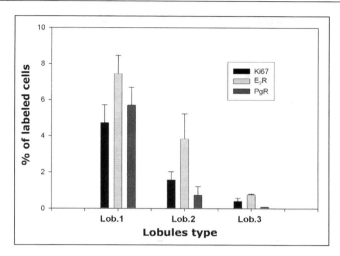

Figure 1. Percentage of positives for estrogen receptor (E2R), progesterone receptor (PgR), proliferative index (Ki-67) in the lobules 1, 2 and 3 of the human breast.

totally devoid of steroid receptor containing cells. The highest number of cells positive for both receptors is found in Lob 1, decreasing progressively in Lob 2 and Lob 3 (Fig. 1).[7]

The content of ERα and PgR in the normal breast tissue varies with the degree of lobular development, in a linear relationship with the rate of cell proliferation of the same structures. The utilization of a double labeling immunocytochemical technique for staining in the same tissue section those cells containing steroid hormone receptors and those that are proliferating, i.e., Ki-67 positive, allowed us to determine that the expression of the receptors occurs in cells other than the proliferating cells, confirming results reported by other authors.[8] Our studies have shown that the proliferative activity and the percentage of ERα and PgR positive cells are highest in Lob 1 in comparison with the various lobular structures composing the normal breast. These findings provide a mechanistic explanation for the higher susceptibility of these structures to be transformed by chemical carcinogens in vitro,[9,10] supporting as well the observations that Lob 1 are the site of origin of ductal carcinomas.[1]

The relationship between ER positive and ER negative breast cancers is not clear. It has been suggested that ER negative breast cancers result from either the loss of the ability of the cells to synthesize ER during clinical evolution of ER positive cancers, or that ER positive and ER negative cancers are different entities. Our data allowed us to postulate that Lob 1 contains at least three cell types, ERα positive cells that do not proliferate, ERα negative cells that are capable of proliferating and a small proportion of ERα positive cells that can also proliferate.[7] Therefore, estrogen might stimulate ERα positive cells to produce a growth factor that in turn stimulates neighboring ERα negative cells capable of proliferating. In the same fashion, the small proportion of cells that are ERα positive and can proliferate could be the source of ERα positive tumors. The findings that proliferating cells in the human breast are different from those that contain steroid hormone receptors explain much of the in vitro data.[11-14] Of interest are the observations that while the ERα positive MCF-7 cells respond to estrogen treatment with increased cell proliferation and that the enhanced expression of the receptor by transfection also increases the proliferative response to estrogen,[11,15] ERα negative cells, such as MDA-MB-468 and others, when transfected with ERα, exhibit inhibition of cell growth under the same type of treatment.[14,15] Although the negative effect of estrogen on those ERα negative cells transfected with the receptor has been interpreted as an interference with the transcription factor used to maintain estrogen independent growth,[16] there is no definitive explanation for their lack of survival. These data can be explained in light of the present work, in which proliferating and ERα positive cells are two separate populations. Furthermore, we have observed that when Lob 1 of normal breast tissue are placed in culture they lose the ERα positive cells, indicating that only proliferating cells, that are also ERα negative, can survive and become stem cells. These observations are supported by the fact that MCF-10F, a spontaneously immortalized human breast epithelial cell line derived from breast tissues containing Lob 1 and Lob 2, is ERα negative.[17] Recently we have shown that 17β-estradiol (E_2), the predominant circulating ovarian steroid, is carcinogenic in human breast epithelial cells and that this process is a nonreceptor mechanism.[18-20] The induction of complete transformation of the estrogen receptor negative human breast epithelial cell (MCF-10F) in vitro confirms the carcinogenicity of E_2, supporting the concept that this hormone could act as an initiator of breast cancer in women. This model provides a unique system for understanding the genomic changes that intervene for leading normal cells to tumorigenesis and for testing the functional role of specific genomic events taking place during neoplastic transformation.[20]

Breast Architecture and Cancer

Despite their architectural similarity, there are important differences between the Lob 1 of the nulliparous woman and the regressed Lob 1 of the parous woman. Lob 1 of nulliparous women has a very active intralobular stroma, whereas those of the parous woman are more hyalinized and indicative of a regressed structure. Another important difference is the higher proliferative activity in the Lob 1 of nulliparous as compared to parous women (Fig. 2). The cells of both Lob 1 and Lob 3 in the parous breast are predominantly in the G_0 phase or resting phase, while in Lob 1 of the nulliparous breast, proliferating cells predominate and the fraction of cells in G_0 is quite low. Thus, parity, in addition to exerting an important influence on the lobular composition of the breast, profoundly influences its proliferative activity.[6,21]

These biologic differences that are influenced by the pattern of breast development may provide some explanation for the increased susceptibility of the breast of nulliparous women to develop breast cancer. It is hypothesized that unlike parous women, the Lob 1 found in the breast of nulliparous women never went through the process of differentiation, seldom reaching the Lob 3 and never the Lob 4 stages.[4] Although the lobules of parous women regress at menopause to Lob 1, they are permanently genetically imprinted by the differentiation process in some way that protects them from neoplastic transformation, even though these changes are no longer morphologically observable.[21-26] In other words, they are biologically different from the Lob 1 of nulliparous women.

Thus, the hypothesis is that parous women who develop breast cancer may do so because they have a defective response to the differentiating influence of the hormones of pregnancy.[1,6,22,27] Developmental differences might not only provide an explanation for the protective effect induced by pregnancy, but also a new paradigm to assess other differences between the Lob 1 of parous and nulliparous women, such as their ability to metabolize estrogens, or repair genotoxic damage. Such differences exist and they have been shown to modulate the response of the rodent mammary gland to chemically induced carcinogenesis. It has been postulated[23] that unresponsive lobules that fail to undergo differentiation under the stimulus of pregnancy and lactation are responsible for cancer development despite the parity history. It stands to reason that having more of these lobules increases the risk of breast cancer. In fact, the extent of age-related menopausal involution of the Lob 1 appears to influence the risk of breast cancer and may modify other breast cancer risk factors, including parity. This postulated and early observations by us[4,5,23] has been confirmed in a recent report[28] focused on breast biopsy specimens from 8736 women with benign breast disease. In this publication, the authors have evaluated not only the Lob 1 or terminal ductal lobular unit but also the atrophic or involuted structures resulting by the normal process of aging in the human breast. The extent of involution of the terminal duct lobular units or Lob 1 was characterized as complete (≥75 percent of the lobules involuted), partial (1 to 74 percent involuted) or none (0 percent involuted). The relative risk of breast cancer was estimated based upon standardized incidence ratios by dividing the observed numbers of incident breast cancers by expected values of population based on incident breast cancers from the Iowa Surveillance,

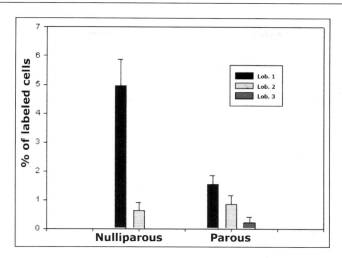

Figure 2. Influence of parity on the proliferative activity of the human breast (Ki-67 staining).

Epidemiology and End Results (SEER) registry. The following findings were noted: 1- Greater degrees of involution were positively associated with advancing age and inversely associated with parity. 2- Overall, the risk of breast cancer was significantly higher for women with no involution, compared to those with partial or complete involution (relative risks [RRs] 1.88, 1.47 and 0.91, respectively). This particular finding is of great interest because it confirms the previous observations of Russo et al[23] indicating that the Lob 1 is a marker of risk. 3- The degree of involution modified the risk of developing breast cancer in women who had atypia in their breast biopsies (RR 7.79, 4.06 and 1.49 for women with none, partial and complete involution, respectively) as well as for those with proliferative disease without atypia (RR 2.94 and 1.11 for those with no and complete involution, respectively). 4- There was an interaction with family history as well; women with a weak or no family history of breast cancer who had complete involution had a risk for breast cancer that was five-fold lower than the risk of those with a strong family history and no involution (RR 0.59 versus 2.77, respectively). This data also confirm the previous observations of Russo et al.[23] 5- Among nulliparous women and those whose age at first birth was over the age of 30, the absence of involution significantly increased the risk of breast cancer. In contrast, for both groups, there was no excess risk if involution was complete.

Altogether the study of Milanese et al[28] provides a powerful confirmation of the risk of Lob 1 or terminal ductal lobular unit in the breast[4,5,23] and denotes an additional morphological parameter like atrophic or involution of the Lob1 or terminal ductal lobular unit as an indication of protection. However, this conclusion must be taken with reservation because in a recent finding of Harvey et al[29] postmenopausal women that have received hormonal replacement therapy have shown an increase in breast density associated with a significant increase in the number of Lob 1 or TDLU. This indicates that reactivation of the so called involuted Lob1 or terminal ductal lobular unit can increase the risk of a woman to develop breast cancer.

References
1. Russo J, Gusterson BA, Rogers AE et al Comparative study of human and rat mammary tumorigenesis. Lab Invest 1991; 62:1-32.
2. Wellings SR. Development of human breast cancer. Adv Cancer Res 1980; 31:287-99.
3. Wellings SR, Jensen HM, Marcum RG. An atlas of subgross pathology of 16 human breasts with special reference to possible precancerous lesions. J Natl Cancer Inst 1975; 55:231-75.
4. Russo J, Rivera R, Russo IH. Influence of age and parity on the development of the human breast. Breast Cancer Res Treat 1992; 23:211-8.

5. Russo J, Romero AL, Russo IH. Architectural pattern of the normal and cancerous breast under the influence of parity. J Cancer Epidemiol Biomarkers & Prevention 1994; 3:219-24.
6. Russo J, Russo IH. Role of differentiation in the pathogenesis and prevention of breast cancer. Endocr Related Cancer 1997; 4:7-21.
7. Russo J, Ao X, Grill C et al. Pattern of distribution for estrogen receptor α and progesterone receptor in relation to proliferating cells in the mammary gland. Breast Cancer Res Treat 1999; 53:217-27.
8. Clarke RB, Howell A, Anderson E. Estrogen sensitivity of normal human breast tissue in vivo and implanted into athymic nude mice: analysis of the relationship between estrogen-induced proliferation and progesterone receptor expression. Breast Cancer Res Treat 1997; 45:121-83.
9. Russo J, Calaf G, Russo IH. A critical approach to the malignant transformation of human breast epithelial cells. CRC Crit Rev Oncol 1993; 4:403-17.
10. Russo J, Reina D, Frederick J et al. Expression of phenotypical changes by human breast epithelial cells treated with carcinogens in vitro. Cancer Res 1988; 48:2837-57.
11. Foster JS, Wimalasena J. Estrogen regulates activity of cyclin-dependent kinases and retinoblastoma protein phosphorylation in breast cancer cells. Mol Endocrinol 1996; 10:488-98.
12. Wang W, Smith R, Burghardt R et al. 17β estradiol-mediated growth inhibition of MDA-MB 468 cells stably transfected with the estrogen receptor: cell cycle effects. Mol Cell Endocrinol 1997; 133:49-62.
13. Levenson AS, Jordan VC. Transfection of human estrogen receptor (ER) cDNA into ER negative mammalian cell lines. J Steroid Biochem Mol Biol 1994; 51:229-39.
14. Weisz A, Bresciani F. Estrogen regulation of proto-oncogenes coding for nuclear proteins. CRC Crit Rev Oncol 1993; 4:361-88.
15. Zajchowski DA, Sager K, Webster L. Estrogen inhibits the growth of estrogen receptor negative, but not estrogen receptor positive, human mammary epithelial cells expressing a recombinant estrogen receptor. Cancer Res 1993; 53:5004-11.
16. Pilat MJ, Christman JK, Brooks SC. Characterization of the estrogen receptor transfected MCF-10A breast cell line 139B6. Breast Cancer Res Treat 1996; 37:253-66.
17. Calaf G, Tahin Q, Alvarado ME et al. Hormone receptors and cathepsin D levels in human breast epithelial cells transformed by chemical carcinogens. Breast Cancer Res Treat 1993; 29:169-77.
18. Russo J, Lareef MH, Balogh G et al. Estrogen and its metabolites are carcinogenic in human breast epithelial cells. J Steroid Biochem Mol Biol 2003; 87:1-25.
19. Fernandez SV, Lareef MH, Russo IH et al. Estrogen and its metabolite 4-hydroxy-estradiol induce mutations in TP53 and LOH in chromosome 13q12.3 near BRCA2 in human breast epithelial cells. Int J Cancer 2006; 118:1862-8.
20. Russo J, Fernandez SV, Russo PA et al. 17-beta estradiol induces transformation and tumorigenesis in human breast epithelial cells. FASEB J 2006; 20:1622-34.
21. Russo J, Russo IH. Development of Human Mammary Gland. In: The Mammary Gland Development, Regulation and Function. MC Neville and CW Daniel, eds. New York: Plenum Press. 1987:67-93.
22. Russo J, Russo IH. Toward a physiological approach to breast cancer prevention. Cancer Epidemiol Biomarkers & Prevention 1994; 3:353-64.
23. Russo J, Lynch H, Russo IH. Mammary gland architecture as a determining factor in the susceptibility of the human breast to cancer. Breast Journal 2001; 7(5):278-91.
24. Russo J, Balogh GA, Chen J et al. The concept of stem cell in the mammary gland and its implication in morphogenesis, cancer and prevention. Frontiers in Bioscience 2006; 11:151-72.
25. Balogh GA, Heulings R, Mailo DA et al. Genomic Signature Induced by Pregnancy in the Human Breast. Int J Oncol 2006; 28:399-410.
26. Russo J, Balogh GA, Heulings R et al. Molecular basis of pregnancy induced breast cancer protection. Eur J Cancer Prev 2006; 15:306-42.
27. Russo J, Russo IH. Development pattern of human breast and susceptibility to carcinogenesis. Eur J Cancer Prev 1993; 2(Suppl 3):85.
28. Milanese TR, Hartmann LC, Sellers TA et al. Age-related lobular involution and risk of breast cancer. J Natl Cancer Inst 2006; 98:1600-7.
29. Harvey JA, Santen RJ, Petroni GR et al. Histology findings of Mammographically Dense—Breast Tissue in Postmenopausal Women with and without Hormone Replacement Therapy. Breast Cancer Res Treat 2004; 88(Suppl 1):S008a.

Chapter 5

Epidemiology of Hormone-Associated Cancers as a Reflection of Age

Svetlana V. Ukraintseva,* Konstantin G. Arbeev and Anatoli I. Yashin

Abstract

In this chapter we review the epidemiology of hormone-associated cancers (prostate, breast, endometrial, ovarian, pancreatic and thyroid) paying special attention to the variability in the age patterns of cancer incidence rate over populations and time periods. We emphasize the comparative analysis of the age specific incidence rate curves as a valuable source of hypotheses about factors influencing cancer risks in populations in addition to the analysis of the age-adjusted rates.

Introduction

Incidence rates of cancer dramatically increased during the 20th century in the US and globally for all sites combined. According to SEER (The Surveillance, Epidemiology and End Results) program data for 2002-2004, cancer is currently the most common (together with heart disease) adult disorder in the US with the life-time risk approaching 45% in men and 38% in women.[1] Over 22 million people in the world were cancer patients in 2003.[2] The global cancer burden is higher in more developed countries and has increased over time.[2-4] This increase in affluent societies refers to three major causes: population aging, an increase in age-specific cancer incidence rates, particularly at old ages, and an improvement in survival of cancer patients. Among these reasons, the increase in incidence rates is the only factor that could potentially be controlled through the cancer prevention. Understanding factors that are responsible for epidemiological trends in cancer incidence rates is, therefore, of great importance for fostering development of successful cancer prophylactics and decreasing the global cancer burden.

In this chapter we overview typical age patterns, place differences and time trends in the incidence and survival rates for selected hormone-associated cancers, including male prostate, female breast, endometrial and ovarian cancers, pancreatic and thyroid cancers for both sexes. Among those, cancers of the breast and prostate are currently among four most common cancer sites (two others are tumors of the lung and colon) in developed regions of the world, mainly responsible for the higher cancer rates in these regions (Fig. 1).

Specifically, we will concentrate on the age patterns of cancer incidence rate and their variability over populations and time periods. This is because comparing the age specific incidence rate curves often provides more information than it can be extracted from the analyses of the age-adjusted rates alone and is a valuable source of additional hypotheses about causative factors of the observed cancer trends. For instance, a simple look on the age patterns of incidence rates for endometrial and ovarian cancers at different periods of time let us suggest that recent declines

*Corresponding Author: Svetlana V. Ukraintseva—Center for Population Health and Aging, Duke University, Durham, NC 27708, USA. Email: svo@duke.edu, svu@mail.ru

Innovative Endocrinology of Cancer, edited by Lev M. Berstein and Richard J. Santen.
©2008 Landes Bioscience and Springer Science+Business Media.

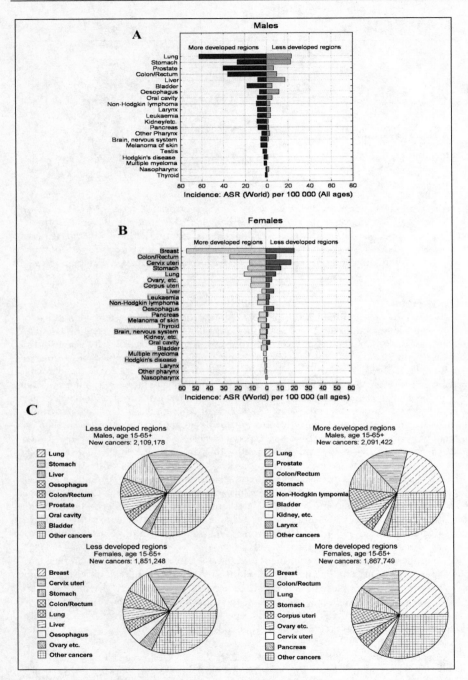

Figure 1. A, B) Age-standardized incidence rates for separate cancer sites in more and less developed regions, by sex. C) Most common adult cancers in more and less developed regions, by sex (GLOBOCAN 1998).[41]

in the age-adjusted rates of these cancers (that seemed consistent) have been driven by fairly different factors (will be discussed below).

Data Sources and Basic Definitions

In this review, we used the data extracted from cancer registries and published by the International Agency for Research on Cancer (IARC), part of the WHO, in the book series Cancer Incidence in Five Continents,[5-7] covering over 200 populations worldwide for the years 1957-2000 and in the monograph series IARC Monographs on the Evaluation of Carcinogenic Risks to Humans.[8,9] We also used statistics on cancer incidence and survival from the National Cancer Institute (NCI) SEER (The Surveillance, Epidemiology and End Results) program[1,10] collecting data from population-based cancer registries covering approximately 26 percent of the US population, as well as from other recognized sources.

The following basic definitions are used in this review. The age-specific cancer incidence rate is defined as the number of new cancer cases (registered for the first time) per 100,000 people in a population of a given age in a particular year or time interval. Age-specific cancer mortality rate stands for the number of cancer deaths per 100,000 people in a population of a given age in a particular year or time interval. The 5-year relative survival from cancer refers to the ratio of the observed survival rate for the patient group to the expected survival rate for persons in the general population similar to the patient group with respect to age, sex, race and calendar year of observation. The 5-year relative survival rate is used to estimate the proportion of cancer patients potentially curable. Because over one-half of all cancers occur in persons 65 years of age and over,[5] many of these individuals die of other causes with no evidence of recurrence of their cancer. The relative survival rate is obtained by adjusting observed survival for the normal life expectancy of the general population of the same age and thus it is an estimate of the chance of surviving the effects of cancer. Cancer burden is broadly characterized by a total number or the proportion of individuals with diagnosed cancer (cancer prevalence) living in general population, no matter when the diagnosis has been made.

Typical Age Patterns of Cancer Incidence and Mortality Rates

There is a prevalent opinion that the shape of the incidence rate curve is a characteristic of a cancer site that is relatively independent on environmental carcinogenicity and best attributed to some intrinsic aspects of a cancer development.[11,12] However, a comparison of incidence rate curves for separate cancer sites over different places and time periods reveals that their shapes substantially vary depending not only on cancer site per se, but also on population and year of study.[5,13] The rates may increase accelerating until very old age (85 and above), or increase almost linearly with age, or manifest decelerated increase with a leveling off at the old ages, or have a wave-like pattern with a peak in middle or late life (see figures in the text as examples). Despite all this variability, the age patterns of overall cancer risk (for all sites combined) do have common features, which include: (i) a peak in early childhood; (ii) the lowest rate in youth; (iii) an increase in the rate, starting at the reproductive period and (iv) the deceleration or decline in cancer rates at the old ages (75 and over) (Fig. 2). These features are recurrent over time and place[5] and can be drawn not only from period data but also from cohort data.[13] The overall cancer mortality rate exhibits a peak at the oldest old ages (90 and over) and then declines, which most probably reflects a decline in the cancer incidence rate observed in earlier years. The mortality peak is lower than the respective peak in the incidence rate and shifts towards older ages (Fig. 2).

Studies of random autopsies from older individuals confirmed diminishing overall cancer risk in advanced years of life.[14,15] Animal experiments revealed remarkable similarity of cancer incidence rate patterns in humans and rodent species—in particular, an intriguing deceleration or decline in overall cancer incidence rate at old ages.[16-18] This is significant finding because it suggests that such deceleration/decline is not simply an artifact of the data and it is unlikely to be due to a diagnostic bias. Two explanations of this phenomenon that are in agreement with both human and animal data have been suggested. First, the differential selection in heterogeneous

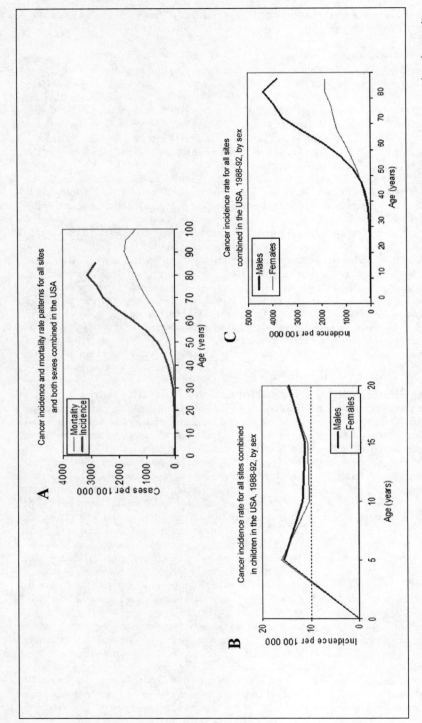

Figure 2. Typical age patterns of overall cancer incidence and mortality rates. Age-specific incidence rates (1988-92), average annual and mortality rate (1990) in the USA (data combined from the sources: IARC, 1997,[42] Smith, 1996,[43] Health US, 1997,[6] Smith, 1999).[44] Figure a is reprinted with permission from: Ukraintseva SV, Yashin AI. Individual aging and cancer risk: How are they related? Demographic Research 2003; 9-8.[21] © 2003 Max-Planck-Gesellschaft.

Table 1. Trends in incidence and patients' survival rates for selected hormone-associated cancers in the US[1,10,40,46]

A. Change in incidence rates between 1950 and 1998 and between 1995 and 2004

Cancer	Change in Incidence Rate 1995-2004 (%)	Change in Incidence Rate 1950-1998 (%)
Prostate	−3	194
Thyroid	53	155
Breast	−8	63
Corpus Uteri	−7	4
Ovary	−13	1
Pancreas	1	14
All cancer sites	−6	60

B. 5-year relative survival rates in 1950 and in 1996-2003

Cancer	5-Year Survival (%) 1996-2003	5-Year Survival (%) 1950
Prostate	99	43
Thyroid	97	80
Breast	90	60
Corpus Uteri	85	72
Ovary	45	30
Pancreas	5	1
All sites	66	35

population may favor the survival of individuals without cancer and increase their share among the elderly that would create the observed decline in the rates.[19] Second, some inherent effects of individual aging may paradoxically oppose cancer development in body and thus contribute to the late deceleration/decline in cancer risk.[17,20,21] For example, the universal decline in rates of basic biological processes in an ageing organism, such as the rates of metabolism and cell proliferation, may contribute to a deceleration of the tumor growth and rates of cancer clinical manifestation at old ages. Metabolic and hormonal changes accompanying ontogenetic transitions in organism (e.g., switching off reproductive function in women) may also play role. Such transitions change the spectrum of internal cancer risk factors, so that it may result in decreasing vulnerability to some cancers (particularly those of female reproductive system, such as ovarian, endometrial and breast cancers) afterwards. For goals of this paper, it is important that the old age decline in cancer risk is a real phenomenon and in case of female hormone associated cancers it could in part be related to the effects of individual aging.[20,21]

Patterns and Trends of Incidence Rates for Hormone Associated Cancers

Prostate Cancer

The age patterns of incidence rate for prostate cancer are typically nonmonotonic with the rate first rapidly increasing during adult life and then declining at the old ages (above 70) (Fig. 3). The low serum testosterone levels as well as elevated estradiol might partially be responsible for the lower risks of prostate cancer in aged men, although results and opinions are not entirely consistent.[22,23]

Both the age-adjusted and age-specific rates of prostate cancer are substantially higher in more developed regions compared to less developed ones (Figs. 1, 3). The rates increased rapidly during

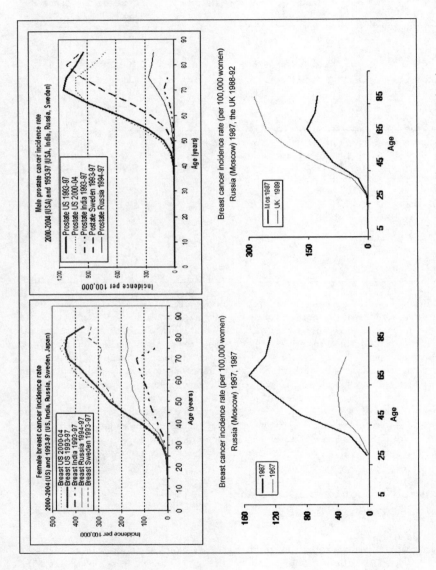

Figure 3. Time and place differences in the age-patterns of incidence rates (average annual) for female breast and male prostate cancers (Aksel and Dvoirin 1991[45]; IARC 1997,[6] IARC 2002[7]; Ries et al 2007[1]).

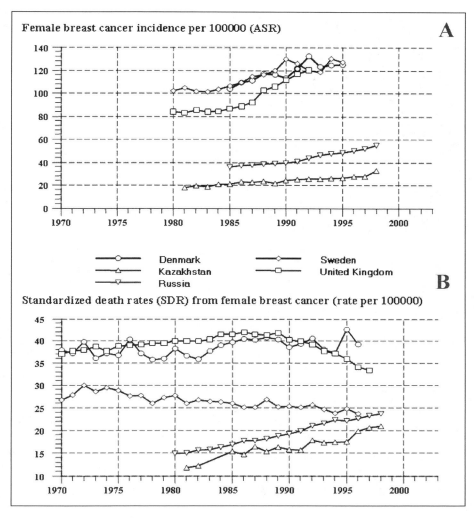

Figure 4. A) Time and place differences in breast cancer age-standardized incidence rates (ASR) (data source: Health for all 2000).[35] The rates are higher in more developed countries (the UK, Sweden, Denmark). B) Time trends and place differences in breast cancer age-standardized death rates (SDR) (Health for all 2000).[35]

second half of 20th century in an association with economic progress and western life style.[1,5] The increase, until recently, was particularly pronounced in the US (Table 1). Exact factors of so dramatic increase in prostate cancer risk remain largely unclear. It could partially be attributed to an increase in early and better detection including that of nonlethal tumors that might be missed from cancer records in the past. Few other factors (both related and not to economic development) have shown a statistically significant association with overall incidence of prostate cancer: African-American race, positive family history, higher tomato products intake (inversely) and alpha-linolenic acid (ALA, the (n-3) fatty acid) in vegetable oils intake.[24,25] Interestingly, high consumption of the ALA is also associated with reduced risk of fatal heart disease.[25] Less statistically supported factors that are associated with the risk of prostate cancer and can also be attributed to western life style include taller height, higher BMI and high total caloric intake. Some studies suggest that tendency to delayed parenthood might be one more potentially important factor contributing to higher prostate cancer risks in male offspring in developed countries. A higher age of father was associated with an elevated risk of prostate cancer in offspring in the Framingham Study.[26]

Relative 5-year survival of prostate cancer patients has dramatically increased for last 50 years (in the US it now practically approached 100 per cent)[40] in an association with improved diagnostic involving both earlier detection and better detection of nonlethal tumors (Table 1).

Breast Cancer

The age patterns of incidence rate for breast cancer are typically decelerating in middle life and declining at the old ages (Fig. 3). The deceleration/decline may in part be related to slowing down metabolism during aging as well as to ontogenetic hormonal changes in body (e.g., ceasing exposure to internal estrogens at menopause) which may reduce breast cancer rates in late life.[21]

Similar to prostate cancer, the breast cancer rates display clear association with economic progress. The incidence rates are generally higher in more developed countries (Figs. 1, 3, 4).

This excess in risk is most probably related to the factors associated with western life style, such as delayed childbirth or use of hormone replacement therapy (HRT) in menopause. As recent

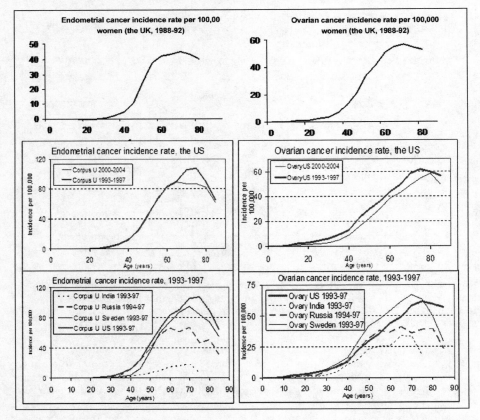

Figure 5. Time and place differences in the age-patterns of incidence rate (average annual) for ovarian and endometrial cancers. The UK, 1988-1992, the US, 1993-1997 and 2000-2004 and different countries, 1993-1997 (data source: IARC 1997,[6] IARC 2002[7]; Ries et al 2007[1]).

studies show, the breast cancer risks rise substantially with age at childbirth for both mothers and female offspring. Women who gave first birth after the age of 35 had a risk increase by 40 percent compared to mothers who experienced their first birth before the age of 20.[27,28] The rate ratios for breast cancer in daughters whose mothers were aged 26 or more years at their birth, relative to women whose mothers were aged 25 years or younger, was 1.3-1.5 in the Framingham Study.[29] Older paternal age may also increase breast cancer risk in female offspring. Women whose fathers were aged 40 or older years at their birth had 1.6-fold increased risk of breast cancer compared with fathers aged less than 30 years.[30]

Another factor, postmenopausal HRT, could contribute to the risk of breast cancer observed primarily at ages over 60. This is particularly true for the US, where postmenopausal HRT was prescribed (until recently) rather often. In a recent study based on SEER data, the notable decline in the rates of new estrogen-receptor-positive breast cancer cases in 2003 was associated with a national-wide reduction in the use of postmenopausal HRT. Age-adjusted incidence rates of breast cancer in women who were 50 years of age or older fell 6.7 percent in the United States in 2003. During this same period, prescriptions for HRT declined rapidly from 61 million prescriptions written in 2001 to 21 million in 2004. This trend followed a highly-discussed 2002 report from the Women's Health Initiative (WHI) study. The latter showed an increased risk of breast cancer and some other disease, such as stroke and pulmonary embolism (but not increased total mortality) among postmenopausal women aged 50-79 (majority were older than 60), who were using HRT including both estrogen and progestin.[31-33] Long-term (but not short-term) exposure to hormonal contraception with estrogens, which is common in developed countries, may also play role in increased risks of breast cancer in premenopausal women. It was shown that premenopausal women who used estrogens during fifteen or more years of life have an increased risk of breast cancer by about 30 percent.[34]

Five-year survival of breast cancer patients varies substantially over populations being generally higher in more developed countries. The best survival rates are currently in the US, where 5-year relative survival approaches 90 per cent (Table 1). The variability in patients' survival can explain diverging trends in cancer mortality among the countries shown on Figure 4. One can see from this figure that while the breast cancer incidence rates increased over time in all the countries compared, mortality from this cancer rose in Russia, Kazakhstan and in less extent, Denmark and declined in Sweden (since 1975) and in the UK (since 1990s). The declining mortality at time of increasing incidence can be explained by a significant improvement in survival of breast cancer patients in the latter countries. It is particularly true for Sweden, where the decline in breast caner mortality is most pronounced, while the incidence rates are among the highest. Respectively, the rise in breast cancer mortality in Russia, Kazakhstan and (less rapidly so) in Denmark most probably reflects an increasing incidence rate on the grounds of relatively poor survival from breast cancer in these countries.[35-37]

Endometrial Cancer

For majority of countries represented in IARC publications[6,7] and also in SEER data,[1] the age pattern of the incidence rate for endometrial (corpus uteri) cancer appears wave-like, with the rate clearly declining at the old ages (above 60) (Fig. 5). Relative stability of this pattern over populations suggests that it may be influenced by ontogenetic factors such as the age-related hormonal changes in a body at menopause, when internal exposure to estrogens ceases. Postmenopausal estrogens are shown to be a risk factor for endometrial cancer. The risk increases with increasing duration of use and decreases with time since last use.[9] One could speculate that ceasing internal exposure to estrogens at menopause would contribute to a decrease in the incidence rates of this cancer later in life in similar way.

The age-adjusted incidence rates of endometrial cancer are in average higher in more developed regions. One reason could again be postmenopausal estrogen therapy that is common in developed countries, while still rare in developing ones. More than 30 case-control studies consistently demonstrated an association between use of postmenopausal estrogens (alone, without progestin)

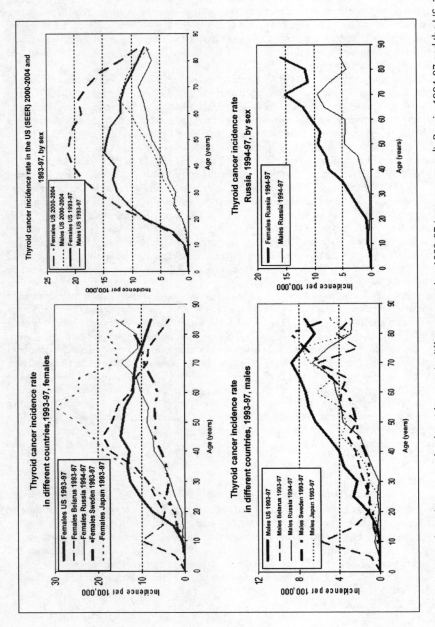

Figure 6. The age-patterns of incidence rates for thyroid cancer in different countries, 1993-97 (average annual), Russia, 1994-97 and the US, 1993-97 and 2000-2004 (average annual) (Ries et al 2007[1]; IARC 2002[2]).

and an increased risk for endometrial cancer.[9] The age-adjusted rates of endometrial cancer were relatively stable in the USA during second half of past century (Table 1); this rate, however, recently declined by about 7 per cent and this decline was almost exclusively attributed to ages above 60. Almost three-fold decline in prescription of postmenopausal HRT (see section on breast cancer for detail) since 2002 might contribute to this trend, similar to that for breast cancer.

For last 50 years the relative 5-year survival of endometrial cancer patients increased from 72 to 85 per cent in the US[1,10] and currently it is one of least deadly cancers contributing to both increasing cancer burden and decreasing cancer mortality.

Ovarian Cancer

The age patterns of ovarian cancer are also wave-like and looking similar in different populations (Fig. 5). This indicates a possible role of internal (e.g., ontogenetic) factors in this cancer development. In the US, the age-adjusted rates of ovarian cancer have recently decreased by about 13 per cent (Table 1). Long-term (more than 10 years) postmenopausal HRT with estrogen alone has been associated with an increase in ovarian cancer risk in separate studies,[38] although this problem is controversial and under discussion. Nevertheless, significant reduction in exposure to postmenopausal HRT since 2002 might, in principle, contribute to a decline in the incidence rates of ovarian cancer, similarly to that for breast and endometrial cancers. Note, however, that a simple look on the age specific incidence rate curves from Figure 5 let us suggest that factor responsible for the decrease in ovarian cancer rates is common for all ages at risk, not only for postmenopausal ones. This decrease looks proportional for the different ages and the incidence rate curve for 2000-2004 appears to be parallel shifted in relation to the 1993-1997 curve. Such trend is completely different from that observed for endometrial cancer and, therefore, requires another explanation. It could be for example some formal changes in diagnostic coding or case registration procedure that lead to the proportional decline in ovarian cancer rates. Increased use of combined oral contraceptives during reproductive period is unlikely to be an explanation since the combined contraceptives are protective against both ovarian and endometrial cancers and were shown to affect their rates in similar way.[9]

Ovarian cancer shows intermediate 5-year survival, compared to other hormone associated sites (Table 1). For 50 years, there was only moderate improvement in the survival rates and ovarian cancer continues to be a deadliest one of female reproductive system. Recently, some advances in this cancer treatment were suggested, which may increase the survival rates in forthcoming years (up to 70 per cent, in average); however, early detection of ovarian cancer remains a major problem. While treatment of the first stage is highly successful, with 5-year survival approaching 90 per cent, most cases of ovarian cancer are detected on late stages, which are poorly curable. Major reason is that this cancer produces very few early stage symptoms (almost none are specific) and attempts to establish the efficient screening program have been not successful so far (more details can be found on NCI web site, www.cancer.gov). Finding solid early diagnostic criteria for ovarian cancer is therefore urgent scientific and clinical oncology task.

Thyroid Cancer

Unlike ovarian cancer, the age patterns of the incidence rate for thyroid cancer vary greatly over populations, particularly in females, being sometimes nearly linear, sometimes decelerating with age, or sometimes declining at the old ages (Fig. 6).

One can see from the Figure 6 that the rates of thyroid cancer can be higher or lower in more compared to less developed countries. In other words, there is no definite correlation between this cancer rates and the level of economic development of a country as it is observed for cancers of breast and prostate. In Belarus, a country that has been significantly exposed to radioactive contamination after Chernobyl disaster in 1986 (the vast majority of the radioactive fallout landed in Belarus), one can see ten years later (1993-1997) a clear peak of childhood morbidity at ages around 10, which probably reflects a particularly negative impact of the radioactive exposure in utero. Such peak is absent on incidence rate curves of other countries (Fig. 6). A large incidence peak, however, can be observed in Japanese women at ages between 50 and 60, who were in uterus

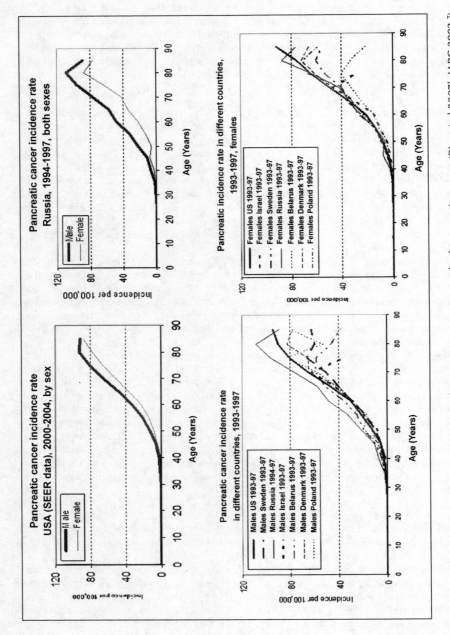

Figure 7. The age-patterns and place differences in the incidence rates (average annual) of pancreatic cancer (Ries et al 2007[1]; IARC 2002[7]).

or young children at time of atomic bombings of Hiroshima and Nagasaki. All this indicates that the age-specific risks of thyroid cancer are greatly influenced by local exposure factors (such as radioactive contamination) and less related to a level of economic development of a country.

Thyroid cancer manifests substantial increase in the incidence rate over time in the US, particularly in females (Table 1, Fig. 6), which probably reflects increasing exposure to factors affecting thyroid vulnerability (for instance, it might be a rise in rates of sporadic goiter linked to spread of lithium treatment for depression, or other factors). Relative 5-year survival of thyroid cancer patients has been one of the best among all cancers since long time: Even in the 1950s this survival approached 80 per cent; nowadays it is nearly a hundred per cent (Table 1).

Pancreatic Cancer

The age patterns of the incidence rate for this cancer are similar for males and females. The incidence rate increases with age until old ages (70+) with the rate that is similar in very different populations (such as the US and Russia) (Fig. 7). These notable similarities suggest that development of pancreatic cancer could be considerably influenced by universal aging-associated changes in a body (which are common for different populations and sexes). Exposures to oxidative stress that accumulate their effects in organism with age or aging-associated insulin resistance might be among these factors.

The age-adjusted incidence rates for pancreatic cancer are generally higher in more developed regions (Fig. 1); contemporary epidemic of diabetes in affluent societies might contribute to this excess. The rates, however, not so dramatically increased in 20th century as it was for some other sites, including prostate, thyroid and breast (IARC 1965-2002[5]; Table 1). The rates of pancreatic cancer have recently stabilized in the US (Table 1, Fig. 7).

5-year relative survival for pancreatic cancer is poorest among the all mentioned cancers (Table 1). It is practically not cured, implying that current diagnostic and treatment strategies for this cancer are not adequate and need fundamental revision. Pancreatic cancer is often missed during routine examination and diagnosed too late due to lack of early symptoms. Even more important is that tumors are very resistant to standard chemotherapy or radiation. One forthcoming option might be novel therapies that target the pancreatic cancer stem cells which have recently been suggested to be mainly responsible for the tumor resistance to conventional treatment.[39]

Conclusions

In this chapter we reviewed typical features of the epidemiology of hormone-associated cancers emphasizing comparison of the age specific incidence rate curves as a valuable source of hypotheses about factors influencing cancer risks. Here the findings are briefly summarized.

Typical Features of the Age Patterns of Cancer Incidence Rate

Typical age patterns of the incidence rate for cancers of the breast, prostate, ovary and endometrium are wave-like, that is, nonmonotonic. Such patterns can be observed over different populations and time periods and also seen in laboratory animals.[5,16-18,21] Differential selection in heterogeneous populations as well as factors of individual aging (such as slow down of metabolism or hormonal changes in an aging body) may play a role in these patterns.[19-21] Thyroid cancer manifests substantial variability of the incidence rate patterns over populations suggesting a predominant contribution of local exposure factors to this cancer risk. Comparing the incidence rate curves for pancreatic cancer allows for assumption that this cancer risk can be influenced by some universal age associated changes in a body that are common for both sexes.

An Association between Cancer Risk and Economic Progress

Age-standardized cancer incidence rates for all sites combined show a clear association with economic progress. The rates are higher in more developed countries and until recently increased over time.[1,5] This is also true for some (but not all) hormone-associated cancers. These cancers substantially vary in their susceptibility to factors associated with economic prosperity and western life style: cancers of the breast, endometrium and prostate display the highest vulnerability to such factors, while cancers of the thyroid and pancreas appear to be least dependent on those.

The incidence rates of female hormone-associated cancers recently declined in the US[1,40] (Table 1). In case of breast and endometrial cancers, this decline can be attributed to reducing exposure to HRT in postmenopausal women; in case of ovarian cancer it is probably related to different factor(s).

Continuing increase of thyroid cancer rates in the US may reflect increasing population exposure to factors affecting thyroid vulnerability, particularly in females.

Variability in Survival of Cancer Patients

The relative 5-years survival of cancer patients greatly improved over last 50 years for most hormone-associated cancers, including thyroid, prostate, breast and endometrial, so that these cancers are nowadays among the least deadly ones (Table 1). Pancreatic cancer does not fit this positive trend and continues to be among the deadliest human malignancies (in both sexes) suggesting that current diagnostic and treatment strategies are not adequately addressing the nature of this cancer. Ovarian cancer shows intermediate survival, with only slight progress happened for past 50 years. It continues to be a most fatal female cancer urgently requiring development of more effective diagnostic and treatment tools.

Acknowledgements

Authors acknowledge support from the NIH research grants 1R01AG027019-01 and 1R01AG02859-01.

References

1. Ries LAG, Melbert D, Krapcho M et al. eds. SEER cancer statistics review, 1975-2004. Bethesda, MD: National Cancer Institute, 2007 (http://seer.cancer.gov/csr/1975_2004/, based on November 2006 SEER data submission, posted to the SEER web site, 2007).
2. Stewart BW, Kleihues P. eds. World cancer report. IARC, 2003.
3. Parkin DM, Bray FI, Devesa SS. Cancer burden in the year 2000. The global picture. Eur J Cancer 2001; 37(Suppl 8):S4-66.
4. Sener SF, Grey N. The global burden of cancer. J Surg Oncol 2005; 92(1):1-3.
5. IARC. Cancer incidence in five continents. Volumes I-VIII. IARC Sci Publ Lyon: IARC Press, 1965-2002.
6. IARC. Cancer incidence in five continents. Parkin DM, Whelan SL, Ferlay J et al. eds. Volume VII. IARC Sci Publ No 143. Lyon: IARC Press, 1997.
7. IARC. Cancer incidence in five continents. Parkin DM, Whelan SL, Ferlay J et al. eds. Cancer incidence in five continents, Vol VIII. IARC Sci Publ No. 155. Lyon: IARC Press, 2002.
8. IARC monographs on the evaluation of carcinogenic risks to humans. Vol 1-88. Lyon: IARC Press, 1972-2006. http://monographs.iarc.fr/ENG/Monographs/allmonos90.php.
9. IARC monographs on the evaluation of carcinogenic risks to humans. Vol 72. Lyon: IARC Press, 1999 (data on hormonal contraception and postmenopausal hormonal therapy).
10. Ries LAG, Eisner MP, Kosary CL et al. eds. SEER cancer statistics review, 1973-1998. Bethesda, MD: National Cancer Institute, 2001, posted to the SEER web site in 2001.
11. Rainsford J, Cohen P, Dix D. On the role of aging in cancer incidence: Analysis of the lung cancer data. Anticancer Res 1985; 5(4):427-30.
12. Volpe EW, Dix D. On the role of aging in cancer incidence: Cohort analyses of the lung cancer data. Anticancer Res 1986; 6(6):1417-20.
13. Ukraintseva SV, Yashin AI. Economic progress as cancer risk factor: Part II. Why is overall cancer risk higher in more developed countries? Max Planck Institute WP-2005-022, 2005. http://www.demogr.mpg.de/papers/working/wp-2005-022.pdf
14. Kuramoto K, Matsushita S, Esaki Y et al. [Prevalence, rate of correct clinical diagnosis and mortality of cancer in 4,894 elderly autopsy cases]Nippon Ronen Igakkai Zasshi 1993; 30(1):35-40. (in Japanese).
15. Stanta G, Campagner L, Cavallieri F et al. Cancer of the oldest old. What we have learned from autopsy studies. Clin Geriatr Med 1997; 13(1):55-68.
16. Pompei F, Polkanov M, Wilson R. Age distribution of cancer in mice: The incidence turnover at old age. Toxicol Ind Health 2001; 17(1):7-16.
17. Anisimov VN, Ukraintseva SV, Yashin AI. Cancer in experimental animals: Does it tell us about cancer in humans? Nature Reviews Cancer 2005; 5(10):807-19.
18. Arbeev KG, Semenchenko AV, Anisimov VN et al. Relationship between cancer and aging: Experimental evidence and mathematical modeling considerations. Presented at: Population Association of America 2004 Annual Meeting. USA: Boston, MA, 2004.

19. Vaupel J, Yashin AI. Cancer Rates over Age, Time and Place: Insights from Stochastic Models of Heterogeneous Populations. WP #88-01-1 of the Center for Population Analysis and Policy, University of Minnesota, 1988.
20. Ukraintseva SV, Yashin AI. How individual aging may influence human morbidity and mortality patterns. Mech Ageing Dev 2001; 122:1447-60.
21. Ukraintseva SV, Yashin AI. Individual aging and cancer risk: How are they related? Demographic Research 2003; 9-8.
22. Kehinde EO, Akanji AO, Memon A et al. Prostate cancer risk: The significance of differences in age related changes in serum conjugated and unconjugated steroid hormone concentrations between Arab and Caucasian men. Int Urol Nephrol 2006; 38(1):33-44.
23. Severi G, Morris HA, MacInnis RJ et al. Circulating steroid hormones and the risk of prostate cancer. Cancer Epidemiol Biomarkers Prev 2006; 15(1):86-91.
24. Giovannucci E, Liu Y, Platz EA et al. Risk factors for prostate cancer incidence and progression in the health professionals follow-up study. Int J Cancer 2007; 121:1571-8.
25. Brouwer IA, Katan MB, Zock PL. Dietary alpha-linolenic acid is associated with reduced risk of fatal coronary heart disease, but increased prostate cancer risk: A meta-analysis. Journal of Nutrition 2004; 134(4):919-22.
26. Zhang Y, Kreger BE, Dorgan JF et al. Parental age at child's birth and son's risk of prostate cancer. The Framingham Study. Am J Epidemiol 1999; 150(11):1208-12.
27. Ewertz M, Duffy SW, Adami HO et al. Age at first birth, parity and risk of breast cancer: a meta-analysis of 8 studies from the Nordic countries. Int J Cancer 1990; 46(4):597-603.
28. Dupont WD, Page DL. Breast cancer risk associated with proliferative disease, age at first birth, and a family history of breast cancer. Am J Epidemiol 1987; 125(5):769-79.
29. Zhang Y, Cupples LA, Rosenberg L et al. Parental ages at birth in relation to a daughter's risk of breast cancer among female participants in the Framingham Study (United States). Cancer Causes Control 1995; 6(1):23-9.
30. Choi JY, Lee KM, Park SK et al. Association of paternal age at birth and the risk of breast cancer in offspring: A case control study. BMC Cancer 2005; 5:143.
31. Ravdin PM, Cronin KA, Howlader N et al. The decrease in breast-cancer incidence in 2003 in the United States. N Engl J Med 2007; 356(16):1670-4.
32. Katalinic A, Rawal R. Decline in breast cancer incidence after decrease in utilisation of hormone replacement therapy. Breast Cancer Res Treat 2007 [Epub ahead of print].
33. Rossouw JE, Anderson GL, Prentice RL et al. Risks and benefits of estrogen plus progestin in healthy postmenopausal women: Principal results from the Women's Health Initiative randomized controlled trial. JAMA 2002; 288:321-333.
34. Steinberg KK, Thacker SB, Smith SJ et al. A meta-analysis of the effect of estrogen replacement therapy on the risk of breast cancer. JAMA 1991; 265(15):1985-90.
35. Health for all. Data Base. WHO Regional Office for Europe, 2000.
36. EUCAN: Cancer incidence, mortality and prevalence in the European Union in 1996, version 3.1. Ferlay J, Bray F, Sankila R et al. IARC Cancer Base No. 4. Lyon: IARC Press, 1999 (a product of European Network of Cancer Registries).
37. Health in Russia. 1999 Statistics. Russian Ministry of Health publication, 2000.
38. Lacey Jr JV, Mink PJ, Lubin JH et al. Menopausal hormone replacement therapy and risk of ovarian cancer. JAMA 2002; 288(3):334-41.
39. Li C, Heidt DG, Dalerba P et al. Identification of pancreatic cancer stem cells. Cancer Res 2007; 67(3):1030-7.
40. Jemal A, Siegel R, Ward E et al. Cancer statistics, 2007. CA Cancer J Clin 2007; 57:43-66.
41. GLOBOCAN: Cancer incidence and mortality worldwide. Ferlay J, Parkin DM, Pisani P. eds. IARC Cancer Base No 3. Lyon: IARC Press, 1998.
42. Health, United States, 1996-97 and Injury Chartbook. National Center for Health Statistics. Hyattsville, Maryland: 1997. http://www.cdc.gov/nchs/hus.htm
43. Smith D. Changing causes of death of elderly people in the United States, 1950-1990. Gerontology 1998; 44:331-5.
44. Smith D. Resistance to causes of death: A study of cancer mortality resistance in the oldest old. In: Robine JM, ed. The paradoxes of longevity. Springer Verlag, 1999:61-71.
45. Aksel E, Dvoirin V. [Statistics of Malignant Neoplasms.]. Moscow: VONTS AMN SSSR, 1991 (in Russian).
46. Jemal A, Tiwari RC, Murray T et al. Cancer statistics, 2004. CA Cancer J Clin 2004; 54:8-29.

CHAPTER 6

Obesity and Diabetes Epidemics:
Cancer Repercussions

Anette Hjartåker, Hilde Langseth and Elisabete Weiderpass*

Abstract

The prevalence of overweight (body mass index, BMI, between 25 and 30 kg/m²) and obesity (BMI of 30 kg/m² or higher) is increasing rapidly worldwide, especially in developing countries and countries undergoing economic transition to a market economy. One consequence of obesity is an increased risk of developing type II diabetes.

Overall, there is considerable evidence that overweight and obesity are associated with risk for some of the most common cancers. There is convincing evidence of a positive association between overweight/obesity and risk for adenocarcinoma of the oesophagus and the gastric cardia, colorectal cancer, postmenopausal breast cancer, endometrial cancer and kidney cancer (renal-cell). Premenopausal breast cancer seems to be inversely related to obesity. For all other cancer sites the evidence of an association between overweight/obesity and cancer is inadequate, although there are studies suggesting an increased risk of cancers of the liver, gallbladder, pancreas, thyroid gland and in lymphoid and haematopoietic tissue.

Far less is known about the association between diabetes mellitus type I (also called insulin dependent diabetes mellitus or juvenile diabetes), type II diabetes (called non-insulin dependent diabetes mellitus or adult onset diabetes mellitus) and cancer risk. The most common type of diabetes mellitus, type II, seems to be associated with liver and pancreas cancer and probably with colorectal cancer. Some studies suggest an association with endometrial and postmenopausal breast cancer. Studies reporting on the association between type I diabetes mellitus, which is relatively rare in most populations and cancer risk are scanty, but suggest a possible association with endometrial cancer.

Overweight and obesity, as well as type II diabetes mellitus are largely preventable through changes in lifestyle. The fundamental causes of the obesity epidemic—and consequently the diabetes type II epidemic—are societal, resulting from an environment that promotes sedentary lifestyles and over-consumption of energy. The health consequences and economic costs of the overweight, obesity and type II diabetes epidemics are enormous. Avoiding overweight and obesity, as well as preventing type II diabetes mellitus, is an important purpose to prevent cancer and other diseases. Prevention of obesity and type II diabetes should begin early in life and be based on the life-long health eating and physical activity patterns. Substantial public investments in preventing overweight, obesity and type II diabetes mellitus are both appropriate and necessary in order to have a major impact on their adverse health effects including cancer.

*Corresponding Author: Elisabete Weiderpass—Cancer Registry of Norway, N-0310 Oslo, Norway. Email: elisabete.weiderpass@kreftregisteret.no

Innovative Endocrinology of Cancer, edited by Lev M. Berstein and Richard J. Santen.
©2008 Landes Bioscience and Springer Science+Business Media.

Introduction

The prevalence of overweight and obesity is increasing rapidly worldwide. The increase in prevalence is especially rapid in developing countries undergoing economic transition. As more people are getting overweight and obese the morbidity patterns change. The first changes are usually an increase in hypertension, hyperlipidemia, glucose intolerance and type II diabetes mellitus. Next emerge increasing rates of cardiovascular diseases and long-term complications of diabetes (e.g., renal failure), followed by increasing rates of various types of cancer.[1]

Diabetes is one of the most common endocrine disorders today. It is caused by both environmental and genetic factors. The environmental factors that may lead to development of diabetes includes obesity, physical inactivity, use of drugs and exposure to toxic agents.[2] There are two main types of diabetes. Type I diabetes—or insulin-dependent diabetes mellitus (IDDM)—is mainly diagnosed during childhood or adolescence and is characterized by a diminished ability of the pancreas to produce insulin. Type II diabetes—or non-insulin dependent diabetes mellitus (NIDDM)—constitutes over 90% of all diabetes cases and has mostly been diagnosed after age forty, although recently much younger cases are being reported. In this type of the disease insulin is usually produced, but cannot be properly utilized due to insulin-resistance in target cells. Advanced cases of NIDDM may need treatment with insulin, which makes the use of the terminology IDDM and NIDDM quite confusing. We will therefore use the terms type I and type II diabetes mellitus in the following text. Both type I and type II diabetes mellitus show strong familial aggregation in all populations. Type II diabetes mellitus is clearly, as was mentioned above, the result of an interaction between genetic susceptibility and environmental factors.[3]

Prevalence of Obesity and Measurement of Body Fat

According to the World Health Organization (WHO) approximately 1.6 billion adults worldwide were overweight in 2005 and at least 400 million adults were obese.[4] The numbers will continue to rise and WHO's projections estimate that by 2015, approximately 2.3 billion adults will be overweight and more than 700 million will be obese.

Obesity refers to excess storage of body fat. In adult men with weight in the acceptable range, the percentage of body fat is around 15-20%, whereas in women it is around 25-30%. Several methods may be used for measuring percentage body fat (e.g., densitometry and dual energy X-ray absorptiometry (DEXA)), but most of them are impractical for use in larger epidemiological studies. As for measures of relative body composition, the body mass index, BMI, is the most common and accepted measure.

BMI is a simple index of weight-for-height used to classify underweight, overweight and obesity in adults. It is calculated as the weight in kilograms divided by the square of the height in meters (kg/m^2). BMI values are age-independent and the same for both sexes. Also, although BMI values may not correspond to the same degree of fatness in different populations (partly

Table 1. Cut-points of body mass index for the classification of weight

BMI	WHO Classification	Description
<18.5 kg/m²	Underweight	Thin
18.5-24.9 kg/m²	-	Healthy, normal or acceptable weight
25.0-29.9 kg/m²	Grade 1 overweight	Overweight
30.0-39.9 kg/m²	Grade 2 overweight	Obesity
≥40.0 kg/m²	Grade 3 overweight	Morbid obesity

Reproduced with permission from: IARC Handbooks of Cancer Prevention, Vol. 6: Weight Control and Physical Activity.1

because of different body proportions) and ethnic-specific BMI definitions have been suggested, a WHO expert consultation has recently recommended the same cut-off values be used worldwide.[5] The cut-points proposed by WHO are given in Table 1. The five different categories are often termed "thin" (BMI < 18.5), "healthy", "normal" or "acceptable" weight (BMI 18.5-24.9 kg/m^2), "overweight" (BMI 25.0-29.9 kg/m^2), "obesity" (BMI 30.0-39.9 kg/m^2) and "morbid obesity" (≥40.0 kg/m^2).

Worldwide prevalence estimates for obesity (BMI >30 kg/m^2) for 2005 and 2015 are given in Figure 1. The figures are based on data from WHO Global InfoBase 2007.[6] Adult mean BMI levels of 22-23 kg/m^2 are found in Africa and Asia, while levels of 25-27 kg/m^2 are prevalent across North America, Europe and in some Latin American, North African and Pacific Island countries.

The average BMI for adult Europeans is nearly 26.5 kg/m^2.[6] A large proportion of the population is overweight and almost a third of the population, some 130 million people, has a BMI over 30.0 kg/m^2. There is a clear upward trend in body weight, not only among adults but also among children.

Data from the 2003-2004 National Health and Nutrition Examination Survey (NHANES) indicate an increase in the proportion of obese in the US population as well.[7] The age-adjusted prevalence among US adults has more than doubled during the last 25 years and is now well above 30%. About two thirds of the adult population have a BMI of 25 or above. The lowest estimates of obesity on the American continent are found in Brazil and Haiti, some 14 and 8% of the population, respectively.[6]

In South-East Asia the prevalence of obesity is around 5%. Particularly low prevalence of obesity is estimated for India (1.3%), Bangladesh (1.5%) and Sri Lanka (0.1%).

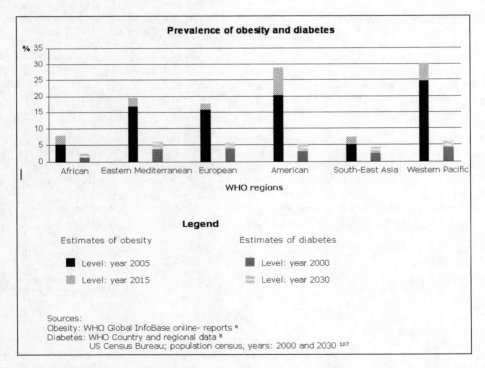

Figure 1. Prevalence of obesity and diabetes worldwide, given as percentages in six different world regions.

The larges variation in obesity within a region is seen in the Western Pacific. The overall prevalence of obesity is estimated to 25%. While very low prevalence is estimated for e.g., Vietnam (0.2%) and Japan (1.6%), remarkably high figures are estimated for Nauru (81%) and Micronesia (70%). In China, the overall prevalence is below 5%, although rates are almost 20% in some cities.

Large variation in obesity prevalence estimates is seen in the Eastern Mediterranean Region as well. Overall, about 17% of the population is estimated to be obese, but the figures range from less than 1% in Afghanistan to more than 40% in Kuwait.

Also, within Africa there is a large variation in obesity prevalence estimates. Very low prevalence (below 0.5%) is estimated for e.g., Zaire, Ethiopia and Eritrea, whereas the obesity prevalence in South Africa is estimated to be 21% and at the Seychelles 28%. In total, the prevalence of obesity in Africa is estimated to 5%. It is expected to rise to about 8% within year 2015.

Prevalence of Diabetes Mellitus

Diabetes mellitus, mostly type II, now affects approximately 6% of the world's adult population with almost 80% of the total residing in developing countries. The number of diabetic patients will reach 300 millions in 2025. More than 97% of those patients will have type II diabetes. Worldwide prevalence estimates for diabetes mellitus in year 2000 and 2030 are given in Figure 1 based on country and regional data from WHO.[8] The region with the highest rates is the Western Pacific where 4.2% of the adult population is affected, followed by European countries with a prevalence of 4%. India leads the global ten in terms of the highest number of people with diabetes with a current figure of 40.9 millions, followed by China with 39.8 millions. Behind them come USA, Russia, Japan, Germany, Pakistan, Brazil, Mexico and Egypt. Developing countries account for seven of the world's top ten.

With the force of globalization and industrialization proceeding at an increasing rate, the prevalence of diabetes is predicted to increase dramatically over the next few decades. The resulting burden of complications and premature mortality will continue to present itself as a major and growing public health problem for most countries.[9]

Association between Obesity and Diabetes Type II

One consequence of obesity is an increased risk of developing type II diabetes. In short, central mechanisms linking increased risk of type II diabetes to obesity include the following: excess body fat and particularly visceral fat release increased amounts of free fatty acids to the blood. Elevation of free fatty acid levels directly affects insulin signaling and causes the liver and skeletal muscles to shift towards greater oxidation of fatty acids for energy production and a relative inhibition of enzymes in the glycolytic cascade. As a result, the capacity of liver and skeletal muscles cells to absorb and metabolize glucose decreases. Also, the tissues capacity to store glucose as glycogen decreases and the cells accumulate more triglycerids instead of glycogen. This state, of reduced responsiveness of muscle, liver and adipose tissue to insulin, is named insulin resistance. To ensure normal glucose and lipid homeostasis the lower response to insulin is compensated by higher than normal secretion of insulin from the beta-cells in the pancreas giving an increased insulin plasma concentration, i.e., hyperinsulinemia. At the extreme, the beta-cells fails to secrete the excess amount of insulin needed and type II diabetes will develop.[10]

Association between Obesity, Diabetes Type II and Risk of Cancer

The global increase in overweight and obesity has a profound impact not only on the prevalence of type II diabetes but also on a wide range of other health aspects such as respiratory and musculoskeletal difficulties, gallbladder disease, cardiovascular diseases and certain types of cancer. The most convincing results regarding an increased BMI and cancer risk are found for oesophageal and gastric cardia adenocarcinomas, colorectal cancer, postmenopausal breast cancer, kidney cancer (renal-cell) and endometrial cancer.[11] Several other types of cancer may also be associated with increased BMI.

Far less is known about type II diabetes' impact on cancer risk. However, it is significant that the greatest risk of cancer in diabetic patients is to the organs in which concentrations of endogenous insulin reach particularly high levels (i.e., liver and pancreas).[12] Some studies have found decreased cancer risk with long lasting type II diabetes which may reflect the inverse relationship between the duration of this type of diabetes and insulin secretion.[13-15] Meta-analyses have indicated that diabetes type II is associated with a 1.2-fold increased risk of bladder cancer, 1.3-fold increased risk of colorectal cancer, 1.7-fold increased risk of pancreatic cancer and 2.5-fold increased risk of hepatocellular carcinoma.[16]

In the next sections we give a broad presentation on what is currently known about obesity, diabetes type I and II and their impact on cancer repercussions. Type II diabetes accounts for the vast majority of all diagnosed cases of diabetes and most of the literature refers to studies on type II diabetes. However, some studies do not distinguished between type I and type II diabetes mellitus. In the following text we will refer to type I and type II diabetes mellitus whenever type is specified in the literature, otherwise the unspecified term diabetes mellitus will be used.

Current Research on the Associations between Obesity and Diabetes and the Risk of Cancer

Obesity

In 2002 The International Agency for Research on Cancer (IARC) published a thorough review on the association between excess body weight and risk of cancer.[1] The report concluded that there was sufficient evidence for a cancer-preventive effect of avoidance of weight gain for cancer of the colon, breast (postmenopausal), endometrium, kidney (renal-cell) and oesophagus (adenocarcinoma). A joint WHO/FAO expert consultation group reached similar conclusions the following year.[11] It has further been suggested that obesity may increase the risk of cancers of the liver, gallbladder and pancreas.[17] Based on prevalence estimates of obesity and overweight in Europe it has been estimated that 3% of all incident cancers in men in the European Union and 6% of all cancers in women may be attributed to excess body weight.[18] In 2001 this corresponded to 27,000 new cancers among men and 45,000 new cancers among women. In the US, overweight and obesity have been estimated to account for as much as 14% of all deaths from cancer in men and 20% in women.[19]

The mechanisms linking obesity to increased cancer risk may vary according to cancer site. Important aspects include hyperlipidemia, impaired glucose tolerance, insulin resistance and subsequent hyperinsulinemia (see below), altered levels of circulating hormones such as growth hormone and sex hormones and increased level of insulin-like growth factor (IGF-1).[17]

An illustration of the central mechanisms and effects of obesity on diabetes 2 and cancer development is given in Figure 2.

Diabetes

Increasing evidence indicates that individuals with type II diabetes are at elevated risk for several common human malignancies, including cancer of the colon, breast, endometrium, pancreas and liver. Laboratory studies have suggested biologically plausible mechanisms. Insulin, for example, is typically at high levels during the development and early stages of diabetes. Activation of the insulin receptor by its ligand, or cross-activation of the insulin-like growth factor 1 receptor, has been shown to be mitogenic and promote tumorigenesis in various model systems.[20] The risk varies according to tumor site: it is the greatest for primary liver cancer, moderately elevated for pancreatic cancer and relatively low for colorectal, endometrial, breast and renal cancers.[12]

Cancer of the Digestive Organs

Oesophageal Cancer

Oesophageal cancer affects nearly half a million people worldwide each year, making it the 6th most common cancer among men and the 9th most common among women.[21] The mortality is high; some 385,000 people die of the cancer every year. The disease affects about twice as many men as women and the rates are several times higher in the less developed regions of the world

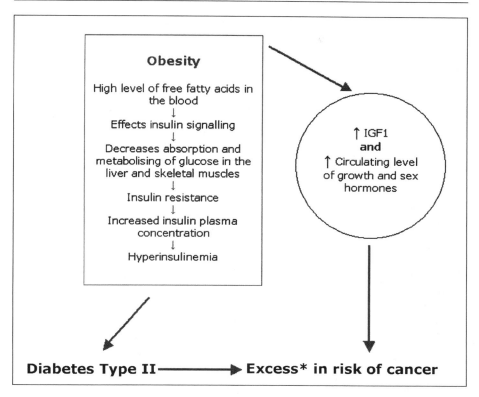

Figure 2. Central mechanisms and effects of obesity on diabetes II and cancer development; *Except for prostate cancer where an inverse association is observed in diabetes patients; ↓ result in; ↑ increased level of IGF1 - insulin-like growth factor.

compared to the more developed parts.[21] The two main histological sub-types of oesophageal cancer are adenocarcinomas and squamous-cell carcinomas.

Obesity
Squamous cell carcinoma of the oesophagus is not found to be related to excess body weight. However, an expert panel stated in 2001 that there is sufficient evidence to conclude that obesity increases the risk of adenocarcinoma of the lower oesophagus.[1] This finding has been confirmed in a recent review.[22] A 2-3 folds increase in risk has been suggested for subjects with a BMI of 25 kg/m^2 or above.[1,22] It has been estimated that more than half of all adenomcarcinomas of the oesophagus in the Unites States of America and more than 40% of the cases in the European Union is attributable to overweight and obesity.[17]

It has been proposed that obesity increases the risk of adenocarcinomas of the oesophagus via increased risk of gastro-oesophageal reflux. However, this pathway is not established.[17]

Diabetes
The relationship between diabetes mellitus and adenocarcinoma of the oesophagus cancer was investigated in a case-control study of US veterans with gastro-oesophageal reflux disease.[23] No association was found. In a Danish study a 30% increase in risk of oesophagus cancer was found in male diabetes patients (95% confidence interval (CI) 1.0-1.6).[24] No increased risk was seen in

women. Except from these studies, reporting contradictory results, little is known about diabetes influence on oesophagus cancer.

Stomach Cancer

Nearly 1 million people are diagnosed with stomach cancer each year.[21] The age-adjusted incidence rate is about twice as high in men as in women (22 and 10 per 100,000, respectively). Generally, there are no overall incidence differences between the more developed parts of the world and the less developed parts. Particularly high age-adjusted incidence rates are seen for men in Korea (69.7 per 100,000) and Japan (62.0 per 100,000). Stomach cancer is the 2nd most common cause of cancer death among men and the 4th most common among women.[21] Cancer of the stomach can be divided in cardia cancer, referring to the upper limit and noncardia cancer. Etiologically cardia cancer seems to be quite similar to cancer of the lower oesophagus.

Obesity

There is scarcity of prospective studies on obesity and stomach cancer. Case-control studies reviewed by an IARC expert panel in 2001 indicate that obesity may double the risk of gastric cardia adenocarcinoma.[1] A recent meta-analysis estimated obese subject to have a 50% (95% CI 20%-80%) increase risk of cardia adenocarcinoma compared to "normal" weight subjects, but the results were heterogeneous between country of origin.[22] No association has been found between obesity and the distal, noncardia type of gastric cancer.[25,26]

Diabetes

Few studies have aimed to investigate a possible association between stomach cancer and diabetes mellitus and the results published show different trends. A reduced risk of stomach cancer overall was observed in diabetes patients in Japan, for both genders,[27] while other studies have found a significant increased risk.[24,28] Results from a cancer incidence study among patients with type I diabetes in Sweden showed a significantly increased risk of stomach cancer overall (standardized incidence rate (SIR) 2.3, 95% CI 1.1-4.1).[29] In a case-control study no evidence of an association was seen between diabetes and cancer of the gastric cardia specifically.[23]

Colorectal Cancer

More than 1 million people worldwide are diagnosed with colorectal cancer every year.[21] Colorectal cancer is the third most common cancer among women and the fourth most common cancer among men. The age-adjusted incidence rate is several times higher in more developed regions of the world (26.6 and 40.0 per 100,000 for women and men, respectively) compared to less developed regions (7.7 and 10.2 per 100,000 for women and men, respectively). More than half a million people worldwide die from colorectal cancer each year.[21]

Obesity

Colorectal cancer is regarded as one of the cancers with greatest prevention potential.[30] Much of the preventive potential ascribes to eating a healthy diet and avoiding physical inactivity. A large number of studies have shown that the risk of colon cancer increases with increasing BMI.[31] Generally, there also seems to be a somewhat increased risk of rectal cancer with increasing BMI, but fewer studies have examined this relationship. An expert panel set down by IARC regarded in 2001 that there is "sufficient evidence" for a colon cancer preventive effect of avoidance of weight gain.[1] More recent studies have confirmed this statement.[32] There is no indication of a threshold effect of obesity; an increased risk of colon cancer has been observed for a wide range of BMI. Overall, cohort studies have shown a 25-100% higher risk of colorectal cancer for overweight and obese subjects compared to leaner ones. For example, in an US study the relative risk (RR) of colorectal cancer for obese men was 1.52 (95% CI 0.9-2.7) compared to "normal" weighted men, whereas obese women had a relative risk of colorectal cancer of 1.26 (95% CI 0.6-2.6) compared to lean peers.[33] In a review paper examining the results from 7 cohort studies and 6 case-control studies the summary relative risk estimate for subjects with a BMI above 28.5 kg/m² compared to subjects with BMI below 22.0 kg/m² was 1.6 for men and 1.3 for women.[34]

It has been estimated that 35% of the colorectal cancer cases among US men and 28% of the colorectal cancer cases among men in the European Union can be attributed to overweight and obesity.[17] For women the corresponding figures are 21% for US women and 14% for women in the European Union.

In order to elucidate the time in colorectal carcinogenesis when obesity might be most important several studies have examined the association between colorectal adenomas, potential precursors of colorectal cancer and obesity. Overall, there seems to be a stronger association between obesity and large adenomas than for obesity and smaller adenomas. Based on this finding it has been suggested that obesity-related factors may act at a later stage in the development of colorectal cancer, i.e., obesity contributes to promotion and progression towards cancer, rather than initiating. An alternative suggestion is that other factors may lead to small adenomas but not to progression and thereby diluting the association between obesity and smaller adenomas.[1]

The association between obesity and colorectal cancer is found for both sexes but is generally stronger among men than among women.[1] The reason for this gender difference is not known, but the findings imply that the effect of obesity is not simply an indicator of energy imbalance. If the positive association between obesity and colorectal cancer were due to energy imbalance one would expect equal results for men and women. One suggestion is that obesity among postmenopausal women may have an offsetting beneficial effect due to high levels of estrogen that may diminish the detrimental effects of obesity.[1]

Diabetes

An increased incidence of colon cancer in diabetes patients has been observed in a number of studies carried out in different parts of the world. A meta-analysis based on results from 6 case-control studies and 9 cohort studies including both type I and type II diabetes showed an increased risk of colorectal cancer in diabetes mellitus patients.[35] Population-based cohort studies in Denmark, Sweden and the US, including a large numbers of diabetes patients, all reported significantly increased incidence of colorectal cancer.[24,36,37] The Danish study reported 30% increased incidence in male patients and 10% increased incidence in female patients.[24] Results from the Swedish study showed an overall standardized mortality ratio (SMR) of 1.6 in men and 1.5 in women. The increased risks were not related to the duration of diabetes prior to the diagnosis of colon cancer.[36] In diabetic patients in the US study the increased risk of developing colorectal cancer accounted for 30% in men and 16% in women.[37] Colorectal cancer was increased by 39% among type II diabetes patients in a population-based retrospective cohort study (95% CI 1.03-1.82) and the risk was particularly high among men.[38]

Primary Liver Cancer

Some 630,000 persons worldwide are diagnosed with liver cancer every year and about 600,000 die from the disease annually.[21] More than 80% of the liver cancer cases occur in the less developed regions of the world.

Obesity

Only a limited number of papers have reported on risk of liver cancer in relation to BMI. A higher risk of liver cancer and higher liver cancer mortality has been reported for obese than for leaner subjects, but the body of evidence is yet too weak to draw any firm conclusions.[17,39]

Diabetes

A possible association between liver cancer (hepatocellular carcinoma—HCC) and diabetes mellitus has been found in several studies. A meta-analysis showed pooled odds ratios (OR) from 13 cohort studies of 2.5 (95% CI 1.9-3.2) and from 13 case-controls studies of 2.5 (95% CI 1.9-3.2).[40] A 4-fold increase in risk of primary liver cancer was observed in male diabetes type II patients in Sweden.[41] The risk for women was increased more than 3-fold compared to the figures for the general population. Patients with diseases predisposing to liver cancer (hepatitis, hepatic cirrhosis, hemochromatosis and alcoholism) were excluded from the analyses, however the risk still remained three times higher.[41] Two case-control studies [42,43] and one cohort study[27] also found a significant increased risk of liver cancer in diabetes patients. In an area with high prevalence of hepatitis virus infection, it was found that type II diabetes increased the risk of developing HCC in those who were hepatitis C virus negative or had a high level of total cholesterol.[44]

Gallbladder Cancer

With some exceptions (e.g., in India, Pakistan, Ecuador), gallbladder cancer occurs quite seldom.[45] The etiology of the disease is sparingly known.

Obesity

The number of studies on gallbladder cancer and obesity is restricted, but the findings seem to be rather consistent in that obesity is associated with an increased risk.[17] In a recent meta-analysis of three case-control studies and eight cohort studies the summary relative risk for gallbladder cancer for obese women was 1.88 (95% CI 1.66-2.13) compared to "normal" weight women.[46] In parallel, obese men had a relative risk of 1.66 (95% CI 1.47-1.88). Overweight women had a 28% (95% CI 4%-57%) increased risk of gallbladder cancer compared to leaner women, whereas only a small and nonsignificant increase in risk was found for overweight men (RR 1.05, 95% CI 0.92-1.19).

In a paper from 2001 it was estimated that 24% of the gallbladder cancer cases in the European Union could be attributed to excess body weight.[18] In 2004 corresponding figures of 36% for the US and 27% for the European Union was published.[17] Further, in 2007, based on prevalence data on obesity and overweight in the US population, it was estimated that 12% of the gallbladder cancer cases among men and 30% of the cases among women could be attributed to a BMI of 25 kg/m^2 or above.[46]

It has been suggested that excess weight increases the risk of gallbladder cancer through increased risk of gallstones that subsequently may cause a chronic inflammation.[45]

Diabetes

Diabetes as a risk factor for gallbladder cancer has been investigated in a few studies. A Swedish study reported a 40% significant increased risk of gallbladder cancer in female diabetes patients (95% CI 1.1-1.6) whereas in male patients a 20% increased risk was found (95% CI 0.9-1.7).[41] Risk of gallbladder cancer was not raised in a cancer incidence and mortality study among type I diabetes patients.[47]

Pancreatic Cancer

More than 230,000 people get pancreas cancer every year.[21] The fatality is high and in developed countries pancreatic cancer contributes significantly to cancer mortality with age-adjusted mortality rate of 8.0 and 5.4 per 100,000 for men and women, respectively. In less developed countries the age-adjusted mortality rate is about 2.0-2.6 per 100,000.[21]

Obesity

It has been suggested that obesity is positively related to pancreatic cancer, but the relation is thought to be modest.[48] While earlier studies have not found any association, more recent studies have indicated a relative risk of 1.7 for obese subjects compared to "normal" weight subject.[17] In a meta-analysis including six case-control studies and eight cohort studies the summary relative risk per unit increase in BMI was 1.02 (95% CI 1.01-1.03), corresponding to a relative risk of 1.19 (95% CI 1.10-1.29) for subjects with a BMI of 30 kg/m^2 or above compared to subject with a BMI of 22 kg/m^2.[49] It has been estimated that about one fourth and one fifth of all pancreatic cancer in the US and in the European Union, respectively, is attributed to excess weight.[17]

Diabetes

Type II diabetes is considered to be an important risk factor for pancreatic cancer, while the relation between type I diabetes and pancreatic cancer is unclear.[29] A large number of studies have been published on the association between type II diabetes and pancreatic cancer. However, it is important to recognize that previous epidemiological studies of the association between diabetes and pancreatic cancer are generally lacking information about the clinical utility of newly identified diabetes as marker for pancreatic cancer. In almost all case-control studies, duration of diabetes is unclear as it has been assessed by self- or proxy report.[50] A meta-analysis of 36 studies on type II diabetes supports a modest causal association.[51] The pooled odds ratio for 17 case-control studies was 1.94 (95% CI 1.53-2.46) and summary estimate for 19 cohort and nested case-control studies was 1.73 (95% CI 1.59-1.88). In 14 of the case-control studies the risk of pancreatic cancer was higher in diabetes patients than in the controls and reached significant level in ten. The combined estimate from all studies was 1.82 (95% CI 1.66-1.99). Results from the cohort studies and the nested case-control studies were remarkably consistent with 15 studies reporting relative risks that were significantly elevated.[51] Similar results were also reported some years ago in another meta-analysis of 11 case-control and 9 cohort studies.[52] The analysis included cases of diabetes diagnosed at least one year prior to the diagnosis or death from pancreatic cancer. The pooled relative risk of pancreatic cancer for the diabetic patients was 2.1 (95% CI 1.6-2.8). The risk was somewhat higher in the cohort studies (RR 2.6, 95% CI 1.6-4.1) than in the case-control studies (OR 1.8, 95% CI 1.1-2.7).[52]

Respiratory Organs

Lung Cancer

Overall, lung cancer is the most frequent type of cancer.[21] Nearly 1.5 million people worldwide get lung cancer every year and about 1.2 millions die of the disease annually. The age-adjusted incidence and mortality rate are about 3 times higher among men than among women (among men 35.5 and 31.2 per 100,000, respectively, among women 12.1 and 10.3 per 100,000, respectively). The age-adjusted incidence and mortality rate are about twice as high in the more developed parts of the world as in the less developed parts.[21]

Obesity

Whether there is an association between BMI and risk of lung cancer is controversial. Several studies have found an inverse association.[1,53] However, as smoking is the primary cause of lung cancer and there is an inverse association between BMI and smoking, an association between BMI and lung cancer may be confounded by smoking habits. Indeed, in nonsmoking populations no association between BMI and lung cancer risk is observed.[17] Also, an increased risk of lung cancer among subjects with a low BMI may be explained by weight loss due to preclinical lung cancer.

Diabetes

Some studies have investigated the hypothesis that the rate of lung cancer is different in diabetic compared with nondiabetic patients but the results are not conclusive. A weak nonsignificant increased risk of lung cancer was seen in female diabetic patients, after adjusting for smoking.[54] Other studies have not found an association between diabetes and risk of lung cancer.[24,27,55,56] However, these studies did not adjust for smoking, the major risk factor for lung cancer and are therefore difficult to interpret. No increased risk of lung cancer in diabetic patients was found in a large UK retrospective study, after adjusting for smoking.[57] In diabetes type I patients a significant increased risk of lung cancer has been observed.[29] A recent study investigated the possible protective effect of diabetes against metastasis in patients with nonsmall cell lung cancer.[58] In fact, they found that stage and diabetes were significant predictors of metastasis.

Skin Melanoma

Nearly 80,000 subjects get malignant melanoma every year.[21] The age-adjusted incidence rate is far higher in the more developed parts of the world than in the less developed parts (8.3 and 0.7 per 100,000, respectively). Particularly, high age-adjusted rates are found in Australia (38.5 per 100,000) and in New Zealand (33.8 per 100,000).[21]

Obesity

Negative, positive and null findings have been reported regarding the association between BMI and malignant melanoma.[1,53,59] It has been suggested that BMI may influence sunbathing habits and hormonal factors, both potentially important for development of malignant melanoma.[1] Overall, no firm conclusion on the association can be drawn.

Diabetes

Little is known about an association between cancer of the skin and diabetes mellitus. Results from one cohort study reported that patients who used insulin therapy to treat type II diabetes had a significantly lower risk of developing nonmelanoma tumor of the skin than patients who used non-insulin anti-diabetics medicines.[60] The protective effect of insulin use became more distinct with increasing age. A study among diabetic patients observed an SIR of 1.0 for melanoma of the skin in both gender and 1.0 and 0.9 for nonmelanoma neoplasms of the skin in men and women, respectively.[24]

Breast Cancer

Breast cancer is by far the most common cancer among women.[21] More than 1.1 million women worldwide are diagnosed with breast cancer every year and more than 400,000 women die from the disease annually. The age-adjusted incidence rate for breast cancer is 67.8 per 100,000 in developed regions of the world and 23.8 per 100,000 in less developed regions.[21]

Obesity

More than 100 epidemiological studies have been conducted to examine the relationship between breast cancer and various measures of obesity. There is convincing evidence that the effect of excess body weight on breast cancer risk varies with menopausal status; the association is negative among premenopausal women and positive among postmenopausal women.

Breast Cancer Risk in Premenopausal Women

The inverse association between BMI and breast cancer risk among premenopausal is modest. Overall, it has been suggested that the risk reduction may be of magnitude 0.6 to 0.7 for women having a BMI of 28 kg/m^2.[1] Two recent prospective studies have shown less impact of excess body weight: in a large study of US nurses obese premenopausal women had a relative risk of breast cancer of 0.81 (95% CI 0.68-0.96) compared to lean women.[61] The risk estimate was more or less the same irrespective of various adjustments for reproductive and lifestyle factors. In a French study overweight premenopausal women had a relative risk of breast cancer of 0.84 (95% CI 0.56-1.27) compared to leaner women.[62]

The mechanism linking BMI to premenopausal breast cancer is not fully known. It has been suggested that excess body weight may be associated with longer or irregular menstrual cycles and polycystic ovary syndrome, increasing the likelihood of anovulation and subsequent decreased levels of estradiol and progesterone. However, this mechanism is still debated.[61]

In contrast to premenopausal breast cancer incidence premenopausal breast cancer mortality does not tend to be higher in lean women than in obese women.[1] That is, obesity worsens the prognosis once breast cancer is established.[63]

Breast Cancer Risk in Postmenopausal Women

After going through the menopause obesity increases both the risk of experiencing breast cancer and the risk of dying from the disease.[1,63] It has been estimated that obese postmenopausal women have a 50% higher risk of breast cancer than lean postmenopausal women.[17,64] When analyzing individual data from eight prospective studies of postmenopausal women performed in developed countries the researchers found a clear significant trend for increasing risk of breast cancer with increasing BMI; compared to women with a BMI of less than 22.5 kg/m^2 the relative risk of breast cancer was 1.10 (95% CI 0.83-1.46) for women with a BMI of 22.5-24.9 kg/m^2, 1.45 (95% CI 1.08-1.95) for women with a BMI of 25.0-27.4 kg/m^2, 1.62 (95% CI 1.17-2.24) for women with a BMI of 27.5-29.9 kg/m^2 and 1.36 (95% CI 1.00-1.85) for women with a BMI of 30.0 or above (p trend = 0.004).[65] It has been estimated that more than one in five postmenopausal breast cancer cases in the US and one in six cases in the European Union can be attributed to overweight and obesity.[17]

The effect of overweight and obesity on postmenopausal breast cancer risk is often found to be strongest among women who have not taken hormone replacement therapy.[65,66] For instance, in an US prospective study no anthropometrical measures were associated with postmenopausal breast cancer among women who had ever used hormone replacement therapy, whereas among non-users both weight, BMI at baseline, changes in BMI since age 18, and maximum BMI were positively associated to breast cancer risk (relative risk for women who were obese at baseline compared to women who were lean at baseline was 2.52, 95% CI 1.62-3.93).[67] The effect of excess body weight on postmenopausal breast cancer risk may also be modified by age.[67,68]

The biological mechanism behind the association between BMI and postmenopausal breast cancer risk is not clearly understood. One suggestion is that overweight and obese women to a greater extent than leaner women convert androgens to estrogens resulting in higher levels of circulating estrogens which in turn may increase the risk of developing breast cancer.[64]

Diabetes

Diabetes mellitus' relationship with breast cancer remains unclear. However, because insulin is a growth factor, it is hypothesized that the chronic hyperinsulinemia seen in individuals with insulin resistance may have cancer-inducing effects on insulin-sensitive tissues such as the breast. High levels of insulin have been shown to be mitogenic for breast tissue,[69] and insulin receptors are frequently over-expressed in breast cancer cells.[70,71] Associations between breast cancer and serum insulin,[72] as well as its metabolic product, C-peptide,[73] have been documented. Insulin resistance may also promote breast cancer via other mechanisms, such as greater estrogen availability due to decreased levels of sex-hormone-binding globulin,[74] or increased circulating levels of insulin-like growth factor 1.[75]

A recent meta-analysis based on results from 5 case-control studies and 15 cohort studies indicated that diabetes mellitus (largely type II) is associated with increased risk of breast cancer.[76] Analysis of all 20 studies showed that women with diabetes had a statistically significant 20% increased risk of breast cancer compared to women without a diabetes diagnosis (RR 1.20, 95% CI 1.12-1.28). The summary estimates for the case-control studies were RR 1.18 (95% CI 1.05-1.32) and cohort studies RR 1.20 (95% CI 1.11-1.30).[76] Wolf and coworkers combined the results of 4 case-control studies and 6 cohort studies and found that diabetes was associated with a 13% and 25% increased risk of breast cancer in case-control and cohort studies, respectively.[77] Results from a recent case-control study support the hypothesis that diabetes may have a role in the development of breast cancer, influencing risk via both sex hormone and insulin pathways.[78] A history of diabetes was associated with breast cancer risk (OR 1.68, 95% CI 1.15-2.47) after adjusting for reproductive and other confounding factors. The researchers found a stronger diabetes-breast cancer association in women with lower BMI (≤22.7 kg/m^2) than in those with higher BMI (>22.7 kg/m^2).[78]

Female Genital Organs

Endometrial Cancer

Nearly 200,000 new cases of endometrial cancer are registered every year, making it the 7th most common cancer site among women worldwide.[21] The age-adjusted incidence rate is more than 4 times higher in the more developed regions of the world than in the less developed regions (13.6 and 3.0 per 100,000, respectively) and is particularly high in the US (22.5 per 100,000).[21]

Obesity

An expert panel concluded in 2001 that there is convincing evidence that obesity increases the risk of endometrial cancer both among pre and postmenopausal women and that the increase in risk is of magnitude 2-3 folds.[1] Others have presented an increased risk of 3- to 10-folds for obese women compared to leaner ones.[79] Further, it has been estimated that 39-45% of all endometrial cancer in the European Union (corresponding to at least 14,000 new cases per year) can be attributed to overweight.[17,18] In the US more than half of all endometrial cancer cases may be attributed to overweight and obesity.[17]

The strong association can be exemplified by a recent prospective US study: obese women had a relative risk of breast cancer of 3.03 (95% CI 2.50-3.68) compared to "normal" weight women.[80] Adult weight gain also increased the risk. Similarly as for breast cancer, hormone replacement therapy may modify the relation between body weight and endometrial cancer risk: that is, a stronger association was revealed for never-users than for former and current users.[80]

The association between obesity and increased risk of endometrial cancer is thought to go through changes in the hormonal milieu that in sum result in an increased effect of unopposed estrogen and thereby increase the risk of cancer in hormonally responsive tissues.[79]

Diabetes

The association between diabetes and endometrial cancer and the possible underlying mechanisms has been widely discussed in the literature. Endometrial cancer is a hormone-related malignancy and diabetes mellitus may cause hormonal alterations that promote the development of the disease. A statistically significant 80% excess incidence of endometrial cancer among patients hospitalized with diabetes mellitus was observed in a large Swedish cohort study (SIR 1.8, 95% CI 1.6-2.0).[36] Similar results were reported in another study from Sweden (RR 1.5, 95% CI 1.2-1.8).[55] Obesity has been reported as increasing the risk of both diabetes and endometrial cancer. In the study by Weiderpass and coworkers[36] the risk estimates for endometrial cancer did not change substantially when excluding patients with a discharge diagnosis of obesity from the analysis, pointing on diabetes as the strongest risk factor. Furthermore, it has been suggested that history of obesity and diabetes may increase the mortality after having an endometrial cancer diagnosis.[81] Results from a population-based case-control study in Sweden showed that recent overweight/obesity and diabetes mellitus (type I and II) are associated with increased endometrial cancer risk.[82] Significant increased risk of endometrial cancer has also been seen in type I diabetes patients specifically.[29] Diabetes has further been found to be one of several risk factors related to endometrial cancer in women younger than 50 years of age.[83]

Ovarian Cancer

Some 205,000 women get ovarian cancer every year and about 125,000 die from the disease annually. The age-adjusted incidence and mortality rate is about twice as high in the more developed parts of the world as in the less developed parts (age-adjusted incidence rate 10.2 and 5.0 per 100,000, respectively).[21]

Obesity

The association between BMI and risk of ovarian cancer has been examined in a relatively limited number of studies and the studies have shown conflicting results.[1,79] In a recent review and meta-analysis it is concluded that obesity is a risk factor for ovarian cancer and it is estimated that obese women have a 30% higher risk (95% CI 10%-50%) of epithelial ovarian cancer than women with a BMI within the "normal" range.[84] It is hypothesized that any association between obesity and ovarian cancer risk may be mediated through adipose tissue's influence on the synthesis and bioavailability of endogenous estrogens, androgens and progesterone.[84] As for other hormone-related cancers menopausal status may modify the impact of obesity on ovarian cancer risk.

Diabetes

Few studies have been performed to investigate a possible association between ovarian cancer and diabetes mellitus. A review of cohort studies on the association between history of diabetes mellitus and occurrence of cancer reported that no cohort studies showed any significantly positive or negative association between diabetes and ovarian cancer.[85] Further, two more recent cohort studies found no association.[28,86] However, one study has found a significant increased risk of ovarian cancer in patients with diabetes type I diagnosed before 30 years old, with greatest risk for those with diabetes diagnosed at ages 10-19 years.[47]

Cervical Cancer

About half a million women worldwide get cervical cancer annually and some 275,000 die of it. More than 400,000 of the new cases and 85% of all deaths occur in the less developed parts of the world.[21]

Obesity

Studies examining risk of cervical cancer in relation to BMI have been inconclusive; both positive association and no associations have been reported.[17,79] It has been suggested that squamous cell carcinoma of the cervix is not associated with BMI, whereas there may be a modest increase of cervical adenocarcinoma with increasing BMI.[79] However, obese women may attend cervical screening more seldom than leaner women and this may confound the findings.[17]

Diabetes

Only a limited number of papers have reported on risk of cervical cancer in relation to diabetes mellitus. Significant increased risk of cervical cancer has been observed in type I diabetes patients specifically.[29] In a population-based cohort study of patients hospitalized with diabetes mellitus the SIR for cervical cancer was 0.9.[24] The incidence rate ratio of cervical cancer was 0.99 in a study among Japanese diabetes patients.[27]

Male Genital Organs

Prostate Cancer

Prostate cancer is the second most common cancer among men; about 680,000 new cases are reported every year. The age-adjusted incidence rate in the more developed parts of the world is 55.6 per 100,000 compared to 9.4 per 100,000 in the less developed parts.[21]

Obesity

The association between BMI and risk of prostate cancer has been examined in a number of studies. In general, body weight does not seem to be strongly associated with prostate cancer. A meta-analysis based on 4 cohort studies and 2 population-based case-control studies gave an 6% increased risk of prostate cancer for overweight men compared to men within the "normal" weight range and a 12% increased risk for obese men.[18] Based on this finding it was further estimated that 4% of the prostate cancer cases in the European Union could be attributed to excess body weight (i.e., about 5000 new cases per year).

It has recently been hypothesized that the nonconclusive findings may, at least in part, be explained by a differential effect of obesity on aggressive and non-aggressive prostate cancer. That is, a negative association between non-aggressive prostate cancer and obesity and a positive association between aggressive prostate cancer and obesity are described.[87] Findings from a recent prospective study support this hypothesis: obese men had a relative risk of non-aggressive prostate cancer of 0.69 (95% CI 0.52-0.93) compared to "normal" weight men, whereas the relative risk of aggressive disease was 1.10 (95% CI 0.83-1.60).[88]

The mechanisms linking obesity to prostate cancer risk are not settled.[89] Androgens have long been thought to increase the risk of prostate, but final confirmation is lacking.[88]

Diabetes

An inverse relationship between diabetes mellitus and prostate cancer has been reported in two large meta-analyses[90,91] and several cohort studies.[92-94] The inverse association is hypothesized to be a result of alterations in sex hormone levels in diabetic patients. In the meta-analysis of Kasper,[91] including 14 studies, diabetic patients showed a statistically significant decrease in the risk of developing carcinoma of the prostate, RR = 0.84 (95 % CI 0.76-0.93). The results were consistent in both cohort and case-control studies.

Testicular Cancer

Worldwide some 49,000 men are diagnosed with testicular cancer every year. The age-adjusted incidence rate is several folds higher in the more developed parts of the world than in the less developed parts (4.5 and 0.8 per 100,000, respectively) and is particularly high in Norway (10.6 per 100,000) and Denmark (10.3 per 100,000).[21]

Obesity

Some studies have reported on an inverse association between BMI and risk of testicular cancer, whereas others have found no relation.[1] The low number of studies and the inconsistent findings makes it impossible to draw any firm conclusions.

Diabetes

Diabetes as a risk factor for testis cancer is investigated in a limited number of studies. Some results indicate no association between diabetes diagnosis overall and testis cancer[24] or between diabetes type I and testis cancer.[47]

Urinary Organs

Kidney Cancer

Some 180,000 new cases of kidney cancer among men and some 80,000 new cases among women arise worldwide every year.[21] Annual mortality numbers are about 100,000. The age-adjusted incidence and mortality is 5 times higher in the more developed regions of the world than in the less developed parts.

Obesity

A high BMI is an established risk factor for kidney cancer.[95] Whereas no association has been seen between BMI and cancer of renal pelvis, there seems to be a does-response relationship between BMI and risk of renal-cell cancer, the main type of adult kidney neoplasms.[1] The association is seen for both sexes. Overall, obese subjects have a more than 2-fold increase in renal-cell cancer risk compared to subjects with a BMI below 25 kg/m^2. In a meta-analysis based on 7 studies from affluent populations it was estimated that the risk of kidney cancer increased by 6% (95% CI 5%-8%) per unit increase in BMI.[18] Compared to a having a "normal" weight this corresponds to a relative risk of 1.36 for overweight subjects and to a relative risk of 1.84 for obese subjects. Further it is estimated that 25-30% of all kidney cancer in the European Union and more than 40% of all kidney cancer in the US can be attributed to excess body weight.[17,18]

The estimates from the meta-analysis referred to above have been confirmed in a large Norwegian prospective study.[96] More than 6450 renal-cell carcinomas were registered among 2 million subjects for whom height and weight had been measured in a standardized manner. In this study, the relative risk of kidney cancer increased by 5% (95% CI 4%-6%) per unit increase in BMI.

Hypertension is an established risk factor for renal-cell cancer. Obesity increases the risk of hypertension, but the increased risk of renal-cell cancer associated with obesity seems to be mediated through a different mechanism.[17] Hormonal changes like increased levels of peptides, steroid hormones and insulin-like growth factor 1 may be involved.[17,97]

Diabetes

A limited number of studies have focused on diabetes mellitus as a risk factor for kidney cancer. However, one considerably large cohort study reported a significantly increased risk of kidney cancer in both male and female diabetes patients.[98] The SIRs were 1.7 (95% CI 1.4-2.0) and 1.3 (95% CI 1.1-1.6) for women and men, respectively.[98] Diabetes mellitus increased the risk of kidney cancer deaths in the Japanese population.[99] Other studies have not confirmed an association.[43]

Bladder Cancer

Worldwide, more than 350,000 subjects are diagnosed with bladder cancer each year. The age-adjusted incidence rate is about 5 times higher for men than for women (10.1 and 2.5 per 100,000, respectively) and is 3-4 times higher in the more developed parts of the world than in the less developed parts.[21]

Obesity

Data from studies on overweight and obesity and subsequent risk of bladder cancer are inconsistent. Generally, there do not seem to be a strong relation. The findings from a recent study among US adults may serve as a typical example: compared to subjects with a BMI of 18.0-22.9 kg/m^2 subjects with a BMI of 30.0 or above had a incidence rate ratio of 1.16 (95% CI 0.89-1.52).[100]

Diabetes

Diabetes mellitus is suspected as a risk factor for urinary bladder cancer. A meta-analysis based on 16 studies concluded that there is a modestly increased risk in diabetes type II patients.[101] In a case-control study among 252 patients with urinary bladder cancer a significant positive association was seen.[102]

Thyroid Cancer

Thyroid cancer is a rather rare disease. It affects strikingly more women than men, 104,000 and 38,000 new cases emerges per year, respectively.[21]

Obesity

A modest increase in thyroid cancer risk with increasing BMI has been suggested based on findings from case-control studies.[1] In a pooled analysis of 12 case-control studies an odds ratio of 1.2 (95% CI 1.0-1.4) was found for women with the high BMI compared to women with low BMI.[103] No association was seen for men. No association was seen in an US cohort study consisting of both sexes.[104]

Diabetes

A possible association between diabetes and thyroid cancer is unclear. A nonsignificant increased risk for thyroid cancer of 30% in men and 20% in women has been reported.[24] A population-based cohort study showed a 20% increased risk of thyroid cancer in diabetes I patients (95% CI 0.6-2.2).[29]

Lymphoid and Haematopoietic Cancers

Worldwide about 690,000 new cases of nonHodgkin's lymphoma, multiple myeloma and leukemia occur every year.[21] Generally, the age-adjusted incidence rates are higher among men than among women and higher in the more developed parts of the world than in the less developed parts.

Obesity

A modest increase in risk of these cancers with increasing BMI has been seen, with relative risk estimates in the range 1.2-2.0.[17,105] A recent review on nonHodgkin's lymphoma concludes that excess body weight probably has a role in the development of the disease.[105] Further, a meta-analysis including 13 cohort studies and nine case-control studies estimated an average relative risk of nonHodgkin's lymphoma of 1.07 (95% CI 1.01-1.14) for overweight subjects and 1.20 (95% CI 1.07-1.34) for obese subjects compared to subjects with a "normal" weight.[106] It is suggested that a high BMI may affect various histological subtypes differently and that it particularly increases the risk of diffuse large B-cell lymphoma.

Diabetes

A limited number of studies have reported on the association between diabetes mellitus and risk of lymphoid and haematopoietic cancers. A cohort study from Japan reported a significant increased risk of nonHodgkins lymphoma among men and nonsignificant increase in women.[27] No association was found for nonHodgkins lymphoma and leukaemia in another study.[47] A borderline significant increased risk of all lymphatic and haematopoietic cancer was found in Danish male and female diabetes patients.[24] The same study reported a nonsignificant 10% increased risk of lymphoma and leukemia specifically, in both genders.

Summary of Findings

The findings on obesity, diabetes and risk of cancer presented in this section are summarized in Table 2.

Concluding Remarks and Recommendations for Further Research

Even though there is a substantial body of literature on the association between obesity and cancer for some cancer sites in humans, such as colon, postmenopausal breast cancer, endometrial cancer, kidney cancer (renal-cell) and oesophagus cancer (adenocarcinoma), further studies on

Table 2. Summary of findings relating obesity and diabetes to risk of various cancers

		Diabetes Mellitus	
Cancer Site	**Obesity**	**Type I**	**Type II**
Oesophagus			
- adenocarcinoma	↑*	..	..
- squamous cell carcinoma	-	..	..
Stomach			
- cardia	↑	..	..
- noncardia	..	..	..
Colorectum	↑*	(↑)	(↑)
Liver	..	(↑)	(↑)
Gallbladder	(↑)	..	..
Pancreas	(↑)	(↑)	↑
Lung	..	..	..
Melanoma of the skin	..	..	..
Breast			
- premenopausal	↓	..	..
- postmenopausal	↑*	..	..
Endometrium	↑*	(↑)	(↑)
Ovary	..	..	..
Cervix	..	..	
Prostate	-	(↓)	(↓)
Testis	..	..	..
Kidney (renal-cell)	↑*	..	..
Bladder	..	(↑)	(↑)
Thyroid gland	..	..	..
Lymphoid and haematopoietic tissue	(↑)	..	..

↑: sufficient data to state an increased risk
-: sufficient data to state no impact on risk
(↑): some data to state an increased risk
(↓): some data to state a decreased risk
..: inconclusive or lack of data
*: sufficient evidence for a cancer-preventive effect of avoidance of weight gain as regarded by the IARC expert panel in 2001.[1]

virtually all other cancer sites in humans are needed. Studies on the association between type I diabetes mellitus and cancer are scarce for all cancer sites and further studies are warranted. Type II diabetes mellitus has been more studied than type I diabetes mellitus in regard to cancer risk, but still our comprehension of its impact is very limited. There is some evidence that persons with type II diabetes mellitus are at an increased risk of liver and pancreas cancer and probably also for bladder, colorectal, endometrial and postmenopausal breast cancer. Further studies are needed for confirming these associations, as well as to clarify possible underlying mechanisms of carcinogenicity.

Overweight, obesity and diabetes mellitus type II are now pandemic in many areas of the world and global trends indicate no evidence of decline in their prevalence. A substantial proportion of cancer cases can be attributable to overweight and obesity. As also stated by the IARC expert panel in 2001[1] other specific topics of research to be further developed include:

- Creation of standardized, validated methods to measure body composition and evaluate the need for ethnic, gender and age-specific body mass index and waist cut points.
- Maintenance and enhancement of systems for monitoring trends in body composition in various populations.
- Development of methods to study environmental factors (physical, economic and socio-cultural) that determine behavioral patterns that lead to obesity and diabetes mellitus type II in populations undergoing various stages of economic development.
- Performance of studies on the relationship between different indicators of body composition and fat distribution and cancer risk.
- Performance of clinical intervention such as dietary modification studies in subgroups of age, sex and ethnicity to alter behavior patterns which may influence weight gain and type II diabetes mellitus.
- Establishment of the effectiveness of various community intervention studies to prevent weight gain and type II diabetes mellitus.
- Performance of studies in humans to establish the mechanisms by which weight gain and diabetes mellitus (type I and type II) are/may be related to cancer development.

Overweight, obesity and type II diabetes mellitus cannot be prevented or managed solely at the level of the individual. Governments, the food industry, the media, communities and individuals all need to work together to modify the environment so that it is less conductive to weight gain/obesity and consequently diabetes mellitus type II development. Most current guidelines indicate a desirable BMI range of 18.5 to 25 kg/m^2, based primarily on the relationships of body weight to the risk of cardiovascular diseases, diabetes and total mortality. The benefits of maintaining weight in this range clearly extend to reduced risks of important cancers. Most individuals will experience lower risks of cardiovascular diseases, diabetes and cancer if they maintain their body weight in the lower part of this range.

Acknowledgements

The authors wish to thank Margrethe Sitek Meo for her secretarial support, especially for compiling the data for Figure 1 and for drawing the figure.

References

1. International Agency for Research on Cancer, World Health Organization. Weight control and physical activity. Vainio H, Bianchini F, editors. 2002. Lyon, IARCPress. IARC Handbooks of Cancer Prevention.
2. Adeghate E, Schattner P, Dunn E. An update on the etiology and epidemiology of diabetes mellitus. Ann NY Acad Sci 2006; 1084:1-29.
3. Trevisan R, Vedovato M, Tiengo A. The epidemiology of diabetes mellitus. Nephrol Dial Transplant 1998; 13 Suppl 8:2-5.
4. World Health Organization. Health topics. 2007; 7-5-2007. Available on: http://www.who.int/topics/obesity/en.
5. WHO Expert Consultation. Appropriate body-mass index for Asian populations and its implications for policy and intervention strategies. Lancet 2004; 363(9403):157-163.

6. World Health Organization. 22-4-2007. WHO Global InfoBase Online 2007. Available on: http://www.who.int/infobase/report.aspx.
7. Ogden CL, Carroll MD, Curtin LR et al. Prevalence of overweight and obesity in the United States, 1999-2004. JAMA 2006; 295(13):1549-1555.
8. World Health Organization. Diabetes Programme. WHO Country and Regional Data 2007. Available on: http://www.who.int/diabetes/facts/world_figures/en.
9. International Diabetes Federation. Diabetes atlas. International Diabetes Federation-Diabetes Atlas. 2007. Available on: http://www.eatlas.idf.org/.
10. Mlinar B, Marc J, Janez A et al. Molecular mechanisms of insulin resistance and associated diseases. Clin Chim Acta 2007; 375(1-2):20-35.
11. World Health Organization, FAO Expert Consultation. Diet, nutrition and the prevention of chronic diseases. 2003. WHO Technical Report Series.
12. Czyzyk A, Szczepanik Z. Diabetes mellitus and cancer. Eur J Intern Med 2000; 11(5):245-252.
13. Hu FB, Manson JE, Liu S et al. Prospective study of adult onset diabetes mellitus (type 2) and risk of colorectal cancer in women. J Natl Cancer Inst 1999; 91(6):542-547.
14. Shoff SM, Newcomb PA. Diabetes, body size and risk of endometrial cancer. Am J Epidemiol 1998; 148(3):234-240.
15. Silverman DT, Schiffman M, Everhart J et al. Diabetes mellitus, other medical conditions and familial history of cancer as risk factors for pancreatic cancer. Br J Cancer 1999; 80(11):1830-1837.
16. Larsson SC, Orsini N, Wolk A. Body mass index and pancreatic cancer risk: A meta-analysis of prospective studies. Int J Cancer 2007; 120(9):1993-1998.
17. Calle EE, Kaaks R. Overweight, obesity and cancer: epidemiological evidence and proposed mechanisms. Nat Rev Cancer 2004; 4(8):579-591.
18. Bergstrom A, Pisani P, Tenet V et al. Overweight as an avoidable cause of cancer in Europe. Int J Cancer 2001; 91(3):421-430.
19. Calle EE, Rodriguez C, Walker-Thurmond K et al. Overweight, obesity and mortality from cancer in a prospectively studied cohort of US adults. N Engl J Med 2003; 348(17):1625-1638.
20. Strickler HD, Wylie-Rosett J, Rohan T et al. The relation of type 2 diabetes and cancer. Diabetes Technol Ther 2001; 3(2):263-274.
21. International Agency for Research on Cancer. Globocan 2002; Cancer Epidemiology Database. Intenational Agency for Research on Cancer 2002.
22. Kubo A, Corley DA. Body mass index and adenocarcinomas of the esophagus or gastric cardia: a systematic review and meta-analysis. Cancer Epidemiol Biomarkers Prev 2006; 15(5):872-878.
23. Rubenstein JH, Davis J, Marrero JA et al. Relationship between diabetes mellitus and adenocarcinoma of the oesophagus and gastric cardia. Aliment Pharmacol Ther 2005; 22(3):267-271.
24. Wideroff L, Gridley G, Mellemkjaer L et al. Cancer incidence in a population-based cohort of patients hospitalized with diabetes mellitus in Denmark. J Natl Cancer Inst 1997; 89(18):1360-1365.
25. Lindblad M, Rodriguez LA, Lagergren J. Body mass, tobacco and alcohol and risk of esophageal, gastric cardia and gastric noncardia adenocarcinoma among men and women in a nested case-control study. Cancer Causes Control 2005; 16(3):285-294.
26. MacInnis RJ, English DR, Hopper JL et al. Body size and composition and the risk of gastric and oesophageal adenocarcinoma. Int J Cancer 2006; 118(10):2628-2631.
27. Khan M, Mori M, Fujino Y et al. Site-specific cancer risk due to diabetes mellitus history: evidence from the Japan Collaborative Cohort (JACC) Study. Asian Pac J Cancer Prev 2006; 7(2):253-259.
28. Inoue M, Iwasaki M, Otani T et al. Diabetes mellitus and the risk of cancer: results from a large-scale population-based cohort study in Japan. Arch Intern Med 2006; 166(17):1871-1877.
29. Zendehdel K, Nyren O, Ostenson CG et al. Cancer incidence in patients with type 1 diabetes mellitus: a population-based cohort study in Sweden. J Natl Cancer Inst 2003; 95(23):1797-1800.
30. Rennert G. Prevention and early detection of colorectal cancer--new horizons. Recent Results Cancer Res 2007; 174:179-187.
31. Gunter MJ, Leitzmann MF. Obesity and colorectal cancer: epidemiology, mechanisms and candidate genes. J Nutr Biochem 2006; 17(3):145-156.
32. Sturmer T, Buring JE, Lee IM et al. Metabolic abnormalities and risk for colorectal cancer in the physicians' health study. Cancer Epidemiol Biomarkers Prev 2006; 15(12):2391-2397.
33. Ahmed RL, Schmitz KH, Anderson KE et al. The metabolic syndrome and risk of incident colorectal cancer. Cancer 2006; 107(1):28-36.
34. Bianchini F, Kaaks R, Vainio H. Overweight, obesity and cancer risk. Lancet Oncol 2002; 3(9):565-574.
35. Larsson SC, Orsini N, Wolk A. Diabetes mellitus and risk of colorectal cancer: a meta-analysis. J Natl Cancer Inst 2005; 97(22):1679-1687.

36. Weiderpass E, Gridley G, Persson I et al. Risk of endometrial and breast cancer in patients with diabetes mellitus. Int J Cancer 1997; 71(3):360-363.
37. Will JC, Galuska DA, Vinicor F et al. Colorectal cancer: another complication of diabetes mellitus? Am J Epidemiol 1998; 147(9):816-825.
38. Limburg PJ, Vierkant RA, Fredericksen ZS et al. Clinically confirmed type 2 diabetes mellitus and colorectal cancer risk: a population-based, retrospective cohort study. Am J Gastroenterol 2006; 101(8):1872-1879.
39. Qian Y, Fan JG. Obesity, fatty liver and liver cancer. Hepatobiliary Pancreat Dis Int 2005; 4(2):173-177.
40. El Serag HB, Hampel H, Javadi F. The association between diabetes and hepatocellular carcinoma: a systematic review of epidemiologic evidence. Clin Gastroenterol Hepatol 2006; 4(3):369-380.
41. Adami HO, Chow WH, Nyren O et al. Excess risk of primary liver cancer in patients with diabetes mellitus. J Natl Cancer Inst 1996; 88(20):1472-1477.
42. Davila JA, Morgan RO, Shaib Y et al. Diabetes increases the risk of hepatocellular carcinoma in the United States: a population based case control study. Gut 2005; 54(4):533-539.
43. La Vecchia C, Negri E, Franceschi S et al. A case-control study of diabetes mellitus and cancer risk. Br J Cancer 1994; 70(5):950-953.
44. Lai MS, Hsieh MS, Chiu YH et al. Type 2 diabetes and hepatocellular carcinoma: A cohort study in high prevalence area of hepatitis virus infection. Hepatology 2006; 43(6):1295-1302.
45. Randi G, Franceschi S, La Vecchia C. Gallbladder cancer worldwide: geographical distribution and risk factors. Int J Cancer 2006; 118(7):1591-1602.
46. Larsson SC, Wolk A. Obesity and the risk of gallbladder cancer: a meta-analysis. Br J Cancer 2007; 96(9):1457-1461.
47. Swerdlow AJ, Laing SP, Qiao Z et al. Cancer incidence and mortality in patients with insulin-treated diabetes: a UK cohort study. Br J Cancer 2005; 92(11):2070-2075.
48. Michaud DS. Epidemiology of pancreatic cancer. Minerva Chir 2004; 59(2):99-111.
49. Berrington dG, Sweetland S, Spencer E. A meta-analysis of obesity and the risk of pancreatic cancer. Br J Cancer 2003; 89(3):519-523.
50. Chari ST, Leibson CL, Rabe KG et al. Probability of pancreatic cancer following diabetes: a population-based study. Gastroenterology 2005; 129(2):504-511.
51. Huxley R, Ansary-Moghaddam A, Berrington de Gonzalez A et al. Type-II diabetes and pancreatic cancer: a meta-analysis of 36 studies. Br J Cancer 2005; 92(11):2076-2083.
52. Everhart J, Wright D. Diabetes mellitus as a risk factor for pancreatic cancer. A meta-analysis. JAMA 1995; 273(20):1605-1609.
53. Samanic C, Chow WH, Gridley G et al. Relation of body mass index to cancer risk in 362,552 Swedish men. Cancer Causes Control 2006; 17(7):901-909.
54. Steenland K, Nowlin S, Palu S. Cancer incidence in the National Health and Nutrition Survey I. Follow-up data: diabetes, cholesterol, pulse and physical activity. Cancer Epidemiol Biomarkers Prev 1995; 4(8):807-811.
55. Adami HO, McLaughlin J, Ekbom A et al. Cancer risk in patients with diabetes mellitus. Cancer Causes Control 1991; 2(5):307-314.
56. Ragozzino M, Melton LJ III, Chu CP et al. Subsequent cancer risk in the incidence cohort of Rochester, Minnesota, residents with diabetes mellitus. J Chronic Dis 1982; 35(1):13-19.
57. Hall GC, Roberts CM, Boulis M et al. Diabetes and the risk of lung cancer. Diabetes Care 2005; 28(3):590-594.
58. Hanbali A, Al Khasawneh K, Cole-Johnson C et al. Protective effect of diabetes against metastasis in patients with nonsmall cell lung cancer. Arch Intern Med 2007; 167(5):513.
59. Gallus S, Naldi L, Martin L et al. Anthropometric measures and risk of cutaneous malignant melanoma: a case-control study from Italy. Melanoma Res 2006; 16(1):83-87.
60. Chuang TY, Lewis DA, Spandau DF. Decreased incidence of nonmelanoma skin cancer in patients with type 2 diabetes mellitus using insulin: a pilot study. Br J Dermatol 2005; 153(3):552-557.
61. Michels KB, Terry KL, Willett WC. Longitudinal study on the role of body size in premenopausal breast cancer. Arch Intern Med 2006; 166(21):2395-2402.
62. Tehard B, Clavel-Chapelon F. Several anthropometric measurements and breast cancer risk: results of the E3N cohort study. Int J Obes (Lond) 2006; 30(1):156-163.
63. Carmichael AR. Obesity and prognosis of breast cancer. Obes Rev 2006; 7(4):333-340.
64. Key TJ, Verkasalo PK, Banks E. Epidemiology of breast cancer. Lancet Oncol 2001; 2(3):133-140.
65. Key TJ, Appleby PN, Reeves GK et al. Body mass index, serum sex hormones and breast cancer risk in postmenopausal women. J Natl Cancer Inst 2003; 95(16):1218-1226.
66. Stephenson GD, Rose DP. Breast cancer and obesity: an update. Nutr Cancer 2003; 45(1):1-16.

67. Morimoto LM, White E, Chen Z et al. Obesity, body size and risk of postmenopausal breast cancer: the Women's Health Initiative (United States). Cancer Causes Control 2002; 13(8):741-751.

68. La Vecchia C, Negri E, Franceschi S et al. Body mass index and post-menopausal breast cancer: an age-specific analysis. Br J Cancer 1997; 75(3):441-444.

69. van der BB, Rutteman GR, Blankenstein MA et al. Mitogenic stimulation of human breast cancer cells in a growth factor-defined medium: synergistic action of insulin and estrogen. J Cell Physiol 1988; 134(1):101-108.

70. Mathieu MC, Clark GM, Allred DC et al. Insulin receptor expression and clinical outcome in node-negative breast cancer. Proc Assoc Am Physicians 1997; 109(6):565-571.

71. Papa V, Belfiore A. Insulin receptors in breast cancer: biological and clinical role. J Endocrinol Invest 1996; 19(5):324-333.

72. Goodwin PJ, Ennis M, Pritchard KI et al. Fasting insulin and outcome in early-stage breast cancer: results of a prospective cohort study. J Clin Oncol 2002; 20(1):42-51.

73. Yang G, Lu G, Jin F et al. Population-based, case-control study of blood C-peptide level and breast cancer risk. Cancer Epidemiol Biomarkers Prev 2001; 10(11):1207-1211.

74. Nyholm H, Djursing H, Hagen C et al. Androgens and estrogens in postmenopausal insulin-treated diabetic women. J Clin Endocrinol Metab 1989; 69(5):946-949.

75. Lawlor DA, Smith GD, Ebrahim S. Hyperinsulinaemia and increased risk of breast cancer: findings from the British Women's Heart and Health Study. Cancer Causes Control 2004; 15(3):267-275.

76. Larsson SC, Mantzoros CS, Wolk A. Diabetes mellitus and risk of breast cancer: A meta-analysis. Int J Cancer 2007; 121(4):856-862.

77. Wolf I, Sadetzki S, Catane R et al. Diabetes mellitus and breast cancer. Lancet Oncol 2005; 6(2):103-111.

78. Wu AH, Yu MC, Tseng CC et al. Diabetes and risk of breast cancer in Asian-American women. Carcinogenesis 2007; 28(7):1561-1566.

79. Modesitt SC, van NJ, Jr. The impact of obesity on the incidence and treatment of gynecologic cancers: a review. Obstet Gynecol Surv 2005; 60(10):683-692.

80. Chang SC, Lacey JV, Jr, Brinton LA et al. Lifetime weight history and endometrial cancer risk by type of menopausal hormone use in the NIH-AARP diet and health study. Cancer Epidemiol Biomarkers Prev 2007; 16(4):723-730.

81. Chia VM, Newcomb PA, Trentham-Dietz A et al. Obesity, diabetes and other factors in relation to survival after endometrial cancer diagnosis. Int J Gynecol Cancer 2007; 17(2):441-446.

82. Weiderpass E, Persson I, Adami HO et al. Body size in different periods of life, diabetes mellitus, hypertension and risk of postmenopausal endometrial cancer (Sweden). Cancer Causes Control 2000; 11(2):185-192.

83. Iatrakis G, Zervoudis S, Saviolakis A et al. Women younger than 50 years with endometrial cancer. Eur J Gynaecol Oncol 2006; 27(4):399-400.

84. Olsen CM, Green AC, Whiteman DC et al. Obesity and the risk of epithelial ovarian cancer: a systematic review and meta-analysis. Eur J Cancer 2007; 43(4):690-709.

85. Mori M, Saitoh S, Takagi S et al. A Review of Cohort Studies on the Association Between History of Diabetes Mellitus and Occurrence of Cancer. Asian Pac J Cancer Prev 2000; 1(4):269-276.

86. Weiderpass E, Ye W, Vainio H et al. Diabetes mellitus and ovarian cancer (Sweden). Cancer Causes Control 2002; 13(8):759-764.

87. Freedland SJ, Giovannucci E, Platz EA. Are findings from studies of obesity and prostate cancer really in conflict? Cancer Causes Control 2006; 17(1):5-9.

88. Littman AJ, White E, Kristal AR. Anthropometrics and Prostate Cancer Risk. Am J Epidemiol 2007; 165(11): 1271-1279.

89. Moyad MA. Is obesity a risk factor for prostate cancer and does it even matter? A hypothesis and different perspective. Urology 2002; 59(4A Suppl):41-50.

90. Bonovas S, Filioussi K, Tsantes A. Diabetes mellitus and risk of prostate cancer: a meta-analysis. Diabetologia 2004; 47(6):1071-1078.

91. Kasper JS, Giovannucci E. A meta-analysis of diabetes mellitus and the risk of prostate cancer. Cancer Epidemiol Biomarkers Prev 2006; 15(11):2056-2062.

92. Calton BA, Chang SC, Wright ME et al. History of diabetes mellitus and subsequent prostate cancer risk in the NIH-AARP Diet and Health Study. Cancer Causes Control 2007; 18(5):493-503.

93. Gonzalez-Perez A, Garcia Rodriguez LA. Prostate cancer risk among men with diabetes mellitus (Spain). Cancer Causes Control 2005; 16(9):1055-1058.

94. Weiderpass E, Ye W, Vainio H et al. Reduced risk of prostate cancer among patients with diabetes mellitus. Int J Cancer 2002; 102(3):258-261.

95. Moore LE, Wilson RT, Campleman SL. Lifestyle factors, exposures, genetic susceptibility and renal cell cancer risk: a review. Cancer Invest 2005; 23(3):240-255.

96. Bjorge T, Tretli S, Engeland A. Relation of height and body mass index to renal cell carcinoma in two million Norwegian men and women. Am J Epidemiol 2004; 160(12):1168-1176.

97. Lipworth L, Tarone RE, McLaughlin JK. The epidemiology of renal cell carcinoma. J Urol 2006; 176(6 Pt 1):2353-2358.

98. Lindblad P, Chow WH, Chan J et al. The role of diabetes mellitus in the aetiology of renal cell cancer. Diabetologia 1999; 42(1):107-112.

99. Washio M, Mori M, Khan M et al. Diabetes mellitus and kidney cancer risk: The results of Japan Collaborative Cohort Study for Evaluation of Cancer Risk (JACC Study). Int J Urol 2007; 14(5):393-397.

100. Holick CN, Giovannucci EL, Stampfer MJ et al. Prospective study of body mass index, height, physical activity and incidence of bladder cancer in US men and women. Int J Cancer 2007; 120(1):140-146.

101. Larsson SC, Orsini N, Brismar K et al. Diabetes mellitus and risk of bladder cancer: a meta-analysis. Diabetologia 2006; 49(12):2819-2823.

102. Kravchick S, Gal R, Cytron S et al. Increased incidence of diabetes mellitus in the patients with transitional cell carcinoma of urinary bladder. Pathol Oncol Res 2001; 7(1):56-59.

103. Dal Maso L, La Vecchia C, Franceschi S et al. A pooled analysis of thyroid cancer studies. V. Anthropometric factors. Cancer Causes Control 2000; 11(2):137-144.

104. Iribarren C, Haselkorn T, Tekawa IS et al. Cohort study of thyroid cancer in a San Francisco Bay area population. Int J Cancer 2001; 93(5):745-750.

105. Skibola CF. Obesity, diet and risk of nonHodgkin lymphoma. Cancer Epidemiol Biomarkers Prev 2007; 16(3):392-395.

106. Larsson SC, Wolk A. Obesity and risk of nonHodgkin's lymphoma: A meta-analysis. Int J Cancer 2007; 121(7):1564-1570.

107. US Census Bureau; population census. IDB data access-display mode. Available on: http://www.census.gov/ipc/www/idbprint.html

CHAPTER 7

Progesterone Receptor Action:
Translating Studies in Breast Cancer Models to Clinical Insights

Carol A. Lange,* Carol A. Sartorius, Hany Abdel-Hafiz,
Monique A. Spillman, Kathryn B. Horwitz and Britta M. Jacobsen

Abstract

P rogesterone receptors (PR) are useful prognostic indicators of breast cancers likely to respond to anti-estrogen receptor (ER) therapies. However, the role of progesterone, therapeutic progestins, or unliganded or liganded PR in breast cancer development or progression remains controversial. PR are ligand-activated transcription factors that act in concert with intracellular signaling pathways as "sensors" of multiple growth factor inputs to hormonally regulated tissues, such as the breast. The recently defined induction of rapid signaling events upon progestin-binding to PR-B provides a means to ensure that receptors and coregulators are appropriately phosphorylated as part of optimal transcription complexes. PR-activated kinase cascades may provide additional avenues for progestin-regulated gene expression independent of PR nuclear action. Herein, we present an overview of progesterone/PR and signaling cross-talk in breast cancer models and discuss the potential significance of progestin/PR action in breast cancer biology using examples from both in vitro and in vivo models, as well as limited clinical data. Kinases are emerging as key mediators of PR action. Cross-talk between PR and membrane-initiated signaling events suggests a mechanism for coordinated regulation of gene subsets by mitogenic stimuli in hormonally responsive normal tissues. Dysregulation of this cross-talk mechanism may contribute to breast cancer biology; further studies are needed to address the potential for targeting PR in addition to ER and selected protein kinases as part of more effective breast cancer therapies.

Introduction

Normal breast development requires estrogen receptor (ERα), progesterone receptor (PR) and peptide growth factors. Estrogen stimulates ductal elongation and progestins induce ductal sidebranching and alveologenesis.[1] Epidermal growth factor (EGF), in addition to promoting the proliferation of terminal end-buds, augments estrogen-induced ductal outgrowth and progesterone-induced sidebranching.[2] Indeed, estrogen induces PR isoform expression only in the presence of EGF,[3] suggesting the existence of important cross-talk between EGFRs and both steroid receptors (SRs). Ligand-activated PRs and ERs are potent mitogens in the developing breast and mammary epithelial cells express PR as well as ERα. Moreover, estrogen is usually required to induce the expression of PR. PR and ER are normally expressed by only ~7-10% of nondividing epithelial cells in the lumen of the mature mammary gland. This nonproliferative condition

*Corresponding Author: Carol A. Lange—Departments of Medicine (Division of Hematology, Oncology and Transplant) and Pharmacology, University of Minnesota Cancer Center, 420 Delaware Street SE, MMC 806, Minneapolis, Minnesota 55455 USA.
Email: Lange047@umn.edu

Innovative Endocrinology of Cancer, edited by Lev M. Berstein and Richard J. Santen.
©2008 Landes Bioscience and Springer Science+Business Media.

appears to be sustained by such inhibitory molecules as TGF-beta or high levels of p27, a CDK inhibitor (reviewed in G.W. Robinson et al [4]). In response to communication between stromal and epithelial compartments, SR-positive epithelial cells express and secrete pro-proliferative molecules, such as Wnts or IGF-II, thereby inducing the proliferation of adjacent SR-negative epithelial cells.[4,5] Recent data indicate that SR-positive cells in the breast may support the activity of nearby stem-like progenitor cells via the expression of secreted factors.[6]

In contrast to the normal breast, where proliferating cells are devoid of SRs, the majority of newly diagnosed breast cancers (~70-80%) express ER and PR. The existence of SR-positive proliferating cells in breast cancer indicates that SR-positive cells may undergo an early switch to autocrine stimulation and/or continue to divide. Breast cancer is not the only setting where PR-containing cells divide. In an in vivo model of the mammary gland during pregnancy, the PR-B isoform colocalizes with cyclin D1 in BrdU-stained (dividing) cells.[7] Thus, signaling pathways involved in normal mammary gland growth and development are likely reactivated during breast cancer progression.

Progestins are recognized as mediators of increased post-menopausal breast cancer risk when taken as part of combined hormone replacement therapy relative to estrogen alone or placebo.[8] Experimental animal models of the effects of hormones on the postmenopausal mammary gland indicate that progestins stimulate proliferation.[9,10] While progestins are not carcinogens, progesterone might induce recently initiated precancerous breast cell populations to inappropriately reenter the cell cycle or stimulate dormant stem cells to undergo self-renewal (discussed below). Breast tumors develop resistance to endocrine-based treatments (anti-estrogens and/or aromatase inhibitors) as they progress. However, the majority (65%) of resistant breast cancers retain high levels of SRs (ERα and PRs). In these resistant, SR-positive cancers, the rapid action of SRs at the membrane might begin to inappropriately trigger the classical transcriptional activities of SRs. In this way, PRs activated by extremely low or sub-threshold concentrations of hormone or PRs phosphorylated in the absence of hormone can activate membrane-associated signaling pathways, including c-Src kinase, EGFR and the p42/p44 MAPK pathway. Elevation of MAPK activity and downstream signaling frequently occurs in breast cancer, providing a strong survival and proliferative stimulus to breast cancer cells. MAPK signaling downstream of EGFR or Her2 (erbB2) is also associated with resistance to endocrine therapies.[11]

This chapter focuses specifically on the role of progesterone and progesterone receptors (PR) in the pathophysiology of breast cancer. We review the literature describing PR-initiated genomic and nongenomic signaling pathways in breast cancer progression with the purpose of highlighting key kinases involved in the integration of rapid cytoplasmic signaling events and PR nuclear actions. We also discuss the clinical findings relevant to the use of PR status in the prediction of breast cancer behavior, evidence for PR action in breast cancer and the potential for PR ligands as therapeutic agents.

Classical Actions of PRs

PRs are activated through binding with the ovarian steroid ligand, progesterone. PRs are classically defined as ligand-activated transcription factors that regulate gene expression by binding directly or indirectly to DNA. Three PR isoforms are the product of a single gene located on chromosome 11 at q22-23 that undergoes transcription via the use of alternate promoters and internal translational start sites.[12] PR isoforms consist of the full length PR-B (116 kDa), N-terminally-truncated PR-A (94 kDa) and PR-C-isoforms (60 kDa). PR-positive cells usually co-express PR-A and PR-B isoforms; these receptors have different transcriptional activities within the same promoter context, but can also recognize entirely different promoters.[13,14] PR-B is required for normal mammary gland development,[15] while PR-A is essential for uterine development and reproductive function.[16] PR-C is devoid of classical transcriptional activity and instead functions as a dominant inhibitor of uterine PR-B in the fundal myometrium during labor.[17] In the absence of progesterone, PRs are complexed with several chaperone molecules including heat shock protein (hsp) 90, hsp70, hsp40, Hop and p23; these interactions are requisite for proper protein folding and assembly of stable PR-hsp90 heterocomplexes that are competent to bind ligand.[18] Hsps also function to connect PRs to protein trafficking systems. After binding to progesterone, the receptors undergo restructuring, dimerization and hsp dissociation. Activated receptors bind directly to specific progesterone response elements (PREs) and PRE-like sequences in the promoter regions of such target genes as *c-myc*,[19] *fatty acid synthetase*,[20] and *MMTV*.[21] Treatment with progestin also results in an upregulation of regulatory molecules without classical PREs in their proximal promoter regions, such as EGFR[22,23], *c-fos*[24,25] and *cyclin D1*.[26,27] PR regulation of genes without canonical PREs can occur through indirect DNA-binding mechanisms, as in the example of PR binding to Specificity protein 1 to promote p21 transcription in the presence of progestin.[28] PRs can also regulate genes by tethering to activating protein 1[29] or signal transducers and activators of transcription (STATs).[25,30]

When either directly or indirectly bound to DNA, PRs regulate the basal transcription machinery in conjunction with nuclear receptor coregulatory molecules. Coregulators modulate transcription through chromatin remodeling and recruitment of transcriptional machinery (e.g., RNA Polymerase-II). Histone acetyl transferases (HATs) and histone deacetylases (HDACs) function as coactivators and corepressors, respectively. Both HATs and HDACs coordinate transcriptional activity with other regulator proteins, including the ATP-dependent chromatin remodeling complexes (SWI/SNF), arginine methyltransferases (CARM1 and PRMT1) and histone kinases (reviewed in N.J. McKenna, B.W. O'Malley[31]).

Direct PR Phosphorylation in Breast Cancer Models

Similar to other SR family members, phosphorylation-dephosphorylation events add multi-functionality to PR action (Fig. 1). Several protein kinases phosphorylate PR isoforms primarily on serine residues within the amino-termini and, to a lesser degree, on serine residues throughout the receptor.[12,32] PR contains a total of 14 known phosphorylation sites (reviewed in C.A. Lange[33]). Serines at positions 81, 162, 190 and 400 appear to be constitutively phosphorylated in the absence of hormone[34] (Fig. 1). One to two hours after progestin treatment, serines at positions 102, 294 and 345 are maximally phosphorylated.[35] Specific kinases have been identified that are responsible for phosphorylation of selected sites. Serines at positions 81 and 294 are phosphorylated by casein kinase II[36] and mitogen-activated protein kinase (MAPK),[37,38] respectively. Progestins can also stimulate Ser294 phosphorylation independently of MAPKs by activation of an unknown kinase(s).[39] Eight of the total 14 sites (i.e., serines 25, 162, 190, 213, 400, 554, 676 and Thr430) are phosphorylated by cyclin A/cyclin-dependent protein kinase 2 (CDK2) complexes in vitro.[34,40] Only five of these sites (i.e., serines 162, 190, 213, 400, 676) are proven in vivo phosphorylation sites.[34,36,40]

While the function of PR phosphorylation is incompletely understood, it might influence aspects of transcriptional regulation, such as interaction with coregulators, as reported for ER-α[41] and recently for PR.[42] PR phosphorylation is also involved in the regulation of ligand-dependent[38] and -independent[43,44] PR nuclear localization, receptor turnover, hormone sensitivity and transcriptional activities.[37,38,45,46] As has been reported for ERα,[47,48] phosphorylated PRs are hypersensitive relative to their underphosphorylated counterparts.[49] For example, following a brief (5-15 min) pretreatment with EGF, phosphorylated nuclear PR-B receptors are transactivated by sub-physiologic progestin levels. EGF and progestins synergistically upregulate mRNA or protein levels for a number of growth regulatory genes,[25] including cyclin D1 and cyclin E;[22] the regulation of cyclins by progestins is MAPK-dependent. Cyclins, in turn, regulate progression of cells through the cell cycle by interaction with cyclin-dependent protein kinases. Progestins activate CDK2,[27] which predominantly phosphorylates PRs at proline-directed (S/TP) sites,[34,40] perhaps allowing for the coordinate regulation of PR transcriptional activity during cell cycle progression. In support of this idea, Narayanan and coworkers[42,50] report that PR activity is highest in the S phase and lower in the G0/G1 phases of the cell cycle, but this activity is impaired during the G2/M phases, concomitant with lowered PR phosphorylation. Overexpression of Cyclin A or CDK2 enhanced PR transcriptional activity. While cyclin A interacts with the N-terminus of PR, CDK2 seems to

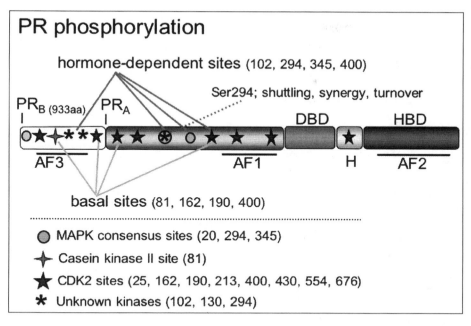

Figure 1. Phosphorylation sites in human PR. PR phosphorylation. Thirteen serine residues and one threonine residue in human PR are shown, to represent basal (constitutive) and hormone-induced phosphorylation sites[40] and may contribute to PR regulation by MAPK,[37-39] casein kinase II,[36] and CDK2.[34,40] Individual PR phosphorylation sites may be regulated by multiple protein kinases[39] and/or in a sequential manner,[143] illustrating the complexity of PR regulation by phosphorylation.

alter PR function indirectly by increasing the phosphorylation and recruitment of steroid receptor coactivator-1 (SRC-1) to liganded PR.

PR Ser294 Phosphorylation in Breast Cancer Models

PR Ser294 is rapidly phosphorylated upon exposure to ligand.[35] Ser294 is also a proline-directed or MAPK consensus site (PXXSP). Progestin-induced Ser294 phosphorylation occurs within 30-60 min independently of MAPK activation, whereas growth factor-induced Ser294 phosphorylation occurs within 3-5 mins in a MAPK-dependent manner.[39] PR Ser294 is considered a significant site for PR regulation by multiple kinases.[37-39,49] Ser294 phosphorylation appears to mediate increased PR nucleo-cytoplasmic shuttling.[39] Rapid nuclear translocation of unliganded PR and nuclear export of liganded PR requires MAPK-dependent phosphorylation of PR Ser294.[39] PR nuclear sequestration in response to MAPK activation might serve to protect inactive or active receptors from degradation in the cytoplasm or upon nuclear export.[39] Following ligand binding, PR undergoes rapid downregulation.[51] Phosphorylation of Ser294 greatly augments PR downregulation by making liganded PR a cytoplasmic target for ubiquitination and degradation by the 26S-proteosome pathway.[37,39] In several recent reports, it has been shown that reversible phosphorylation of PR Ser294 couples increased transcriptional activity to rapid down-regulation of the PR protein by the ubiquitin-proteosome pathway.[37-39,49,52] Further investigation is required to determine whether the link between these events involves regulation of transcriptional events by components of the ubiquitin pathway and/or participation of nucleo-cytoplasmic shuttling factors or chaperones.

In the absence of progestins, however, EGF-induced nuclear accumulation of PR is required for transcriptional activation. Labriola et al[43] report that exposure of T47D breast cancer cells to the EGF family member, heregulin, can stimulate PR nuclear localization, DNA binding and transcriptional activity in the absence of hormone. Heregulin exposure also resulted in activation of MAPK and PR Ser294 phosphorylation. Qiu et al[39] report that PR Ser294 phosphorylation results in similar nuclear activity. However, growth factors alone failed to stimulate PR transcriptional activity or alter PR downregulation in T47D cell variants.[38] However, in the presence of ligand, MAPK activation greatly augmented both of these events.[38,39] One explanation for these apparently conflicting results is that differential expression of EGFR family members expressed on the cell surface between T47D cell line clones might lead to differences in the activation of downstream intracellular kinases, such as CDK2.[44] Indeed, regulation of PR by alternate signaling pathways may contribute to dysregulated gene expression and changes in cell growth and/or survival. For example, PR-B regulation of IRS-2 expression in breast cancer cells requires phosphorylation of PR Ser294 and occurs in the absence of ligand.[49] In any case, these exciting data[39,43] suggest a continuum between PR hypersensitivity to extremely low ligand concentrations and complete ligand-independence, a phenomenon that is well-documented for androgen receptor (AR) and ERα.

Extranuclear Actions of PR

While the genomic effects of steroid hormone treatment are delayed by several minutes to hours (i.e., following transcription and translation), the extranuclear or nongenomic effects occur rapidly in only a few minutes. Progestin treatment of breast cancer cells causes a rapid and transient activation of MAPK signaling that is ER-dependent, but independent of PR transcriptional activity.[53,54] Migliaccio et al were the first to report that estradiol activates p60-Src kinase and MAPK in MCF-7 cells[55] and that PR and ERα interact to stimulate p60-Src kinase in T47D cells.[53] Maximal activation of p60-Src kinase is observed within 2-5 minutes and downstream activation of p42/p44 MAPKs occurs within 5-10 minutes of progestin treatment.[53,54]

Human PR contains a proline-rich (PXXP) motif that mediates direct binding to the Src-homology three (SH3) domains of signaling molecules in the p60-Src kinase family in a ligand-dependent manner.[54] In vitro experiments demonstrate that purified liganded PR-A and PR-B activate the c-Src-related protein kinase, HcK; PR-B but not PR-A activates c-Src and MAPKs in vivo. PR-B with a mutated PXXP sequence prevents c-Src/PR interaction and blocks progestin-induced activation of c-Src (or HcK) and p42/p44 MAPKs. Furthermore, mutation of the PR-B DNA-binding domain (DBD) abolished PR transcriptional activity without affecting progestin-induced c-Src or MAPK kinase activation. Therefore, nongenomic MAPK activation by progestin/PR-B/c-Src complexes probably occurs by way of a c-Src-dependent mechanism involving Ras activation via phosphorylation of the c-Src substrate adaptor proteins p190 and/or Shc and followed by Grb-2 and Sos binding (Fig. 2).

Ballare et al[56] report that MAPK activation by progestins is blocked by antiprogestins and antiestrogens in COS-7 cells transfected with PR and ERα. They propose that c-Src/MAPK activation by PR is mediated indirectly by the interaction of the Src-homology two (SH2) domain of c-Src with phosphotyrosine 537 of ERα.[56] In their model, activation of c-Src and the MAPK pathway by progestins depends upon the presence of unliganded ERα, which interacts constitutively with PR-B via two domains that flank the proline-rich sequence of PR. Deletion of either of these two ER-interacting domains in PR-B blocked c-Src/MAPK activation by progestins in the presence of ERα.[56] Mutation of PR-B's PXXP domain had no effect. In contrast, Boonyaratanakornkit et al[54] report that ectopic PR expression increased basal c-Src activity in COS-7 cells in the absence of progestins and independently of added ER; co-expression of both PR-B and ERα reduced basal levels of c-Src activity. Under these conditions (i.e., low basal c-Src activity), progestin binding to PR-B clearly activated c-Src. In addition, progestins activated c-Src in PR-null MCF12A cells transduced with wild-type PR but not the PXXP-mutant PR adenoviruses. Both groups found

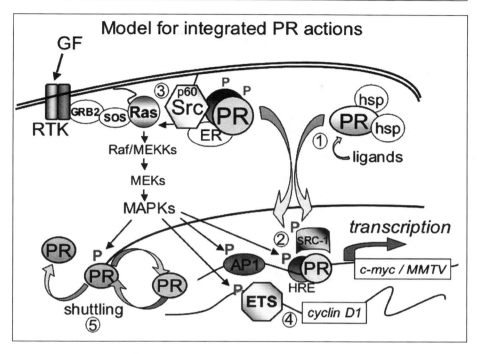

Figure 2. Functional significance of PR phosphorylation. Phosphorylation (P) of specific sites in PRs couple multiple receptor functions, including transcription, nuclear-cytoplasmic shuttling and PR downregulation. 1) Ligand-binding mediates dissociation of heat-shock proteins and nuclear accumulation of PR dimers. 2) Nuclear PRs mediate gene regulation; phosphorylated PRs recruit regulatory molecules that include phospho-proteins and likely function in inter-connected processes (transcription, elongation, localization and turnover). 3) PRs and growth factors activate MAPKs independently via a c-Src kinase-dependent pathway, resulting in positive regulation of PR action via "feed-back" regulation (i.e., direct phosphorylation of liganded PRs or coactivators). 4) Activation of MAPKs by PRs provides for regulation of gene targets whose promoters do not contain PREs and are otherwise independent of PR-transcriptional activities but utilize PR or SR-activated MAPKs. 5) MAPK regulation of PRs mediates nuclear accumulation/shuttling and nuclear export coupled to regulation of PR transcription.

that ERα interacts with the SH2-domain of c-Src, but neither group tested the effects of estrogen on the ability of progesterone to activate c-Src or MAPKs.[54,56]

Although discrepancies between these two models must be resolved, it is possible that overexpression of SRs in COS-7 cells leads to concentration-dependent effects resulting in the formation of different signaling complexes depending on the presence of other signaling and adaptor molecules. In support of this idea, Wong et al[57] identified an additional ER-interacting "adaptor" protein, termed MNAR (modulator of nongenomic activity of estrogen receptor), that contains both LXXLL (nuclear receptor binding) and PXXP (SH3-domain binding) motifs. MNAR is essential for ER-Src interaction, but it is not required for progestin/PR-dependent activation of c-Src (D.P. Edwards, personal communication). Taken together, these data indicate that multiple interactions contribute to direct protein kinase activation by SRs and suggest that at least some nongenomic signaling functions of amphibian PR have been conserved in mammals. Interestingly, a separate gene product encoding the putative mammalian homologue of membrane progesterone receptor (mPR), a progesterone-binding G-protein coupled receptor first identified in spotted sea trout oocytes,[58] has been described. Further studies are needed to determine if mPR plays a role in progestin-induced "rapid" signaling or if mPR interacts with classical PRs. However, studies with mPR underscore the important concept that binding proteins other than classical steroid receptors may regulate some nongenomic steroid-mediated signaling events.

Integration of Rapid Signaling and Nuclear SR Actions

While its role in mammalian physiology remains unclear, SR-mediated activation of cytoplasmic signaling molecules could theoretically serve to potentiate several nuclear functions of activated SRs (Fig. 2). One mechanism by which amplification of SR nuclear functions might occur is through rapid, direct phosphorylation of SRs and/or their coregulators in response to activation of SR-induced cytoplasmic pathways that coincide with ligand binding. Clearly, such a positive feedback loop would explain the dramatic influence of activated signaling pathways on PR nuclear function. For example, several progestin-dependent functions of PR are MAPK-dependent, including upregulation of cyclins D1 and E, CDK2 activation and S-phase entry.[22,38,44,59]

Following ligand-binding, most SRs stimulate a transient (3-10 min) activation of MAPKs. However, mitogenic signaling requires sustained (hrs to days) MAPK activation in fibroblast cell models.[60] Recently, Faivre et al[61] found that in addition to rapid and transient activation of MAPK by progestin/PR-B (5-15 min), progestin-bound PR-B induced subsequent oscillations in MAPK activity that culminated in a sustained (hrs to days) phase of MAPK activation that was EGFR- and c-Src-dependent. Further studies revealed the creation of an autocrine signaling loop, in which PR-B triggered transcriptional upregulation of Wnt-1, leading to activation of frizzled-dependent MMPs and shedding of EGF ligands from the cell surface. This signaling cascade implicates Wnt-1-dependent transactivation of EGFR in response to progestins; PR induced transcriptional upregulation of Wnt-1 and EGFR mRNA was sensitive to inhibition of MAPKs. Additional experiments demonstrated that progestin-induced cyclin D1 upregulation, S-phase entry, or soft-agar growth of T47D breast cancer cells was either blocked by shRNA targeted to Wnt-1 or inhibitors of MAPK, c-Src and EGFR. Finally, progestins failed to stimulate S-phase entry in MCF-7 cells that stably express a PXXP-mutant PR-B, which is unable to bind to the SH3-domain of c-Src and activate MAPK.[59] Soft-agar growth of T47D cells stably expressing the same PR mutant (PXXP) was greatly attenuated.[61] In addition to c-Src and MAPKs, STATs are important effectors downstream of EGFR signaling. Progestins induce tyrosine phosphorylation and nuclear translocation of Stat5[25] and Stat3.[30] Proietti et al[30] demonstrate that Stat3 phosphorylation and activation by the nongenomic actions of PR is a critical event for breast cancer cell growth; T47D cell growth and tumor growth of progestin-induced mammary adenocarcinomas in BALB/c mice was dependent on PR activation of Jak1 and Jak2, c-Src and Stat3. Taken together, these data indicate that progesterone, via robust PR-B/c-Src signaling to MAPK in combination with PR-dependent transcriptional events, upregulates and activates EGFR signaling to induce cell proliferation. Dysregulation of either arm of this pathway may contribute to uncontrolled proliferation of breast cancer cells.

The extranuclear actions of PRs may contribute to deregulated breast cancer cell growth[59] and/or increased breast cancer risk,[8] perhaps by linking steroid hormone action to the regulation of MAPK-regulated genes (i.e., transcription factor targets of MAPK). Similarly, the extranuclear actions of liganded ERα are thought to induce a state of "adaptive hypersensitivity" during endocrine therapy in which growth factor signaling pathways are co-opted by upregulated ERα.[62] In this model of ER-dependent MAPK activation, liganded ERα associated with the cell membrane interacts with the adapter protein Shc and induces its phosphorylation, leading to recruitment of Grb-2 and Sos, followed by activation of Ras and the Raf-1/MEK/MAPK module. ERα activation of MAPK may explain why many tumors respond well to aromatase inhibitors, yet fail to respond to selective estrogen receptor modulators (SERMS) designed to inhibit ER transcriptional activity. SERMs can act as partial transcriptional agonists of phosphorylated receptors and may not block ER-dependent MAPK activation.[62] In theory, PR-B or AR in SR-positive breast cancers could participate in MAPK-activating complexes, perhaps bypassing anti-estrogen therapies. Few groups have studied membrane-associated or cytoplasmic signaling complexes containing both ERα and

PR-B or AR.[63,64] However, AR is frequently (70%) expressed in metastatic breast cancer,[65] and expression of functional AR defines a sub-set of ER/PR-negative breast cancers.[66] These studies suggest that it will be important to target SRs that may substitute for ERα in the activation of c-Src-dependent mitogenic signaling cascades.

PR Action and Breast Cancer Cell Growth, Apoptosis and Aggressiveness in Vitro

Among the most controversial issues regarding the role of progestins in breast cancers is their influence, or lack thereof, on tumor cell proliferation. Complicating the interpretation of the results utilizing in vitro breast cancer models of receptor function is the use, in addition to progesterone, of a myriad of different synthetic progestins with activities unrestricted to PR. For example, while the 19-nor progestins—norgestrel and gestodene—enhance MCF-7 cell proliferation, this effect is inhibitable by antiestrogens but not antiprogestins,[67,68] indicating the lack of involvement of PR signaling. Indeed, cross-reactivity of synthetic progestins at pharmacologic doses with ER has been reported.[69,70] One explanation of these confusing results is that progestin may interact with different PR isoforms to carry out inhibitory or proliferative functions. Sumida et al demonstrate the growth inhibitory effects of progestins with either PR isoform,[71] and McGowan et al show that overexpression of PR-A sensitized breast cancer cells to progestin-mediated growth inhibition.[72] In contrast, Moore et al report prolonged proliferative and survival effects of progestins on breast cancer cells.[73,74]

Flow cytometric studies have also addressed questions of progestin-mediated proliferation by using a single physiological progestin pulse under transiently estrogen deprived conditions. These studies show biphasic effects of progestins in vitro, with cells accelerating through the first mitotic cell cycle then arresting in late G1 of the next cycle.[27,75] Cycle arrest is associated with decreases in cyclins D1, D3 and E, loss of cyclin A and B and induction of the cell cycle inhibitors p21 and p27. Pulsing with progesterone did not restart proliferation; rather it delayed p21 depletion.[27] Similarly, Lin et al[76] report decreased cell proliferation in response to progesterone in conjunction with upregulation of p21, decreased cyclins A, B1 and D1 expression and downregulation of phosphorylated p42/44 MAPK. Thus, these studies suggest that progestins tend to be anti-proliferative in vitro in mono-layer cell cultures.

Equally confusing are conflicting reports of the effects of PR and progestins on apoptosis in vitro. Several studies report pro-apoptotic effects of progestins concomitant with decreases in expression levels of the anti-apoptotic genes bcl-2 and bcl-X_L.[77-80] Antiprogestin/partial agonists, such as RU486, have also been shown to promote apoptosis,[81] but dosage effects confound the interpretation of results.[82] On the other hand, recent studies suggest that unliganded PR[83] and/ or progestin-occupied PR[84] protect cells from damage and apoptosis induced by radiation[84] or chemotherapeutic agents, such as taxanes,[83] doxorubicin or 5-fluorouracil.[85] Moore et al[74] report progestin-induced protection of breast cancer cell death accompanied by upregulation of bcl-X_L, but loss of bcl-2. These contradictory in vitro data prevent a definitive conclusion regarding the apoptotic effects of progestins.

Similarly, the effects of progesterone on invasiveness of breast cancer cells in vitro are poorly understood. Many studies show that progestins increase cell invasiveness[72,83,86] with PR-A exaggerating this phenotype. Sumida et al, however, report that treatment with progestins reduce cell invasiveness.[71]

Notably, studies using human breast cancer cell line models (T47D or MCF-7) grown in soft-agar (i.e., as 3-D colonies) clearly demonstrate a proliferative role for synthetic progestins (R5020) or progesterone in response to PR-dependent transcriptional upregulation of Wnt-1.[87] These results suggest that breast epithelial cells may require a specific architecture (i.e., polarity) for the mitogenic and other "appropriate" gene expression effects of progestins to occur. This architecture is not modeled on plastic surfaces in vitro (i.e., mono-layer cultures). Differences in cell behavior when grown using plastic as mono-layer cultures vs. 3D models have clearly contributed to the controversial area of PR action as a breast cancer cell mitogen. Therefore, we recommend that future investigations into the effects of progestins on tumor cell behavior utilize 3-D models or in vivo models of PR-positive breast cancer.

Expression Profiling in Vitro

Results from expression profiling of breast cancer cells in vitro are consistent with the results from experimental mouse models, which suggest that the two PR isoforms subserve different functions. In mice—where the PR-A to PR-B ratio is 3:1 compared to humans where it is 1:1—ablation of one or the other PR isoform leads to divergent effects on the mammary gland. PR-A knockout (leaving only PR-B) leads to normal early development,[16] while PR-B knockout (leaving only PR-A) leads to reduced pregnancy-associated lobuloalveolar development and reduced side-branching.[15] On the other hand, overexpression of PR-B causes precocious ductal arrest and inappropriate ductal development,[88] while overexpresison of PR-A causes mammary epithelial cell hyperplasia, excessive ductal branching and a disorganized basement membrane.[89] To explain these isoform-specific differences, gene profiling studies have been performed in vitro using human breast cancer cells expressing PR-A or PR-B. The first such study used 6 hrs of progesterone treatment in an attempt to identify direct PR target genes.[14,90] Of 94 genes identified, 65 were regulated only by PR-B, 4 only by PR-A and 25 by both PR isoforms. This regulatory pattern was confirmed in subsequent studies using breast cancer cells with inducible PR-A vs. PR-B treated 6 hrs with progesterone.[83] The latter studies also demonstrate that unliganded PR can regulate transcription; CDK2 mediates ligand-independent activation of PR-B via Ser400 phosphorylation (44).

More recent studies used progesterone-treated breast cancer cells that express both PR isoforms.[91-93] Analysis of the protein pathways indicate that progesterone suppresses genes involved in proliferation and metastasis,[91] supporting an anti-proliferative role for this hormone. However, a remarkable number of the genes upregulated by progestins encode proteins involved in signal transduction and cell adhesion,[83,14] lending some support to the concept that progestins/PR may contribute to the dysregulation of pathways important for breast cancer progression that are perhaps not well modeled in vitro. Additionally, the above studies address gene regulation in response to unliganded or liganded PRs (i.e., single hormone exposure). We propose that PR isoforms act as sensors for signal transduction pathways (discussed above) and thus promoter selectivity is predicted to be highly sensitive to phosphorylation events. Further studies will be needed to address alterations in the signature of PR regulated genes in the context of the high kinase activities characteristic of aggressive breast cancer.

Progestins and Antiprogestins in Breast Tumor Models

Antiprogestins

For a time, therapeutic interest in antiprogestins led to many more studies on these drugs than on the biology of progestins themselves in breast tumors. Several rodent and human tumor models have been used to study the efficacy of antiprogestins for endocrine therapy. These include carcinogen- (DMBA or MNU) induced mammary tumors in the rat, serially transplantable MXT (+) mouse and human T61 mammary tumors and MCF7 human tumor xenografts. Tumors in each of these models are ER+ and PR+. Several different antiprogestins, including mifepristone (RU 38.486; Roussel), the Schering compounds onapristone (ZK 98.299 and ZK 112.993) and the ORG compounds (31710 and 31806) effectively inhibit tumor growth 40 to >90%, depending on the drug, dose and model.[94-103] Antiprogestins were at least as effective as tamoxifen as a single-line therapy. Combination treatment of established tumors in both the rodent and human tumor models with an antiprogestin and an antiestrogen (tamoxifen or ICI164384) had an additive effect on inhibition of tumor growth.[95,100] These studies led to speculation that antiprogestins would be useful for endocrine therapies and fueled the notion that progestins induced proliferation. Indeed, several small clinical studies investigated the potential of mifepristone and onapristone as first- or third-line therapies (reviewed in J.G. Klijn et al[104]). However, because of apparent liver toxicity (onapristone), discrepancies among results and the abortifacient properties of these hormones, the testing of antiprogestins for breast cancer therapy has generally been discontinued.

Only two of the above studies examined progestins alone. Megestrol acetate or MPA had no effect on MXT mouse tumors or slightly inhibited DMBA rat tumor growth.[94,101] This suggests that antiprogestins do not directly antagonize progesterone-mediated tumor growth, even though PR expression was required for inhibition.[102] It is possible that they exert a PR-dependent antiestrogenic effect through ER transrepression[105] or that they suppress effects of unliganded PR.[83]

Progestins

Human tumor models utilize immune-compromised mice as hosts for "xenografted" breast cancer cell lines. Several ER+ and PR+ human breast cancer cell lines (MCF7, ZR-75, T47D) are grown as solid tumors in this manner.[106] Tumors derived from each of these cell lines are estrogen-dependent and require continuous estradiol administration for growth. They have been widely used as models for studying estrogen-suppression based therapies, such as antiestrogens and aromatase inhibitors.[107,108] Only a few studies, however, have assessed effects of progestins in these models. Neither MCF7 nor T47D cells grow in response to progesterone in ovariectomized female mice[109-111] in the absence or presence of estradiol.

In our experience, progesterone or MPA had negligible, nonsignificant growth inhibitory effects in ovariectomized mice bearing T47D xenografts in an estrogenized background.[111] These data suggest that in hormone-dependent models of human breast cancer, progestins are neither mitogenic nor effective at suppressing estrogen-dependent growth. ER^{neg} and PR^{neg} MDA-231 human breast cancer cells form hormone-independent tumors in vivo. If PR was expressed in these cells, progesterone treatment reduced tumor formation.[86]

There is one example of progestin-dependent murine mammary tumor growth. Long-term (10-12 months) chronic treatment of female BALB/c mice with MPA leads to the formation ER+ and PR+ mammary tumors.[112,113] They are maintained by serial transplantation and have a growth requirement for progestins (either progesterone or MPA) rather than estrogens.[114] After serial passage, some tumors acquire progestin independence. Both progestin-dependent and -independent tumors can be inhibited by antiprogestins and antisense oligonucleotides to PR.[115,116] Whereas most clinical human tumors are ER+ and PR+ and respond to antiestrogen therapies, it is possible that some tumors that originate during long-term HRT or in association with pregnancy may have developed in response to progestins. The BALB/c mice would serve as potential models for these rare tumors.

Progesterone Regulation of BRCA1

Carriers of mutations in the breast cancer susceptibility genes BRCA1 and BRCA2 exhibit a 10-fold higher risk of developing tumors in hormonally responsive tissues, such as the breast and ovaries (cumulative risk of 85-90% by age 70) compared to the general population.[117] BRCA1 mutant breast tumors have a poor nuclear grade, high frequency of p53 mutations and are more often ER- and PR-negative compared to sporadic cancers. Because oophorectomy of premenopausal women reduces breast cancer risk substantially (>40%),[118] linkages between steroid hormones and BRCA1 tumor types have been sought since their discovery.[119-121] Fibroblasts from Brca$^{-/-}$ knockout mice that are also p53$^{-/-}$ exhibit ligand-independent activation of ER and PR-dependent transcription;[122] see also Rosen et al.[117] Haploinsufficiency of BRCA1 may be a deleterious state that initiates alterations in steroid hormone receptor expression and tumor mitogenic response.[123] Poole et al[124] report the accumulation of lateral branching and extensive alveologenesis in the mammary glands of nulliparous BRCA1/p53-deficient mice. PR, but not ER, were overexpressed due to a defect in their proteasome-dependent degradation. Notably, treatment of these mice with the PR antagonist mifepristone (RU486) blocked mammary tumorigenesis. These provocative studies suggest that antiprogestin therapy may help prevent the development of breast cancer in individuals with BRCA1 mutations.

General Steroid Receptors and Breast Cancer

A recent study[125] described the steroid receptor assay results of 54,865 patients with stage I–IIIA breast cancers. Their biopsy or mastectomy specimens were sent to two central laboratories that performed identical assays, monitored with tightly controlled quality control procedures. The authors report that ~82% of breast cancers were ER+ and of these ~71% were also PR+. Thus among all breast cancers, ~58% expressed both ER and PR. It is now well established that independent of treatment modalities, women with steroid receptor positive tumors live longer than their receptor negative counterparts. Large studies with long-term follow-up, such as those from San Antonio or the NSABP, indicate a 10% survival advantage for patients with receptor positive disease.[126] Positive hormone receptor status is an independent predictor of outcome and augurs a more favorable prognosis even after controlling for patient age, disease stage, tumor grade, histology, race/ethnicity and US geographical distribution.

Progesterone Receptors and Tamoxifen Responsiveness

The independent role of ER-positivity as a marker of good prognosis and responsiveness to endocrine therapies has been appreciated since the early 1970s. Resistance of a subset of ER+ tumors to endocrine therapies may be due to aberrant estrogen signaling in ER+ tumors that lack PR.[127] Indeed, compared to ER+ and PR− tumors, pretreatment PR-positivity in ER+ tumors is associated with improved outcome prediction as shown by 5 year disease survival rates[128] and by improved response to such adjuvant endocrine therapies as tamoxifen.[128-133] However, not all studies have demonstrated a value for PR, due perhaps to assay variability.[134] The presence of both ER and PR in metastatic disease has also been shown to predict improved response to tamoxifen treatment.[131,135]

Clinical Significance of PR-A vs. PR-B:
Two Subsets of ER+, PR+ Tumors?

We first showed that human breast cancer cells express two forms of PR, the PR-A and PR-B isoforms.[136] Despite having a similar primary amino acid structure over the majority of their length, these receptors regulate entirely different gene subsets.[83,14] The clinical implications of this remain under investigation. Studies using monoclonal antibodies show that PR-A and PR-B colocalize in the same cells in normal endometrium[137] and breast cancers,[138] further adding to the complexity of analyzing expression ratios of the two isoforms by IHC. By immunoblotting, their ratio changes during malignant progression, with approximately equimolar levels of PR-A and PR-B in normal human tissues, but aberrant PR-A:PR-B ratios in breast cancers. An immunoblotting study by Graham et al[139] of 202 PR+ breast cancers showed a median PR-A:PR-B ratio of ~1.3 (close to equimolar), but with outliers ranging between 0.04 (essentially PR-B+) to ~180 (essentially PR-A+) in a significant number of tumors. These authors concluded that when ratios are aberrant, the PR-A isoform tends to be in excess,[140,141] and tumors tend to be less differentiated.[141] We[142] studied the association between PR-A:PR-B ratios and clinical outcome in 297 ER+, axillary node-positive patients, using MAb 1294 for immunoblotting. Eighteen percent of tumors had more than a 2-fold excess of PR-B over PR-A; 10% had more than a 2-fold excess of PR-A over PR-B. We concluded that high PR-A levels were due to loss of PR-B. Our studies also included clinical data showing that tamoxifen-treated patients with high PR-A:PR-B ratios were 2.76 times more likely to relapse. Thus, clinical studies that have addressed the issue of PR isoforms agree that an excess of PR-A is harmful. We suggest that patients with PR-A rich tumors may represent an ER+/PR+ subgroup with intrinsic insensitivity to tamoxifen and perhaps to other selective ER modulators. Growth factor signaling is tightly linked to tamoxifen resistance. Notably, Ser294 phosphorylated PR-B is hypersensitive to low progesterone concentrations and thus degrades very rapidly relative to PR-A, which is hypo-phosphorylated at this site (discussed above); hyperactive but unstable PR-B relative to PR-A may contribute to increased PR-A/PR-B ratios in a subset of breast cancers. In this setting, targeting PR-B and relevant kinases would seem appropriate, but remains untested clinically.

Concluding Remarks

Studies aimed at defining a proliferative role for progestins in breast cancer models remain controversial, but have perhaps been hindered by observations made with liganded receptors in the absence of controlled inhibition or activation of alternate signaling pathways. In the context of multiple signaling inputs, PR clearly coordinates receptor responses to growth factors and steroid hormones. The newly discovered ability of SRs to activate kinase pathways classically defined as key regulators of cell growth underscores the concept that activation of signal transduction pathways is an integral feature of SR action. This aspect of SR function is likely to play an important role in cancer progression and the development of resistance to endocrine therapies.[62] Targeting the relevant protein kinases (c-Src, MAPKs and CDKs) as an integral feature of SR (PR, ER) action should provide significant improvements over the use of traditional SR-blocking strategies for advanced or progressive breast cancers.

Acknowledgements

We thank Michael Franklin for editorial comments and Dean Edwards (Baylor College of Medicine) and Natalie Ahn (University of Colorado, Boulder) for generous gifts of reagents. Studies contributed by Carol Lange's laboratory were supported by NIH grants DK53825/CA123763 and CA116790. These studies were also supported by grants to Britta Jacobsen (Department of Defense 06-1-0503), Carol Sartorius (Susan G. Komen Foundation: BCTR0402682) and grants to Kathryn Horwitz from the NIH (CA26869), the Avon Foundation, the Breast Cancer Research Foundation and the National Foundation for Cancer Research.

References

1. Hovey RC, Trott JF, Vonderhaar BK. Establishing a framework for the functional mammary gland: from endocrinology to morphology. J Mammary Gland Biol Neoplasia 2002; 7(1):17-38.
2. Haslam SZ, Counterman LJ, Nummy KA. Effects of epidermal growth factor, estrogen and progestin on DNA synthesis in mammary cells in vivo are determined by the developmental state of the gland. J Cell Physiol 1993; 155(1):72-78.
3. Ankrapp DP, Bennett JM, Haslam SZ. Role of epidermal growth factor in the acquisition of ovarian steroid hormone responsiveness in the normal mouse mammary gland. J Cell Physiol 1998; 174(2):251-60.
4. Robinson GW, Hennighausen L, Johnson PF. Side-branching in the mammary gland: the progesterone-Wnt connection. Genes Dev 2000; 14(8):889-94.
5. Rosen JM. Hormone receptor patterning plays a critical role in normal lobuloalveolar development and breast cancer progression. Breast Dis 2003; 18:3-9.
6. Li Y, Rosen JM. Stem/progenitor cells in mouse mammary gland development and breast cancer. J Mammary Gland Biol Neoplasia 2005; 10(1):17-24.
7. Aupperlee MD, Smith KT, Kariagina A et al. Progesterone receptor isoforms A and B: temporal and spatial differences in expression during murine mammary gland development. Endocrinology 2005; 146(8):3577-88.
8. Chlebowski RT, Hendrix SL, Langer RD et al. Influence of estrogen plus progestin on breast cancer and mammography in healthy postmenopausal women: the Women's Health Initiative Randomized Trial. JAMA 2003; 289(24):3243-53.
9. Haslam SZ. Experimental mouse model of hormonal therapy effects on the postmenopausal mammary gland. Breast Dis 2005; 24:71-8.
10. Haslam SZ, Osuch JR, Raafat AM et al. Postmenopausal hormone replacement therapy: effects on normal mammary gland in humans and in a mouse postmenopausal model. J Mammary Gland Biol Neoplasia 2002; 7(1):93-105.
11. Schiff R, Massarweh SA, Shou J et al. Advanced concepts in estrogen receptor biology and breast cancer endocrine resistance: implicated role of growth factor signaling and estrogen receptor coregulators. Cancer Chemother Pharmacol 2005; 56 Suppl 1:10-20.
12. Horwitz KB, Sheridan PL, Wei LL et al. Human progesterone receptors: synthesis, structure and phosphorylation. Prog Clin Biol Res 1990; 322(41):41-52.
13. Jacobsen BM, Richer JK, Schittone SA et al. New human breast cancer cells to study progesterone receptor isoform ratio effects and ligand-independent gene regulation. J Biol Chem 2002; 277(31):27793-800.

14. Richer JK, Jacobsen BM, Manning NG et al. Differential gene regulation by the two progesterone receptor isoforms in human breast cancer cells. J Biol Chem 2002; 277(7):5209-18.
15. Mulac-Jericevic B, Lydon JP, DeMayo FJ et al. Defective mammary gland morphogenesis in mice lacking the progesterone receptor B isoform. Proc Natl Acad Sci USA 2003; 100(17):9744-9.
16. Mulac-Jericevic B, Mullinax RA, DeMayo FJ et al. Subgroup of reproductive functions of progesterone mediated by progesterone receptor-B isoform. Science 2000; 289(5485):1751-4.
17. Condon JC, Hardy DB, Kovaric K et al. Up-regulation of the progesterone receptor (PR)-C isoform in laboring myometrium by activation of nuclear factor-kappaB may contribute to the onset of labor through inhibition of PR function. Mol Endocrinol 2006; 20(4):764-75.
18. Pratt WB, Toft DO. Regulation of signaling protein function and trafficking by the hsp90/hsp70-based chaperone machinery. Exp Biol Med (Maywood) 2003; 228(2):111-33.
19. Moore MR, Zhou JL, Blankenship KA et al. A sequence in the 5' flanking region confers progestin responsiveness on the human c-myc gene. J Steroid Biochem Mol Biol 1997; 62(4):243-52.
20. Chalbos D, Chambon M, Ailhaud G et al. Fatty acid synthetase and its mRNA are induced by progestins in breast cancer cells. J Biol Chem 1987; 262(21):9923-6.
21. Krusekopf S, Chauchereau A, Milgrom E et al. Co-operation of progestational steroids with epidermal growth factor in activation of gene expression in mammary tumor cells. J Steroid Biochem Mol Biol 1991; 40(1-3):239-245.
22. Lange CA, Richer JK, Shen T et al. Convergence of progesterone and epidermal growth factor signaling in breast cancer. Potentiation of mitogen-activated protein kinase pathways. J Biol Chem 1998; 273(47):31308-16.
23. Brass AL, Barnard J, Patai BL et al. Androgen up-regulates epidermal growth factor receptor expression and binding affinity in PC3 cell lines expressing the human androgen receptor. Cancer Res 1995; 55(14):3197-203.
24. Church DR, Lee E, Thompson TA et al. Induction of AP-1 activity by androgen activation of the androgen receptor in LNCaP human prostate carcinoma cells. Prostate 2005; 63(2):155-68.
25. Richer JK, Lange CA, Manning NG et al. Convergence of progesterone with growth factor and cytokine signaling in breast cancer. Progesterone receptors regulate signal transducers and activators of transcription expression and activity. J Biol Chem 1998; 273(47):31317-26.
26. Gregory CW, Johnson RT Jr, Presnell SC et al. Androgen receptor regulation of G1 cyclin and cyclin-dependent kinase function in the CWR22 human prostate cancer xenograft. J Androl 2001; 22(4):537-48.
27. Groshong SD, Owen GI, Grimison B et al. Biphasic regulation of breast cancer cell growth by progesterone: role of the cyclin-dependent kinase inhibitors, p21 and p27(Kip1). Mol Endocrinol 1997; 11(11):1593-607.
28. Owen GI, Richer JK, Tung L et al. Progesterone regulates transcription of the p21(WAF1) cyclin-dependent kinase inhibitor gene through Sp1 and CBP/p300 J Biol Chem 1998; 273(17):10696-701.
29. Tseng L, Tang M, Wang Z et al. Progesterone receptor (hPR) upregulates the fibronectin promoter activity in human decidual fibroblasts. DNA Cell Biol 2003; 22(10):633-40.
30. Proietti C, Salatino M, Rosemblit C et al. Progestins induce transcriptional activation of signal transducer and activator of transcription 3 (Stat3) via a Jak- and Src-dependent mechanism in breast cancer cells. Mol Cell Biol 2005; 25(12):4826-40.
31. McKenna NJ, O'Malley BW. Combinatorial control of gene expression by nuclear receptors and coregulators. Cell 2002; 108(4):465-74.
32. Takimoto G, Horwitz K. Progesterone receptor phosphorylation—Complexities in defining a functional role. Trends Endocrinol Metab 1993; 4:1-7.
33. Lange CA. Making sense of cross-talk between steroid hormone receptors and intracellular signaling pathways: who will have the last word? Mol Endocrinol 2004; 18(2):269-78.
34. Zhang Y, Beck CA, Poletti A et al. Phosphorylation of human progesterone receptor by cyclin-dependent kinase 2 on three sites that are authentic basal phosphorylation sites in vivo. Mol Endocrinol 1997; 11(6):823-32.
35. Zhang Y, Beck CA, Poletti A et al. Identification of a group of Ser-Pro motif hormone-inducible phosphorylation sites in the human progesterone receptor. Mol Endocrinol 1995; 9(8):1029-40.
36. Zhang Y, Beck CA, Poletti A et al. Identification of phosphorylation sites unique to the B form of human progesterone receptor. In vitro phosphorylation by casein kinase II. J Biol Chem 1994; 269(49):31034-40.
37. Lange CA, Shen T, Horwitz KB. Phosphorylation of human progesterone receptors at serine-294 by mitogen-activated protein kinase signals their degradation by the 26S proteasome. Proc Natl Acad Sci USA 2000; 97(3):1032-7.

38. Shen T, Horwitz KB, Lange CA. Transcriptional hyperactivity of human progesterone receptors is coupled to their ligand-dependent down-regulation by mitogen-activated protein kinase-dependent phosphorylation of serine 294. Mol Cell Biol 2001; 21(18):6122-31.

39. Qiu M, Olsen A, Faivre E. Mitogen-activated protein kinase regulates nuclear association of human progesterone receptors. Mol Endocrinol 2003; 17(4):628-42.

40. Knotts TA, Orkiszewski RS, Cook RG et al. Identification of a phosphorylation site in the hinge region of the human progesterone receptor and additional amino-terminal phosphorylation sites. J Biol Chem 2001; 276(11):8475-83.

41. Font de Mora J, Brown M. AIB1 is a conduit for kinase-mediated growth factor signaling to the estrogen receptor. Mol Cell Biol 2000; 20(14):5041-7.

42. Narayanan R, Adigun AA, Edwards DP et al. Cyclin-dependent kinase activity is required for progesterone receptor function: novel role for cyclin A/Cdk2 as a progesterone receptor coactivator. Mol Cell Biol 2005; 25(1):264-77.

43. Labriola L, Salatino M, Proietti CJ et al. Heregulin induces transcriptional activation of the progesterone receptor by a mechanism that requires functional ErbB-2 and mitogen-activated protein kinase activation in breast cancer cells. Mol Cell Biol 2003; 23(3):1095-111.

44. Pierson-Mullany LK, Lange CA. Phosphorylation of progesterone receptor serine 400 mediates ligand-independent transcriptional activity in response to activation of cyclin-dependent protein kinase 2. Mol Cell Biol 2004; 24(24):10542-57.

45. Takimoto GS, Hovland AR, Tasset DM et al. Role of phosphorylation on DNA binding and transcriptional functions of human progesterone receptors. J Biol Chem 1996; 271(23):13308-16.

46. Takimoto GS, Tasset DM, Eppert AC et al. Hormone-induced progesterone receptor phosphorylation consists of sequential DNA-independent and DNA-dependent stages: analysis with zinc finger mutants and the progesterone antagonist ZK98299. Proc Natl Acad Sci USA 1992; 89(7):3050-4.

47. Migliaccio A, Di Domenico M, Green S et al. Phosphorylation on tyrosine of in vitro synthesized human estrogen receptor activates its hormone binding. Mol Endocrinol 1989; 3(7):1061-1069.

48. Ali S, Metzger D, Bornert JM et al. Modulation of transcriptional activation by ligand-dependent phosphorylation of the human oestrogen receptor A/B region. EMBO J 1993; 12(3):1150-1160.

49. Qiu M, Lange CA. MAP kinases couple multiple functions of human progesterone receptors: degradation, transcriptional synergy and nuclear association. J Steroid Biochem Mol Biol 2003; 85:147-157.

50. Narayanan R, Edwards DP, Weigel NL. Human progesterone receptor displays cell cycle-dependent changes in transcriptional activity. Mol Cell Biol 2005; 25(8):2885-98.

51. Nardulli AM, Katzenellenbogen BS. Progesterone receptor regulation in T47D human breast cancer cells: analysis by density labeling of progesterone receptor synthesis and degradation and their modulation by progestin. Endocrinology 1988; 122(4):1532-1540.

52. Daniel AR, Qiu M, Faivre EJ et al. Linkage of progestin and epidermal growth factor signaling: phosphorylation of progesterone receptors mediates transcriptional hypersensitivity and increased ligand-independent breast cancer cell growth. Steroids 2007; 72(2):188-201.

53. Migliaccio A, Piccolo D, Castoria G et al. Activation of the Src/p21ras/Erk pathway by progesterone receptor via cross-talk with estrogen receptor. EMBO J 1998; 17(7):2008-18.

54. Boonyaratanakornkit V, Scott MP, Ribon V et al. Progesterone receptor contains a proline-rich motif that directly interacts with SH3 domains and activates c-Src family tyrosine kinases. Mol Cell 2001; 8(2):269-80.

55. Migliaccio A, Di Domenico M, Castoria G et al. Tyrosine kinase/p21ras/MAP-kinase pathway activation by estradiol-receptor complex in MCF-7 cells. EMBO J 1996; 15(6):1292-300.

56. Ballare C, Uhrig M, Bechtold T et al. Two domains of the progesterone receptor interact with the estrogen receptor and are required for progesterone activation of the c-Src/Erk pathway in mammalian cells. Mol Cell Biol 2003; 23(6):1994-2008.

57. Wong C, McNally C, Nickbarg E et al. Estrogen receptor-interacting protein that modulates its nongenomic activity-crosstalk with Src/Erk phosphorylation cascade. Proc Natl Acad Sci USA 2002; 99(23):14783-14788.

58. Zhu Y, Bond J, Thomas P. Identification, classification and partial characterization of genes in humans and other vertebrates homologous to a fish membrane progestin receptor. Proc Natl Acad Sci USA 2003; 100(5):2237-42.

59. Skildum A, Faivre E, Lange CA. Progesterone receptors induce cell cycle progression via activation of mitogen-activated protein kinases. Mol Endocrinol 2005; 19(2):327-39.

60. Murphy LO, Blenis J. MAPK signal specificity: the right place at the right time. Trends Biochem Sci 2006; 31(5):268-75.

61. Faivre E, Lange C. Progesterone receptors upregulate Wnt-1 to induce EGFR transactivation and c-Src-dependent sustained activation of Erk1/2 MAP Kinase in breast cancer cells. Mol Cell Biol 2006; 27(2):466-80.

62. Santen R, Jeng MH, Wang JP et al. Adaptive hypersensitivity to estradiol: potential mechanism for secondary hormonal responses in breast cancer patients. J Steroid Biochem Mol Biol 2001; 79(1-5):115-25.

63. Migliaccio A, Castoria G, Di Domenico M et al. The progesterone receptor/estradiol receptor association and the progestin-triggered S-phase entry. Ernst Schering Res Found Workshop 2005(52):39-54.

64. Migliaccio A, Castoria G, Di Domenico M et al. Steroid-induced androgen receptor-oestradiol receptor beta-Src complex triggers prostate cancer cell proliferation. EMBO J 2000; 19(20):5406-17.

65. Schippinger W, Regitnig P, Dandachi N et al. Evaluation of the prognostic significance of androgen receptor expression in metastatic breast cancer. Virchows Arch 2006; 449(1):24-30.

66. Doane AS, Danso M, Lal P et al. An estrogen receptor-negative breast cancer subset characterized by a hormonally regulated transcriptional program and response to androgen. Oncogene 2006; 29; 25(28):3994-4008.

67. Catherino WH, Jeng MH, Jordan VC. Norgestrel and gestodene stimulate breast cancer cell growth through an oestrogen receptor mediated mechanism. Br J Cancer 1993; 67(5):945-52.

68. Jeng MH, Parker CJ, Jordan VC. Estrogenic potential of progestins in oral contraceptives to stimulate human breast cancer cell proliferation. Cancer Res 1992; 52(23):6539-46.

69. Kalkhoven E, Kwakkenbos-Isbrucker L, de Laat SW et al. Synthetic progestins induce proliferation of breast tumor cell lines via the progesterone or estrogen receptor. Mol Cell Endocrinol 1994; 102(1-2):45-52.

70. van der Burg B, Kalkhoven E, Isbrucker L et al. Effects of progestins on the proliferation of estrogen-dependent human breast cancer cells under growth factor-defined conditions. J Steroid Biochem Mol Biol 1992; 42(5):457-65.

71. Sumida T, Itahana Y, Hamakawa H et al. Reduction of human metastatic breast cancer cell aggressiveness on introduction of either form a or B of the progesterone receptor and then treatment with progestins. Cancer Res 2004; 64(21):7886-92.

72. McGowan EM, Clarke CL. Effect of overexpression of progesterone receptor A on endogenous progestin-sensitive endpoints in breast cancer cells. Mol Endocrinol 1999; 13(10):1657-71.

73. Moore MR, Hagley RD, Hissom JR. Progestin effects on lactate dehydrogenase and growth in the human breast cancer cell line T47D. Prog Clin Biol Res 1988; 262:161-79.

74. Moore MR, Conover JL, Franks KM. Progestin effects on long-term growth, death and Bcl-xL in breast cancer cells. Biochem Biophys Res Commun 2000; 277(3):650-4.

75. Musgrove EA, Lee CS, Sutherland RL. Progestins both stimulate and inhibit breast cancer cell cycle progression while increasing expression of transforming growth factor alpha, epidermal growth factor receptor, c-fos and c-myc genes. Mol Cell Biol 1991; 11(10):5032-43.

76. Lin VC, Woon CT, Aw SE et al. Distinct molecular pathways mediate progesterone-induced growth inhibition and focal adhesion. Endocrinology 2003; 144(12):5650-7.

77. Gompel A, Somai S, Chaouat M et al. Hormonal regulation of apoptosis in breast cells and tissues. Steroids 2000; 65(10-11):593-8.

78. Kandouz M, Lombet A, Perrot JY et al. Proapoptotic effects of antiestrogens, progestins and androgen in breast cancer cells. J Steroid Biochem Mol Biol 1999; 69(1-6):463-71.

79. Franke HR, Vermes I. Differential effects of progestogens on breast cancer cell lines. Maturitas 2003; 46(Suppl 1):S55-8.

80. Formby B, Wiley TS. Progesterone inhibits growth and induces apoptosis in breast cancer cells: inverse effects on Bcl-2 and p53 Ann Clin Lab Sci 1998; 28(6):360-9.

81. Bardon S, Vignon F, Montcourrier P et al. Steroid receptor-mediated cytotoxicity of an antiestrogen and an antiprogestin in breast cancer cells. Cancer Res 1987; 47(5):1441-8.

82. Horwitz KB. The antiprogestin RU38 486: receptor-mediated progestin versus antiprogestin actions screened in estrogen-insensitive T47Dco human breast cancer cells. Endocrinology 1985; 116(6):2236-45.

83. Jacobsen BM, Schittone SA, Richer JK et al. Progesterone-independent effects of human progesterone receptors (PRs) in estrogen receptor-positive breast cancer: PR isoform-specific gene regulation and tumor biology. Mol Endocrinol 2005; 19(3):574-87.

84. Vares G, Ory K, Lectard B et al. Progesterone prevents radiation-induced apoptosis in breast cancer cells. Oncogene 2004; 23(26):4603-13.

85. Moore MR, Spence JB, Kiningham KK et al. Progestin inhibition of cell death in human breast cancer cell lines. J Steroid Biochem Mol Biol 2006; 98(4-5):218-27.

86. Lin VC, Eng AS, Hen NE et al. Effect of progesterone on the invasive properties and tumor growth of progesterone receptor-transfected breast cancer cells MDA-MB-231. Clin Cancer Res 2001; 7(9):2880-6.

87. Faivre EJ, Lange CA. Progesterone receptors upregulate Wnt-1 to induce epidermal growth factor receptor transactivation and c-Src-dependent sustained activation of Erk1/2 mitogen-activated protein kinase in breast cancer cells. Mol Cell Biol 2007; 27(2):466-80.
88. Shyamala G, Yang X, Cardiff RD et al. Impact of progesterone receptor on cell-fate decisions during mammary gland development. Proc Natl Acad Sci USA 2000; 97(7):3044-9.
89. Shyamala G, Yang X, Silberstein G et al. Transgenic mice carrying an imbalance in the native ratio of A to B forms of progesterone receptor exhibit developmental abnormalities in mammary glands. Proc Natl Acad Sci USA 1998; 95(2):696-701.
90. Jacobsen BM, Richer JK, Sartorius CA et al. Expression profiling of human breast cancers and gene regulation by progesterone receptors. J Mammary Gland Biol. Neoplasia 2003; 8(3):257-68.
91. Leo JC, Wang SM, Guo CH et al. Gene regulation profile reveals consistent anticancer properties of progesterone in hormone-independent breast cancer cells transfected with progesterone receptor. Int J Cancer 2005; 117(4):561-8.
92. Ghatge RP, Jacobsen BM, Schittone SA et al. The progestational and androgenic properties of medroxy-progesterone acetate: gene regulatory overlap with dihydrotestosterone in breast cancer cells. Breast Cancer Res 2005; 7(6):R1036-50.
93. Graham JD, Yager ML, Hill HD et al. Altered progesterone receptor isoform expression remodels progestin responsiveness of breast cancer cells. Mol Endocrinol 2005; 19(11):2713-35.
94. Bakker GH, Setyono-Han B, Henkelman MS et al. Comparison of the actions of the antiprogestin mifepristone (RU486), the progestin megestrol acetate, the LHRH analog buserelin and ovariectomy in treatment of rat mammary tumors. Cancer Treat Rep 1987; 71(11):1021-7.
95. Bakker GH, Setyono-Han B, Portengen H et al. Endocrine and antitumor effects of combined treatment with an antiprogestin and antiestrogen or luteinizing hormone-releasing hormone agonist in female rats bearing mammary tumors. Endocrinology 1989; 125(3):1593-8.
96. Bakker GH, Setyono-Han B, Portengen H et al. Treatment of breast cancer with different antiprogestins: preclinical and clinical studies. J Steroid Biochem Mol Biol 1990; 37(6):789-94.
97. El Etreby MF, Liang Y. Effect of antiprogestins and tamoxifen on growth inhibition of MCF-7 human breast cancer cells in nude mice. Breast Cancer Res Treat 1998; 49(2):109-17.
98. Michna H, Schneider MR, Nishino Y et al. Antitumor activity of the antiprogestins ZK 98.299 and RU 38.486 in hormone dependent rat and mouse mammary tumors: mechanistic studies. Breast Cancer Res Treat 1989; 14(3):275-88.
99. Michna H, Schneider MR, Nishino Y et al. The antitumor mechanism of progesterone antagonists is a receptor mediated antiproliferative effect by induction of terminal cell death. J Steroid Biochem 1989; 34(1-6):447-53.
100. Nishino Y, Schneider MR, Michna H. Enhancement of the antitumor efficacy of the antiprogestin, onapristone, by combination with the antiestrogen, ICI 164384. J Cancer Res Clin Oncol 1994; 120(5):298-302.
101. Schneider MR, Michna H, Nishino Y et al. Antitumor activity of the progesterone antagonists ZK 98.299 and RU 38.486 in the hormone-dependent MXT mammary tumor model of the mouse and the DMBA- and the MNU-induced mammary tumor models of the rat. Eur J Cancer Clin Oncol 1989; 25(4):691-701.
102. Schneider MR, Michna H, Habenicht UF et al. The tumour-inhibiting potential of the progesterone antagonist Onapristone in the human mammary carcinoma T61 in nude mice. J Cancer Res Clin Oncol 1992; 118(3):187-9.
103. Schneider MR, Michna H, Nishino Y et al. Tumor-inhibiting potential of ZK 112.993, a new progesterone antagonist, in hormone-sensitive, experimental rodent and human mammary tumors. Anticancer Res 1990; 10(3):683-7.
104. Klijn JG, Setyono-Han B, Foekens JA. Progesterone antagonists and progesterone receptor modulators in the treatment of breast cancer. Steroids 2000; 65(10-11):825-30.
105. Sathya G, Jansen MS, Nagel SC. Identification and characterization of novel estrogen receptor-beta-sparing antiprogestins. Endocrinology 2002; 143(8):3071-82.
106. Clarke R. Human breast cancer cell line xenografts as models of breast cancer. The immunobiologies of recipient mice and the characteristics of several tumorigenic cell lines. Breast Cancer Res Treat 1996; 39(1):69-86.
107. Yue W, Wang J, Savinov A et al. Effect of aromatase inhibitors on growth of mammary tumors in a nude mouse model. Cancer Res 1995; 55(14):3073-7.
108. Osborne CK, Coronado E, Allred DC et al. Acquired tamoxifen resistance: correlation with reduced breast tumor levels of tamoxifen and isomerization of trans-4-hydroxytamoxifen. J Natl Cancer Inst 1991; 83(20):1477-82.
109. Shafie SM, Grantham FH. Role of hormones in the growth and regression of human breast cancer cells (MCF-7) transplanted into athymic nude mice. J Natl Cancer Inst 1981; 67(1):51-6.

110. Osborne CK, Hobbs K, Clark GM. Effect of estrogens and antiestrogens on growth of human breast cancer cells in athymic nude mice. Cancer Res 1985; 45(2):584-90.
111. Sartorius CA, Harvell DM, Shen T et al. Progestins initiate a luminal to myoepithelial switch in estrogen-dependent human breast tumors without altering growth. Cancer Res 2005; 65(21):9779-88.
112. Lanari C, Molinolo AA, Pasqualini CD. Induction of mammary adenocarcinomas by medroxyprogesterone acetate in BALB/c female mice. Cancer Lett 1986; 33(2):215-23.
113. Lanari C, Kordon E, Molinolo A et al. Mammary adenocarcinomas induced by medroxyprogesterone acetate: hormone dependence and EGF receptors of BALB/c in vivo sublines. Int J Cancer 1989; 43(5):845-50.
114. Kordon E, Lanari C, Meiss R et al. Hormone dependence of a mouse mammary tumor line induced in vivo by medroxyprogesterone acetate. Breast Cancer Res Treat 1990; 17(1):33-43.
115. Montecchia MF, Lamb C, Molinolo AA et al. Progesterone receptor involvement in independent tumor growth in MPA-induced murine mammary adenocarcinomas. J Steroid Biochem Mol Biol 1999; 68(1-2):11-21.
116. Lamb CA, Helguero LA, Giulianelli S et al. Antisense oligonucleotides targeting the progesterone receptor inhibit hormone-independent breast cancer growth in mice. Breast Cancer Res 2005; 7(6): R1111-21.
117. Rosen EM, Fan S, Isaacs C. BRCA1 in hormonal carcinogenesis: basic and clinical research. Endocr Relat Cancer 2005; 12(3):533-48.
118. Rebbeck TR, Levin AM, Eisen A et al. Breast cancer risk after bilateral prophylactic oophorectomy in BRCA1 mutation carriers. J Natl Cancer Inst 1999; 91(17):1475-9.
119. Gudas JM, Nguyen H, Li T et al. Hormone-dependent regulation of BRCA1 in human breast cancer cells. Cancer Res 1995; 55(20):4561-5.
120. Marks JR, Huper G, Vaughn JP et al. BRCA1 expression is not directly responsive to estrogen. Oncogene 1997; 14(1):115-21.
121. Spillman MA, Bowcock AM. BRCA1 and BRCA2 mRNA levels are coordinately elevated in human breast cancer cells in response to estrogen. Oncogene 1996; 13(8):1639-45.
122. Zheng WQ, Lu J, Zheng JM et al. Variation of ER status between primary and metastatic breast cancer and relationship to p53 expression*. Steroids 2001; 66(12):905-10.
123. King TA, Gemignani ML, Li W et al. Increased progesterone receptor expression in benign epithelium of BRCA1-related breast cancers. Cancer Res 2004; 64(15):5051-3.
124. Poole AJ, Li Y, Kim Y et al. Prevention of Brca1-mediated mammary tumorigenesis in mice by a progesterone antagonist. Science 2006; 314(5804):1467-70.
125. Arpino G, Weiss H, Lee AV et al. Estrogen receptor-positive, progesterone receptor-negative breast cancer: association with growth factor receptor expression and tamoxifen resistance. J Natl Cancer Inst 2005; 97(17):1254-61.
126. Grann VR, Troxel AB, Zojwalla NJ et al. Hormone receptor status and survival in a population-based cohort of patients with breast carcinoma. Cancer 2005; 103(11):2241-51.
127. Horwitz KB, Costlow ME, McGuire WL. MCF-7; a human breast cancer cell line with estrogen androgen, progesterone and glucocorticoid receptors. Steroids 1975; 26(6):785-95.
128. Bardou VJ, Arpino G, Elledge RM et al. Progesterone receptor status significantly improves outcome prediction over estrogen receptor status alone for adjuvant endocrine therapy in two large breast cancer databases. J Clin Oncol 2003; 21(10):1973-9.
129. Clark GM, McGuire WL, Hubay CA et al. Progesterone receptors as a prognostic factor in Stage II breast cancer. N Engl J Med 1983; 309(22):1343-7.
130. McGuire WL, Clark GM. The prognostic role of progesterone receptors in human breast cancer. Semin Oncol 1983; 10(4 Suppl 4):2-6.
131. Ravdin PM, Green S, Dorr TM et al. Prognostic significance of progesterone receptor levels in estrogen receptor-positive patients with metastatic breast cancer treated with tamoxifen: results of a prospective Southwest Oncology Group study. J Clin Oncol 1992; 10(8):1284-91.
132. Muss HB. Endocrine therapy for advanced breast cancer: a review. Breast Cancer Res Treat 1992; 21(1):15-26.
133. Osborne CK, Schiff R, Arpino G et al. Endocrine responsiveness: understanding how progesterone receptor can be used to select endocrine therapy. Breast 2005; 14(6):458-65.
134. Tamoxifen for early breast cancer: an overview of the randomised trials. Early Breast Cancer Trialists' Collaborative Group. Lancet 1998; 351(9114):1451-67.
135. Allegra JC, Lippman ME, Thompson EB et al. Estrogen receptor status: an important variable in predicting response to endocrine therapy in metastatic breast cancer. Eur J Cancer 1980; 16(3):323-31.
136. Horwitz KB, Alexander PS. In situ photolinked nuclear progesterone receptors of human breast cancer cells: subunit molecular weights after transformation and translocation. Endocrinology 1983; 113(6):2195-201.

137. Mote PA, Balleine RL, McGowan EM et al. Colocalization of progesterone receptors A and B by dual immunofluorescent histochemistry in human endometrium during the menstrual cycle. J Clin Endocrinol Metab 1999; 84(8):2963-71.

138. Mote PA, Bartow S, Tran N et al. Loss of co-ordinate expression of progesterone receptors A and B is an early event in breast carcinogenesis. Breast Cancer Res Treat 2002; 72(2):163-72.

139. Graham JD, Yeates C, Balleine RL et al. Characterization of progesterone receptor A and B expression in human breast cancer. Cancer Res 1995; 55(21):5063-8.

140. Graham JD, Yeates C, Balleine RL et al. Progesterone receptor A and B protein expression in human breast cancer. J Steroid Biochem Mol Biol 1996; 56(1-6 Spec No):93-8.

141. Bamberger A, Milde-Langosch K, Schulte H et al. Progesterone receptor isoforms, pr-b and pr-a, in breast cancer: correlations with clinicopathologic tumor parameters and expression of ap-1 factors. Horm Res 2000; 54(1):32-7.

142. Hopp TA, Weiss HL, Hilsenbeck SG et al. Progesterone Receptor (PR) A and B in Breast Cancer: PR-A Rich Tumors have poorer disease-free survival. Clin Cancer Res 2004; 10(8):2751-60.

143. Clemm DL, Sherman L, Boonyaratanakornkit V et al. Differential hormone-dependent phosphorylation of progesterone receptor A and B forms revealed by a phosphoserine site-specific monoclonal antibody. Mol Endocrinol 2000; 14(1):52-65.

CHAPTER 8

Aromatase Expression in Women's Cancers

Serdar E. Bulun* and Evan R. Simpson

Abstract

Estrogen has been positively linked to the pathogenesis and growth of three common women's cancers (breast, endometrium and ovary). A single gene encodes the key enzyme for estrogen biosynthesis named aromatase, inhibition of which effectively eliminates estrogen production in the entire body. Aromatase inhibitors successfully treat breast cancer, whereas their roles in endometrial and ovarian cancers are less clear. Ovary, testis, adipose tissue, skin, hypothalamus and placenta express aromatase normally, whereas breast, endometrial and ovarian cancers overexpress aromatase and produce local estrogen exerting paracrine and intracrine effects. Tissue specific promoters distributed over a 93 kilobase regulatory region upstream of a common coding region alternatively control aromatase expression. A distinct set of transcription factors regulates each promoter in a signaling pathway- and tissue-specific manner. In cancers of breast, endometrium and ovary, aromatase expression is primarily regulated by increased activity of the proximally located promoter I.3/II region. Promoters I.3 and II lie 215 bp from each other and are coordinately stimulated by PGE_2 via a cAMP-PKA-dependent pathway. In breast adipose fibroblasts exposed to PGE_2 secreted by malignant epithelial cells, activation of PKC potentiates cAMP-PKA-dependent induction of aromatase. Thus, inflammatory substances such as PGE_2 may play important roles in inducing local production of estrogen that promotes tumor growth.

Introduction

In this chapter, we will review the pathologic significance and regulation of aromatase in ovarian hormone-related women's cancers (breast, endometrium and ovary). We will first provide a relevant brief overview of physiologic and genetic concepts regarding aromatase expression in human tissues.

The Aromatase Enzyme

The aromatase enzyme is localized in the endoplasmic reticulum of estrogen-producing cells.[1,2] Aromatase enzyme complex is comprised of two polypeptides. The first of these is a specific cytochrome P450, namely aromatase cytochrome P450 (the product of the *CYP19* gene).[1] The second is a flavoprotein, NADPH-cytochrome P450 reductase and is ubiquitously distributed in most cells. Thus, cell-specific expression of aromatase P450 (P450arom) determines the presence or absence of aromatase activity. For practical purposes, we will refer to "P450arom" as "aromatase" throughout this text. Since only a single gene (*CYP19*) encodes aromatase in mice and humans, targeted disruption of this gene or inhibition of its product effectively eliminates estrogen biosynthesis in these species.[1]

*Corresponding Author: Serdar E. Bulun—Department of Obstetric and Gynecology, Northwestern University, 303 E. Superior Street, Suite 4-123 Chicago, IL 60611, USA. Email: sbulun@northwestern.edu

Innovative Endocrinology of Cancer, edited by Lev M. Berstein and Richard J. Santen. ©2008 Landes Bioscience and Springer Science+Business Media.

In the human, aromatase is expressed in a number of cells including the ovarian granulosa cell, the placental syncytiotrophoblast, the testicular Leydig cell, as well as various extraglandular sites including the brain and skin fibroblasts.[3] The principal product of the ovarian granulosa cells during the follicular phase is estradiol. Additionally, aromatase is expressed in human adipose tissue. Whereas the highest levels of aromatase are in the ovarian granulosa cells in premenopausal women, the adipose tissue becomes the major aromatase expressing body site after menopause (Fig. 1).[4,5] Although aromatase level per adipose tissue fibroblast may be small, the sum of estrogen arising from billions of adipose tissue fibroblasts in the entire body makes a physiologic impact. In adipose tissue, estrogenically weak estrone is produced from androstenedione of adrenal origin in relatively large quantities. However, at least half of this peripherally produced estrone is eventually converted to estradiol in extraovarian tissues (Fig. 1).[6]

The CYP19 (Aromatase) Gene

The aromatase gene is transcribed from the telomere to the centromere and the region encoding the aromatase protein spans 30 kb of the 3'-end and contains 9 exons (II-X).[7] The ATG translation start site is located in coding exon II. The upstream (telomeric) 93 kb of the gene contains a number of promoters.[2,3] The most proximal gonadspecific promoter II and two other proximal

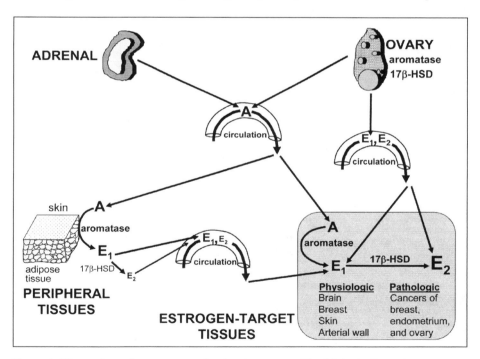

Figure 1. Tissue sites of estrogen production in women. The biologically active estrogen, estradiol (E_2) is produced at least in three major sites: 1-direct secretion from the ovary in reproductive age women; 2-by conversion of circulating androstenedione (A) of adrenal and/or ovarian origins to estrone (E_1) in peripheral tissues; and 3-by conversion of A to E_1 in estrogen target tissues. In the latter two instances, estrogenically weak E_1 is further converted to E_2 within the same tissue. The presence of the enzyme aromatase and 17βhydroxysteroid dehydrogenase (17β-HSD) is critical for E_2 formation at these sites. E_2 formation by peripheral and local conversion is particularly important for postmenopausal women and for estrogen-dependent diseases such as breast cancer, endometriosis and endometrial cancer. Figure used with permission from Bulun SE, Lin Z, Imir G. et al. Pharmacol Rev 2005; 57:359-383.[15]

promoters, I.3 (expressed in adipose tissue and breast cancer) and I.6 (expressed in bone) are found to be located within the 1-kb region upstream of the ATG translation start site in exon II, as expected (Fig. 2). Promoter I.2, the minor placenta-specific promoter, is located approximately 13 kb upstream of the ATG site in exon II. The promoters specific for the brain (I.f), endothelial cells (I.7), fetal tissues (I.5), adipose tissue (I.4) and placenta (2a and I.1) are localized in tandem order at ~3, 36, 43, 73, 78 and 93-kb, respectively, upstream of the first coding exon, the exon II (Fig. 2).[2,8] In addition to promoter II specific sequences, transcripts containing two other unique sequences, untranslated exons I.3 and I.4, are present in adipose tissue and in adipose tissue fibroblasts maintained in culture.[8] Transcription initiated by use of each promoter gives rise to a transcript with a unique 5'-untranslated end that contains the sequence encoded in the first exon immediately downstream of this particular promoter (Fig. 2). Therefore, the 5'-untranslated region of aromatase mRNA is promoter specific and may be viewed as a signature of the particular promoter used. It should be emphasized again that all of these 5'-ends are spliced onto a common junction 38 bp upstream of the ATG translation start site.[8] Consequently, the sequence encoding the open reading frame is identical in each case. Thus, the expressed protein is the same regardless of the splicing pattern (Fig. 2).

Normal Hormonal Pathways that Regulate Aromatase Expression

The primary site of aromatase expression in premenopausal women is the ovarian follicle, where FSH induces aromatase and thus estradiol production in a cyclic fashion.[3] Ovarian aromatase expression is mediated primarily by FSH receptors, cAMP production and activation of the proximal promoter II (Fig. 3).[3] Men and postmenopausal women also produce estrogen by aromatase that resides in extragonadal tissues such as adipose tissue and skin (Fig. 3).[3] Estrogen produced in these extragonadal tissues are of paramount importance for the closure of bone plates

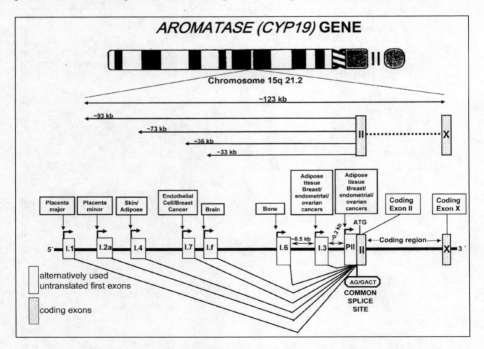

Figure 2. CYP19 (aromatase) gene. Expression of the aromatase gene is regulated by the tissue-specific activation of a number of promoters via alternative splicing. Figure used with permission from: Bulun SE, Lin Z, Imir G et al. Pharmacol Rev 2005; 57:359-383.[15]

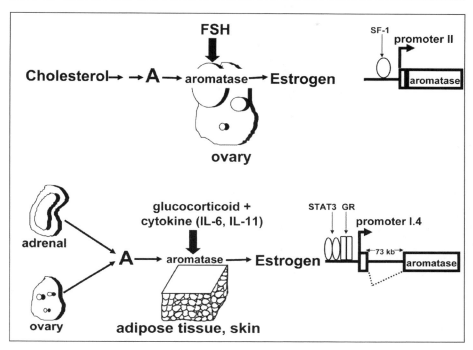

Figure 3. Physiological regulation of aromatase expression. FSH induces aromatase expression via through a cAMP-dependent pathway in ovarian granulosa cells via promoter II. Steroidogenic factor-I (SF-1) mediates this action of FSH. On the other hand, a combination of a glucocorticoid and a member of the class I cytokine family induces aromatase expression in skin and adipose tissue fibroblasts via promoter I.4 located 70 kb upstream of the coding region. Binding of signal transducers and activators of transcription (STAT)-3 and glucocorticoid receptor (GR) upstream of promoter I.4 mediate regulation of aromatase expression in these fibroblasts. Figure used with permission from: Bulun SE, Lin Z, Imir G et al. Pharmacol Rev 2005; 57:359-383.[15]

and bone mineralization in both men and postmenopausal women, since the phenotype of men with defective genes of aromatase or estrogen receptor-α include severe osteoporosis and extremely tall stature with growth into adulthood.[9] A distal promoter (I.4) located 73 kilobases upstream of the coding region directs as was mentioned aromatase expression in adipose tissue and skin fibroblasts. Promoter I.4 in these tissues is regulated by combined action of a glucocorticoid and a member of the class I cytokine family [e.g., interleukin (IL)-6, IL-11, leukemia inhibitory factor (LIF), oncostatin-M] (Fig. 3).[10]

The alternative use of promoters comprises the basis for differential regulation of aromatase expression by various hormones, growth factors and cytokines in a tissue specific manner. For example, extremely high baseline levels of the placental promoter I.1 activity are maintained constitutively in the syncytiotrophoblast and a consequence of decreasing levels of inhibitory transcription factors as cytotrophoblasts differentiate to a syncytiotrophoblast.[11,12] On the other hand, extremely low baseline levels of promoter II in the ovary are stimulated strikingly by FSH via a cAMP dependent pathway in the developing follicle (Fig. 3).[3] Serum, cytokines and growth factors are inhibitory to promoter II. In case of adipose and skin fibroblasts, promoter I.4 is used in vivo and activated as was said above coordinately by a glucocorticoid in the presence of a cytokine (IL-6, IL-11, LIF, oncostatin M). Glucocorticoid receptors and the Jak-1/STAT-3 pathway mediate this induction.[10]

Promoter use in cultured adipose tissue fibroblasts is a function of hormonal treatments. For example, in vitro studies showed that PGE_2 or cAMP analogs stimulate aromatase expression strikingly via proximally located promoters II and I.3, whereas treatment with a glucocorticoid plus a member of the class I cytokine family switches promoter use to I.4.[10,13]

Pathological Expression of Aromatase in Women's Cancers

Breast and endometrial cancers are highly responsive to estrogen for growth evident by high concentrations of estrogen receptors in these tissues.[14] Malignant breast and endometrial tumors also produce large amounts of estrogen locally via overexpressing aromatase compared to their normal counterparts.[15] In particular, aromatase overexpression in breast cancer tissue has been shown to be critical, since the use of aromatase inhibitors is clearly therapeutic in breast cancer. Aromatase is also overexpressed in endometrial cancer.[16] Although preliminary trials showed promising results, the therapeutic role of aromatase inhibitors in endometrial cancer is not as clear yet.[17,18]

Experimental and epidemiological evidence suggest that estrogen and progesterone are implicated in ovarian carcinogenesis. New data have indicated that estrogen favors neoplastic transformation of the ovarian surface epithelium while progesterone offers protection against ovarian cancer development.[19-23] Since a subset of ovarian cancers was linked to endometriosis and, aromatase is a key molecular target in endometriosis, aromatase expression in ovarian cancer may also be targeted for treatment in selected patients.[15] In fact, recent pilot studies employing aromatase inhibitors have shown various degrees of clinical benefit for patients with advanced stages of ovarian cancer.[24-27]

Aromatase and Breast Cancer

Paracrine interactions between malignant breast epithelial cells, proximal adipose fibroblasts and vascular endothelial cells are responsible for estrogen biosynthesis and lack of adipogenic differentiation in breast cancer tissue. It appears that malignant epithelial cells secrete factors that inhibit the differentiation of surrounding adipose fibroblasts to mature adipocytes and also stimulate aromatase expression in these undifferentiated adipose fibroblasts.[28] The in vivo presence of malignant epithelial cells also enhances aromatase expression in endothelial cells in breast tissue.[29] We developed a model in breast cancer, which reconciles the inhibition of adipogenic differentiation and estrogen biosynthesis in a positive feedback cycle.

The desmoplastic reaction (formation of the dense fibroblast layer surrounding malignant epithelial cells) is essential for structural and biochemical support for tumor growth. In fact, the some pathologists refer to 70% of breast carcinomas as "scirrhous" type indicating the rock-like consistency of these tumors.[30] This consistency comes from the tightly packed undifferentiated adipose fibroblasts around malignant epithelial cells. Malignant epithelial cells achieve this by secreting large quantities of TNF and IL-11 that inhibit the differentiation of fibroblasts to mature adipocytes. Thus, large numbers of these estrogen producing cells are maintained proximal to malignant cells.[28,29] At the same time, a separate set of factors secreted by malignant epithelial cells activates aromatase expression in surrounding adipose fibroblasts.[28,29]

Malignant epithelial cells induce aromatase via activation of aberrant promoters in breast cancer tissue and adipose fibroblasts proximal to tumor (Fig. 4). The breast adipose tissue in disease-free women maintains low levels of aromatase expression primarily via promoter I.4 that lies 73 kb upstream of the common coding region (Fig. 4).[8] The proximal promoters I.3 and II are used only minimally in normal breast adipose tissue.[8] Transcription via activity of promoters II and I.3 in the breast tumor fibroblasts and malignant epithelial cells, however, is strikingly increased (Fig. 4).[31-34] Additionally, the endothelial-type promoter I.7 is also upregulated in breast tumor tissue (Fig. 4).[35] Thus, it appears that the prototype estrogen-dependent malignancy (breast cancer) takes advantage of four promoters utilized in various cell types for aromatase expression (Fig. 4). The sum of aromatase mRNA species arising from these four promoters markedly increase total aromatase mRNA levels in breast cancer compared with the normal breast that uses almost exclusively promoter I.4 (Fig. 4).

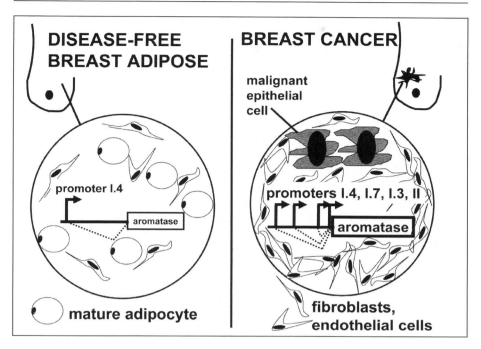

Figure 4. Promoter use for aromatase expression in normal and malignant breast tissues. The levels of total aromatase mRNA levels in breast cancer tissue are strikingly higher than normal breast tissue. The normal breast adipose tissue maintains low levels of aromatase expression primarily via promoter I.4. Promoters I.3 and II are used only minimally in normal breast adipose tissue. Promoter II and I.3 activities in the breast cancer, however, are strikingly increased. Additionally, the endothelialtype promoter I.7 is also upregulated in breast cancer. Thus, it appears that the prototype estrogendependent malignancy (breast cancer) takes advantage of four promoters (II, I.3, I.7 and I.4) for aromatase expression. The sum of aromatase mRNA species arising from these four promoters markedly increase total aromatase mRNA levels in breast cancer compared with the normal breast. Figure used with permission from: Bulun SE, Lin Z, Imir G et al Pharmacol Rev 2005; 57:359-383.[15]

Tissue Origins of Estrogen in Postmenopausal Women with Breast Cancer

Estrogen arises from two sources in a postmenopausal woman with breast cancer. First, estrogen that arises from extraovarian body sites such as subcutaneous adipose tissue and skin reaches breast cancer by way of circulation in an endocrine manner. Second, estrogen locally produced in breast cancer tissue makes an impact via paracrine or intracrine mechanisms.

Endocrine Effect

Aromatase in adipose tissue and skin. The potential roles of extraovarian aromatase in human physiology and pathology were also recognized initially in the 1960s.[36] These studies demonstrated that the conversion rate of plasma androstenedione to estrone in humans increased as a function of obesity and aging.[5,37] These same studies also revealed the importance of extraovarian tissues (primarily adipose tissue and skin) as the origin of estrogen in postmenopausal women (see Fig. 1). Extraovarian estrogen formation was shown to be correlated positively with excess body weight in both pre and postmenopausal women and may be increased as much as ten-fold in morbidly obese postmenopausal women.[5,37] This elevation in association with both obesity and aging bears a striking relationship to the incidence of endometrial hyperplasia and cancer, which are more commonly observed in elderly obese women.[38] It is now recognized that the continuous production of estrogen by the adipose tissue in these women is one of the risk factors of endometrial hyperplasia and cancer.

Evidence is also suggestive of a role of estrogens produced by adipose tissue in the pathogenesis of the breast cancer. For example, breast cancer incidence correlates positively with the body fat content or serum estradiol levels in postmenopausal women suggesting that estrogens collectively produced in all extraovarian sites reach the breast tissue by circulation in an endocrine fashion and stimulate tumor growth.[39,40] A role for adipose tissue estrogen biosynthesis in promoting the growth of breast cancer is implied because of the palliative effects of adrenalectomy in the past. As estrone production by adipose tissue is dependent on plasma androstenedione secreted by the adrenal cortex as substrate, the role of adrenalectomy is explicable in terms of the denial of substrate precursor for adipose tissue estrogen biosynthesis. Today, reduction of estrogen biosynthesis in the adipose tissue is accomplished by the use of aromatase inhibitors in the treatment of breast cancer (Fig. 5).[41,42]

Paracrine/Intracrine Effect

Local aromatase in breast cancer tissue. Mechanisms giving rise to increased local concentrations of estrogen in breast cancer via aromatase overexpression within the tumor tissue has been demonstrated by a number investigators.[43-45] These studies showed strikingly increased local levels of estrone, estrone sulfate and eastradiol in breast tumor tissue compared with circulating estrogen levels.[43-45]

A series of paracrine interactions between malignant breast epithelial cells and surrounding adipose stroma were uncovered and explained increased local estrogen levels in the breast bearing a cancer. For example, independent studies from at least six different laboratories were indicative of striking increases in aromatase enzyme activity and mRNA levels in breast fat adjacent to cancer compared with those in distal fat or disease free breast adipose tissue (Fig. 5).[32-34,46-49] We also found that an elevation in aromatase expression in adipose stroma surrounding malignant epithelial cells is regulated by complex cellular, molecular and genomic mechanisms.[29,31,47] Interestingly, the overall aromatase expression in breast adipose tissue in mastectomy specimens bearing a breast tumor was significantly higher than that in benign breast tissue removed for reduction mammoplasty.[31,50,51]

Estrogens can act both directly or indirectly on human breast cancer cells to promote proliferation. Breast cancer cells in culture elaborate a number of growth stimulants in response to estrogen, which can act in an autocrine and paracrine manner to stimulate their growth. However, there is also evidence that estrogens can directly induce proliferation of breast cancer cells.

The pathologic significance of local aromatase activity in breast cancer was recognized based on the following in vitro data. MCF-7 breast cancer cells, which were stably transfected to express an MMTV-promoter-driven human aromatase cDNA and inoculated into oophorectomized nude mice, remained dependent on circulating androstenedione for their rapid growth.[52] Another evidence for the importance of local aromatase expression in the breast tissue came from an in vivo mouse model demonstrating that aromatase overexpression in breast tissue is sufficient for maintaining hyperplasia in the absence of circulating estrogen and that aromatase inhibitors abrogated hyperplasia.[53] These transgenic mice with MMTV-promoter-driven local aromatase in breast tissue are more prone for breast cancer development.[54]

Role of Adipose Tissue in Aromatase Expression in Malignant Breast Tumor Tissue

Cell Types That Express Aromatase in Breast Cancer

Breast adipose tissue is primarily comprised of mature lipid containing cells and other stromal elements. This latter group of cells in the breast adipose tissue was characterized using immunohistochemical methods.[55] Ninety percent of these resident cells of adipose tissue are fibroblasts, i.e., the potential precursors of mature adipocytes and another 7% represented by endothelial cells. The majority (80-90%) of aromatase transcripts in adipose tissue was demonstrated to reside in fibroblasts compared with mature adipocytes.[55] Moreover, aromatase enzyme activity was found to reside primarily in the fibroblast component of the adipose tissue in a previous study from the same laboratory.[56]

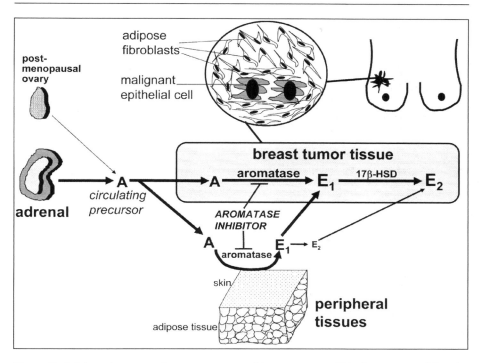

Figure 5. Origins of estrogen in postmenopausal breast cancer. This figure exemplifies the important pathologic roles of extraovarian (peripheral) and local estrogen biosynthesis in an estrogen-dependent disease in postmenopausal women. The estrogen precursor androstene-dione (A) originates primarily from the adrenal in the postmenopausal woman. Aromatase expression and enzyme activity in extraovarian tissues such as fat increases with advancing age. The aromatase activity in skin and subcutaneous adipose fibroblasts gives rise to formation of systemically available estrone (E_1) and to a smaller extent estradiol (E_2). The conversion of circulating A to E_1 in undifferentiated breast adipose fibroblasts compacted around malignant epithelial cells and subsequent conversion of E_1 to E_2 in malignant epithelial cells provide high tissue concentrations of E_2 for tumor growth. The clinical relevance of these findings is exemplified by the successful use of aromatase inhibitors to treat breast cancer. Figure used with permission from: Bulun SE, Lin Z, Imir G et al. Pharmacol Rev 2005; 57:359-383.[15]

Immunoreactive aromatase was localized to both the malignant epithelial cells and surrounding fibroblasts in breast tumor tissues.[57-59] Different antibodies, however, showed variable affinity to malignant epithelial cells vs fibroblasts.[60] Immunoreactive aromatase was also observed in endothelial cells in normal breast tissue and breast tumors. Recently published data using RNA from lasercaptured breast tumor cells showed aromatase mRNA in both stromal and malignant epithelial cells in tumor tissues from 3 patients.[60] Markedly high levels of aromatase enzyme activity have been consistently detected in breast adipose fibroblasts freshly isolated from breast tissue with or without cancer.[55,56] Aromatase enzyme activity in malignant breast epithelial cells, on the other hand, in experimental conditions is either undetectable or extremely low.[61]

Adjacent adipose tissue including the dense fibroblast layer seems to account for the majority of aromatase expression in breast tumors for the following reasons. First, the quantity of adjacent adipose tissue surrounding a clinically detectable breast tumor is comparatively very large, e.g., the volume of adipose tissue within 1-inch radius of a 1 ml breast tumor is 129 ml. Second, the most intense aromatase immunostaining was observed in the adipose tissue fibroblasts located in and around the fibrous capsule (i.e., desmoplastic reaction) surrounding malignant cells.[48]

Third, levels of aromatase expression and activity in fibroblasts isolated from breast adipose tissue or tumor are 10-15 times higher than those found in malignant epithelial cells or cell lines.[61]

Impaired Adipogenic Differentiation in Breast Cancer

Link to aromatase overexpression. Extraordinarily large quantities of TNF and IL-11 are produced and secreted by malignant breast epithelial cells[28] (Fig. 6).[28] These two cytokines mediate one of the most commonly observed biological phenomena in breast tumors, namely the desmoplastic reaction. Desmoplastic reaction or accumulation of fibroblasts around malignant epithelial cells serves to maintain the strikingly hard consistency in many of these tumors (i.e., the traditional macroscopic description of malignant breast tumors as "scirrhous cancer") and increased local concentrations of estrogen via aromatase overexpression localized to these undifferentiated fibroblasts. The inhibition of differentiation of fibroblasts to mature adipocytes mediated by TNF and IL-11 is the key event responsible for desmoplastic reaction, because neither malignant cell-conditioned media nor these cytokines caused the proliferation of adipose tissue fibroblasts.[28] Moreover, blocking both TNF and IL-11 in cancer cell-CM conditioned medium using neutralizing antibodies is sufficient to reverse this antidifferentiative effect of cancer cells completely (Fig. 6).[28] In summary, desmoplastic reaction primarily occurs via the action of cytokines (TNF and IL-11) secreted by the malignant epithelial cells to inhibit the differentiation of adipose tissue fibroblasts to mature adipocytes. This tumor-induced block in adipocyte differentiation is mediated by the selective inhibition of expression of the essential adipogenic transcription factors, namely, C/EBPα and PPARγ (Fig. 6).[28]

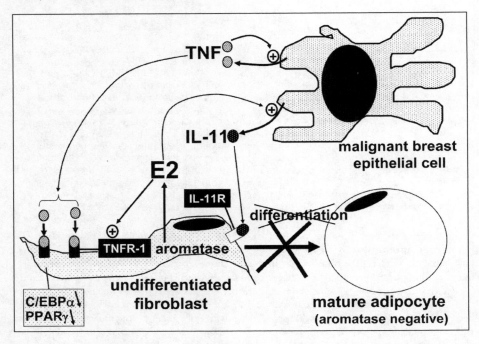

Figure 6. Detail of epithelial-stromal interaction via estrogen and cytokines in breast cancer. Estradiol (E_2) increases secretion of antiadipogenic cytokines (IL-11) from malignant epithelial cells and upregulates their antiadipogenic-type receptors (TNF-receptor type 1, TNFR1) in undifferentiated fibroblasts. These redundant mechanisms give rise to accumulation of undifferentiated fibroblasts around malignant epithelial cells (desmoplastic reaction), which express aromatase and form E_2. Figure used with permission from: Bulun SE, Lin Z, Imir G et al. Pharmacol Rev 2005; 57:359-383.[15]

Estrogen per se seems to potentiate this antiadipogenic action via indirect mechanisms. For example, treatment of T47D breast cancer cells with estradiol increased the mRNA levels of IL-11 by 3-fold.[62] Moreover, the cellular actions of TNF are mediated by two distinct receptors TNFR1 (also known as p60 in humans) and TNFR2 (p80). TNFR1 but not TNFR2 was found to be responsible for the inhibition of adipocyte differentiation using mutants of TNF specific for the stimulation of either receptor type.[63] We recently demonstrated that TNFR1 is responsible for inhibition of adipocyte differentiation in breast cancer.[64] Interestingly, estradiol enhances this anti-adipogenic effect by inducing TNFR1 levels in adipose fibroblasts (Fig. 6).[64]

Thus, large amounts of antiadipogenic cytokines (e.g., TNF and IL-11) secreted by malignant epithelial cells serve to maintain increased numbers of the aromatase-expressing cell type, i.e., undifferentiated adipose fibroblast, in breast tumor tissue. This is further enhanced by stimulatory effects of estrogen on IL-11 production in cancer cells and on the TNF receptor type that mediates adipogenic inhibition (Fig. 6).

Transcriptional Mechanisms Responsible for Elevated Aromatase Expression in Breast Cancer

Alternative promoter use is a major mechanism that mediates increased aromatase expression in breast cancer. The normal breast adipose tissue maintains low levels of aromatase expression primarily via promoter I.4 that lies 73 kb upstream of the common coding region (see Fig. 4). The proximally located promoters I.3 and II are used only minimally in normal breast adipose tissue. Promoter II and I.3 activities in the breast cancer, however, are strikingly increased.[31-34] Additionally, the endothelial-type promoter I.7 is also upregulated in breast cancer.[35] Thus, as was mentioned above it appears that the prototype estrogen-dependent malignancy breast cancer takes advantage of four promoters (II, I.3, I.7 and I.4) for aromatase expression (see Fig. 4). The sum of aromatase mRNA species arising from these four promoters markedly increase total aromatase mRNA levels in breast cancer compared with the normal breast that uses almost exclusively promoter I.4 (see Fig. 4)

Upregulation of Promoters I.3 and II

Using an in vivo approach, we and two other groups demonstrated by quantitative exon specific RT-PCR that the use of the proximal promoters II/I.3 are strikingly upregulated in adipose tissue adjacent to breast cancer and in breast cancer tissue per se.[31,33,34] As noted earlier, promoters II and I.3 are located within 215 bp from each other and are coordinately induced by cAMP-dependent or independent mechanisms in adipose fibroblasts in breast tumors. These promoters possibly share common regulatory DNA motifs.

Increased promoter I.3/II activity is in part, the basis for increased aromatase expression in peri- and intratumoral adipose tissue fibroblasts (see Fig. 4).[31] Over the past several years, others and we sought to elucidate the mechanisms underlying this cancer-induced increase in promoters I.3/II activity in adipose tissue fibroblasts.

PGE$_2$ induces aromatase via promoters I.3 and II employing both cAMP/PKA- and PKC-dependent pathways.[13] In this model, PGE$_2$ stimulates binding activity of an orphan nuclear receptor LRH-1 to a nuclear receptor half-site (-136/-124 bp) upstream of promoter II.[65,66] Treatment with PGE$_2$ strikingly increased both LRH-1 expression and its binding activity to the aromatase promoter II in cultured adipose fibroblasts. LRH-1 overexpression significantly increased aromatase promoter II activity and aromatase enzyme activity in cultured adipose fibroblasts (Fig. 7). From an in vivo perspective, LRH-1 was upregulated in undifferentiated fibroblasts in breast tumor tissue compared with those in disease-free breast tissue. The recently reported increases in COX-2 expression and beneficial effects of nonsteroidal anti-inflammatory in breast cancer support this model.[67,68] In vivo evidence for increased PGE$_2$ formation in breast cancer, however, is still lacking at this time.

In addition to the LRH-1-binding site, we isolated two *cis*-acting elements that conferred stimulation of promoter I.3/II use in response to cAMP plus or minus PKC activation, the signaling pathways induced by PGE$_2$.[29,69] Two critical elements were determined as a C/EBP site

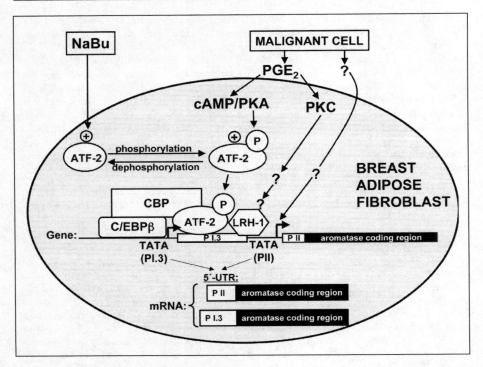

Figure 7. Effects of PGE$_2$, PKA, PKC and sodium butyrate (NaBu) on aromatase expression in breast adipose fibroblasts. We recently found that NaBu profoundly decreased promoter I.3/II-specific aromatase mRNA expression induced by PGE$_2$ or a surrogate hormomonal cocktail made of dibutyryl cAMP (Bt$_2$cAMP) plus the PKC activator phorbol diacetate (PDA). MCM, Bt$_2$cAMP+PDA or NaBu regulated aromatase mRNA levels or enzyme activity only specifically via promoters I.3/II but not other promoters. Recruitment of phosphorylated ATF-2 by a CRE (-211/-199) in the promoter I.3/II region conferred the response to malignant epithelial cells conditioned medium, PGE$_2$ or Bt$_2$cAMP+PDA. Malignant cell-conditioned medium, PGE$_2$ or Bt$_2$cAMP+PDA stabilized a complex comprised of phosphorylated ATF-2, C/EBPβ and CBP in the common regulatory region of promoters I.3/II. The inhibitory effect of NaBu on transcription was not accompanied by comparable changes in overall histone acetylation patterns of promoters I.3/II. NaBu treatment, however, consistently decreased ATF-2 phosphorylation and disrupted the activating complex. Taken together, these findings represent a novel mechanism of NaBu action and provide evidence that aromatase activity can be attenuated in a signaling pathway and tissue specific fashion. Our data also suggested that malignant cells secreted substances other than PGE2. These unknown substances were associated with signaling pathways other than cAMP-PKA in the activation of aromatase promoters I.3 and II.

(-317/-304) and a CRE (-211/-197), since mutation of either element abolished cAMP-induced promoter activity (Fig. 7).[69]

PGE2 or a cAMP analog (plus or minus PKC activator) induced phosphorylation of ATF-2 and its binding to the CRE (Fig. 7).[69] This CRE is occupied by nonphosphorylated ATF-2 in fibroblasts treated with benign epithelial cell-conditioned medium associated with inactivation of promoters I.3 and II. Moreover, chromatin immunoprecipitation PCR showed that the activator transcriptional complex in a malignant environment contains C/EBPβ, phosphorylated ATF-2 and p300/CBP, whereas the inactivator complex (benign environment) contained nonphosphorylated ATF-2 (Fig. 7).[69]

We recently found that sodium-butyrate (NaBu) profoundly decreased cAMP analog (plus or minus PKC activator)-induced promoter I.3/II-specific aromatase mRNA expression. A cAMP analog (plus or minus a PKC activator) or NaBu regulated aromatase mRNA levels or enzyme activity only via promoters I.3/II but not promoters I.1 or I.4 in breast, ovarian, placental and hepatic cells. Mechanistically, recruitment of phosphorylated ATF2 by a CRE (-211/-199) in the promoter I.3/II region conferred the response to a cAMP analog (plus or minus PKC activator). Treatment with a cAMP analog (plus or minus PKC activator) stabilized a complex comprised of phosphorylated ATF-2, C/EBPβ and CBP in the common regulatory region of promoters I.3/II (Fig. 7). The inhibitory effect of NaBu on transcription was not accompanied by comparable changes in overall histone acetylation patterns of promoters I.3/II. NaBu treatment, however, consistently decreased ATF-2 phosphorylation and disrupted the activating complex (Fig. 7). Together, these findings represent a novel mechanism of NaBu action and provide evidence that aromatase activity can be attenuated in a signaling pathway- and tissue-specific fashion.[69]

In an alternative experimental model, we found that conditioned medium from malignant breast epithelial cells (MCF-7 or T47D) markedly induced aromatase expression in adipose tissue fibroblasts via promoters I.3 and II (Fig. 7).[29,69] Malignant epithelial cell-conditioned medium also induced phosphorylation of ATF-2 and its binding activity to the promoter I.3/II region. As in the case of treatment with a cAMP analog (plus or minus a PKC activator), incubation of breast adipose fibroblasts with malignant epithelial cell-conditioned medium stabilized a complex made of phosphorylated ATF-2, C/EBPβ and CBP at the *aromatase* promoter I.3/II region.[69] NaBu also disrupts this transcriptional complex assembled in response to malignant epithelial cell conditioned medium.[69] We hypothesize that a hormonal cocktail secreted from malignant epithelial cells induces aromatase in undifferentiated adipose fibroblasts via redundant pathways. Although PGE$_2$ seems to be an important component of this cocktail, other substances can also induce aromatase expression via promoters I.3/II.[29] For example, the addition of a COX2 inhibitor or an adenylyl cyclase inhibitor does not reverse induction of aromatase expression by malignant epithelial cellconditioned medium.[29]

A unified model for promoter II/I.3 activation in breast cancer therefore predicts that malignant epithelial cells secrete a number of factors including PGE$_2$ (Fig. 7). These factors induce a number of signaling pathways in a redundant fashion to activate the transcription of the aromatase gene via promoter I.3/II in adipose fibroblasts. PGE$_2$ possibly arising from malignant epithelial cells is a candidate factor for activation of promoters I.3 and II in breast cancer. This, however, has not been demonstrated in vivo. Neither PGE$_2$ nor its downstream regulators cAMP or LRH-1-binding site in promoter II were found to be essential for activation of promoters II in adipose fibroblasts treated with malignant cell-conditioned medium.[29] In disease-free breast tissue, incorporation of a number of transcriptional repressors into the multimeric complex that occupies promoter I.3/II region is associated with inhibition of transcription. Malignant epithelial cell conditioned medium, on the other hand, gives rise to replacement of this inhibitory complex by an activator transcriptional complex comprised of distinct factors such as phosphorylated ATF-2, C/EBPβ, p300/CBP and possibly LRH-1 (Fig. 7).[69]

In summary, the proximal promoters II and I.3 clustered within a 215 bp region are coordinately regulated. They remain quiescent in fibroblasts of normal breast tissue via redundant binding of multiple transcriptional inhibitors (Fig. 7). In a malignant breast environment, however, these promoter regions are occupied by multiple transcriptional enhancers as a result of activation of multiple signaling pathways in a fail-safe fashion to increase aromatase expression in breast fibroblasts (Fig. 7).

Regulation of Promoters II and I.3 in MCF-7 Cells

A group of investigators studied the regulation of a number of gene reporter constructs of the promoter II/I.3 region.[70] They found that ERR alpha-1 and CREB1 upregulate and EAR2, COUP-TFI, RAR gamma, Snail and Slug proteins downregulate this promoter region.[70] The in vivo relevance of these findings will become clearer in future, once the relative significance of aromatase enzyme activity and estrogen biosynthesis is demonstrated in malignant epithelial cells.

Upregulation of Promoter I.7 in Breast Cancer

Studies summarized above employed exon specific RT-PCR analysis of 5'-untranslated ends of aromatase mRNA in breast cancer tissues. This limited strategy permitted only the detection of promoters previously identified from healthy tissues.[31,33,34] Discovery-driven approaches designed to identify novel promoter regions in breast cancer or adjacent adipose tissues, however, have not been published until recently. To identify novel promoter regions in cancer tissues and proximal fat, we employed the 5'-rapid amplification of cDNA ends (RACE) procedure using total RNA isolated from breast cancer and proximal adipose tissue samples. We cloned a novel 101bp untranslated first exon (I.7) that comprises the 5'-end of 29-54% of aromatase mRNA isolated from breast cancer tissues.[35] The levels of aromatase mRNA with exon I.7 were significantly increased in breast cancer tissues and adipose tissue adjacent to tumors. We identified a promoter immediately upstream of exon I.7 and mapped this to about 36 kb upstream of ATG translation start site of the aromatase gene.[35] Promoter I.7 is a TATA-less promoter containing *cis*-regulatory elements found in megakaryocytic and endothelial type promoters. Maximal promoter activity could be demonstrated in human microvascular endothelial cells. Binding of the transcription factor GATA-2-to a specific GATA cisregulatory element in this promoter was critical for its regulation in endothelial cells.[35] In conclusion, promoter I.7 is a GATA-2-regulated endothelial type promoter of the human aromatase gene and may increase estrogen biosynthesis in vascular endothelial cells of breast cancer. The activity of this promoter may also be important for intracrine and paracrine effects of estrogen on blood vessel physiology.

Summary of Regulation of Aromatase Expression in Breast Cancer

Several alternative cellular and molecular mechanisms serve to maintain excessive levels of aromatase activity in breast stroma proximal to malignant epithelial cells. First, malignant epithelial cell derived factors induce aromatase over expression via the transcription factors LRH-1, C/EBPβ and phosphorylated ATF-2 (see Fig. 5). These factors are incorporated into a multimeric transcriptional complex that occupies the aromatase promoter I.3/II region in adipose tissue fibroblasts adjacent to epithelial cells. Second, aromatase is overexpressed in vascular endothelial cells of tumor tissue via binding of GATA2 and other endothelial type transcription factors to promoter I.7. These factors may also mediate angiogenesis in tumor tissue. Moreover, estrogen is known to induce the angiogenic factor VEGF in cancer cells (see Fig. 5).[71-74] Third, we demonstrated recently that antiadipogenic cytokines IL-11 and TNF secreted by malignant epithelial cells block the differentiation of the aromatase-expressing cells (fibroblasts) to mature adipocytes that do not express aromatase (see Fig. 5). Thereby, these cytokines secreted abundantly by malignant epithelial cells serve to maintain a dense layer of aromatase-expressing fibroblasts proximal to malignant epithelial cells to provide structural and hormonal support. Fourth, the expression of IL-11 in malignant epithelial cells and antiadipogenic type TNF receptors in adjacent adipose tissue fibroblasts are upregulated by estrogen produced as a consequence of elevated aromatase activity in breast tumors. This positive feedback involving complex epithelial-stromal interactions favor higher numbers of undifferentiated fibroblasts, angiogenesis and increased local estrogen concentrations in breast tumors (see Fig. 5). These four mechanisms interact to maintain high levels of estrogen production in a breast tumor.[74]

Aromatase Inhibitors in the Treatment of Breast Cancer

Today, aromatase inhibitors are the most effective endocrine-treatment of estrogen-responsive breast cancer (Fig. 7).[75] Six recent head to head randomized clinical trials published since 2000 demonstrated the superiority of aromatase inhibitors to tamoxifen in the treatment of breast cancer.[76-83] Longterm side effect profiles of these agents will determine whether aromatase inhibitors will replace tamoxifen or other selective estrogen receptor modulators in the long run.

There are two intriguing implications of these results. First, it is pharmacologically more efficacious to block estrogen formation rather than its action at least by currently approved estrogen antagonists or SERMs. Second, the local effect of aromatase inhibitors at the target tissue level to block local estrogen formation possibly represents the most critical mechanism for the superior therapeutic potential of aromatase inhibitors (Fig. 7).

Targeting aromatase in breast cancer as a therapeutic strategy was first conceptualized in the 1960s.[75] Aminoglutethimide was the first aromatase inhibitor tested for this purpose. Although the first generation aromatase inhibitor aminoglutethimide was as efficacious as tamoxifen in the treatment of breast cancer, its adverse side effects precluded its widespread use.[75] Tamoxifen was introduced in the 1970s and became the gold standard for hormonal treatment of breast cancer.[75] Second generation aromatase inhibitors were tested in Europe in the 1980s and were found to be as efficacious as tamoxifen.[75] Finally, the third generation aromatase inhibitors were approved in the U.S. to treat postmenopausal breast cancer in the 1990s and proven to be superior to tamoxifen.[76-85] These new inhibitors have a benign side effect profile and suppress estrogen production in extraovarian tissues and within the breast cancer tissue itself. This effectively blocks estrogenic action, reduces recurrences and prolongs disease free survival in postmenopausal women with breast cancer.[76,77] Aromatase inhibitors are also effective in the treatment of breast cancer that became resistant to treatment with tamoxifen.[80]

In these studies, tumors that express estrogen receptor (ER) were more responsive to aromatase inhibitors compared with the tumors with an unknown receptor status.[76,77] Future studies are required to determine whether aromatase inhibitors might be beneficial in ER-negative tumors via ER-independent mechanisms.

Aromatase and Endometrial Cancer

The role of aromatase expression and the therapeutic use of aromatase inhibitors have been well defined for breast cancer and endometriosis. Aromatase is also expressed in endometrial cancer tissue and aromatase inhibitors have been used to treat endometrial cancer.[16-18,86] The pathologic significance of local estrogen biosynthesis via aromatase expression in endometrial cancer tissue or the therapeutic value of aromatase inhibitors in its management, however, is not clear at the moment.

Endometrial cancer is the most common gynecological malignancy found in women.[87] These tumors rather often have high concentrations of estrogen receptors, their growth is clearly enhanced by estrogen and unopposed estrogen exposure (in the absence of progesterone) predisposes women to development of endometrial cancer.[87] Although there is no consistent evidence of increased concentrations of circulating estrogen in women with endometrial cancer, the local concentration of estradiol in endometrial cancer tissues was reported to be higher than that in blood and in the endometrium of cancer-free women.[88-92] It is therefore conceivable that endometrial cancer itself synthesizes estradiol in situ, which then contributes to growth and possibly carcinogenesis.

A conversion study demonstrated significant conversion of androstenedione to estrone in endometrial cancer tissue.[93] Aromatase protein and mRNA were detected in endometrial cancer using immunohistochemistry and RTPCR, whereas aromatase expression was low or undetectable in endometrial hyperplasia (a precursor lesion of endometrial cancer).[16,94] These observations are suggestive that intratumoral aromatase may play a role in the pathology of endometrial cancer. Immunoreactive aromatase was found in malignant epithelial, endometrial stromal and myometrial cells. Aromatase in stromal but not epithelial cells correlated positively with advanced surgical stage and poor survival (Dr. Makio Shozu, personal communication).

Currently available 3rd generation aromatase inhibitors may be used for endocrine treatment of endometrial cancer.[95] Treatment of endometrial cancer tissues in vitro with aromatase inhibitors demonstrated that in situ depletion of estrogen results in decreased cell proliferation of tumor cells.[96] Treatment of women with endometrial cancer with aromatase inhibitors blocked estrogen production in vivo in tumor tissue.[97] Safety data from the clinical trials of postmenopausal women with breast cancer indicated a preventive role of aromatase inhibitors in that an aromatase inhibitor reduced the risk of endometrial cancer.[98]

On the other hand, the therapeutic efficacy of aromatase inhibitors in advanced endometrial cancer is not clear. The Gynecologic Oncology Group (GOG) performed a phase II trial of anastrozole in advanced, recurrent, or persistent endometrial cancer.[18] Twenty-three patients were entered, all with grade 2 or 3 cancers. Two partial responses were noted.[18] In a recent report, two cases of reproductive-aged women with grade 1 endometrial cancer who were treated with medroxyprogesterone acetate and anastrozole daily for 3 and 6 months subsequently reverted to normal endometrium. A progestin combined with the elimination of production of estrogen may be an effective therapy in well differentiated endometrial cancer in the obese premenopausal woman.[17] Thus, there are some early preliminary encouraging results. It is, however, too early to predict whether aromatase inhibitors will be used widely in the treatment of endometrial cancer.

Aromatase and Ovarian Cancer

Estrogen, Progesterone and Ovarian Cancer

Since premenopausal ovary contains large amounts of estrogen and progesterone and ovarian cancer largely develops in postmenopausal women, it was hypothesized that ovarian cancer was not an ovarian steroid-responsive disease. In view of the protective effect of oral contraceptives and pregnancy, the disruptive and inflammatory effects of incessant ovulation on the surface epithelium were hypothesized to represent the primary mechanism of ovarian carcinogenesis.[19,20,23]

Accumulating evidence, however, are suggestive of significant roles of estrogen and progesterone in ovarian cancer. A retrospective 1979-1998 cohort study of 44,241 postmenopausal women revealed that estrogen only hormone replacement therapy (HRT), particularly for 10 or more years, significantly increased risk of ovarian cancer. Relative risks for 10 to 19 years and 20 or more years were 1.8 (95% CI, 1.1-3.0) and 3.2 (95% CI, 1.7-5.7), respectively (p-value for trend <0.001). This study did not show an increased risk in women who used short-term estrogen plus progestin HRT, but authors suggested that risk associated with longer-term estrogen plus progestin HRT warrants further investigation.[99] The estrogen plus progestin WHI HRT study found a trend for increased ovarian cancer risk, which though was not significant.[100] These are some of the first pieces of important epidemiological evidence supporting that estrogen might plays a critical role in the pathophysiology of ovarian cancer. This has also been supported by other epidemiological and experimental data.[19,20,23]

Estrogens appear to favor neoplastic transformation of the ovarian surface epithelium while progesterone offers protection against ovarian cancer development.[21,22] Specifically, estrogens, particularly those present in ovulatory follicles, are both genotoxic and mitogenic to ovarian surface epithelial cells. In contrast, pregnancy-equivalent levels of progesterone are highly effective as apoptosis inducers for ovarian epithelial and ovarian cancer cells. In this regard, high-dose progestin may exert an exfoliation effect and rid an aged ovarian surface epithelium of premalignant cells. A limited number of clinical studies have demonstrated efficacies of antiestrogens, aromatase inhibitors and progestins alone or in combination with chemotherapeutic drugs in the treatment of ovarian cancer. As a result of increased life expectancy in most countries, the number of women taking HRT in general continues to grow. Since in the U.S. after WHI a serious drop in the number of HRT prescriptions was registered. Therefore, knowledge of the mechanism of action of steroid hormones on the ovarian surface epithelium and ovarian cancer is of paramount significance to HRT risk assessment and to the development of novel therapies for the prevention and treatment of ovarian cancer.[19,20,23]

A Possible Link between Endometriosis, Ovarian Cancer, Aromatase and Prostaglandin Formation

Another piece of evidence regarding the role of estrogen in ovarian carcinogenesis comes from the biological and epidemiological links of endometrioid ovarian cancer to endometriosis.[19,20,23] It was proposed that endometrioid and/or undifferentiated ovarian cancer may develop from the endometriotic implants seeded on the ovarian surface epithelium.[19,20,23] Endometriosis is an estrogen-dependent disease that affects 6-10% of U.S. women of reproductive age (approximately 4-7 million).[101] Endometriosis is a systemic disorder that is characterized by the presence of endometrium like tissue in ectopic sites outside the uterus, primarily on pelvic peritoneum and ovaries.[101]

Local estrogen formation via aromatase expression in endometriosis is extraordinarily important for its pathogenesis and treatment.[86,102-106] In fact, work from our laboratory and other investigators over the past 10 years uncovered a molecular link between inflammation and estrogen production in endometriosis.[86] This is mediated by a positive feedback cycle that favors expression of aromatase and COX-2 and continuous local production of estradiol and PGE_2 in endometriotic tissue.[107-109] In this vicious cycle, PGE_2 induces aromatase, whereas the product of aromatase enzyme, i.e., estradiol, induces COX-2 and thus PGE_2 formation. It is possible that PGE_2-induced aromatase expression may also play a biological role and represent a therapeutic target in a subset of ovarian carcinomas related to endometriosis.

Aromatase Inhibitors for the Treatment of Ovarian Cancer

Ovarian cancer is the fourth most common cause of cancer death in women. Most patients present at an advanced stage and the disease commonly relapses after primary surgery and chemotherapy. Relapsed ovarian cancer is not curable in the majority of women and responses to salvage chemotherapy are often sustained for less than a year at the expense of toxicities that may diminish quality of life.

In experimental models of ovarian cancer, it was demonstrated that moderate-high expression of ERα is associated with a growth response to estrogen and these models are growth-inhibited by antiestrogen strategies both in vitro and in vivo.[110-112] In addition, a number of proteins are estrogen regulated and these include the PR, the EGF receptor and HSP27.[113-116]

Clinical studies of tamoxifen in chemoresistant ovarian cancer have suggested that a subset of unselected patients respond to tamoxifen treatment, but the characteristics of responding tumors have not been defined. In one study, 105 patients in first relapse received tamoxifen and an overall response rate of 17% was reported.[117] This was later reanalyzed to give a 13% response rate in cisplatin-resistant disease and 15% in cisplatin-sensitive disease.[118] Another trial of tamoxifen reported a 17% response rate in chemoresistant disease.[119] ERα has been suggested to be linked with clinical response, but to date no significant association has been demonstrated.[117]

The therapeutic role of aromatase inhibitors have recently been explored in advanced ovarian cancer. Phase II studies suggested that aromatase inhibitors are at least as effective as other hormonal treatments in advanced ovarian cancer.[24-27] Because of the significant epidemiological association of estrogen with ovarian cancer, the minimal side effects of aromatase inhibitors and demonstrated activity of hormonal therapies in other endocrine associated malignancies, further study is needed.

Conclusion

Estrogen is positively linked to the pathogenesis and growth of three common women's cancers (breast, endometrium and ovary). A single gene encodes the key enzyme for estrogen biosynthesis named aromatase, inhibition of which effectively eliminates estrogen production in the entire body. Aromatase inhibitors successfully treat breast cancer, whereas their roles in endometrial and ovarian cancers are less clear and need further exploration.

Acknowledgement

This research work was supported, in part, by the NIH grants CA67167, HD38691 and HD46260 and grants from the AVON Foundation, Northwestern Memorial Foundation, Lynn Sage Cancer Research Foundation and the Friends of Prentice (to SEB).

References

1. Simpson ER, Clyne C, Rubin G et al. Aromatase—a brief overview. Annu Rev Physiol 2002; 64:93-127.
2. Sebastian S, Bulun SE. A highly complex organization of the regulatry region of the human CYP19 (aromatase) gene revealed by the human genome project. J Clin Endocrinol Metab 2001; 86:4600-4602.

3. Simpson ER, Mahendroo MS, Means GD et al. Aromatase cytochrome P450, the enzyme responsible for estrogen biosynthesis. Endocr Rev // 1994; 15:342-355.
4. Bulun SE, Simpson ER. Competitive RT-PCR analysis indicates levels of aromatase cytochrome P450 transcripts in adipose tissue of buttocks, thighs and abdomen of women increase with advancing age. J Clin Endocrinol Metab 1994; 78:428-432.
5. Grodin JM, Siiteri PK, MacDonald PC. Source of estrogen production in postmenopausal women. J Clin Endocrinol Metab 1973; 36:207-214.
6. MacDonald PC, Madden JD, Brenner PF et al. Origin of estrogen in normal men and in women with testicular feminization. J Clin Endocrinol Metab 1979; 49:905-916.
7. Shozu M, Sebastian S, Takayama K et al. Estrogen excess associated with novel gainoffunction mutations affecting the aromatase gene. N Engl J Med 2003; 348(19):1855-1865.
8. Mahendroo MS, Mendelson CR, Simpson ER. Tissuespecific and hormonallycontrolled alternative promoters regulate aromatase cytochrome P450 gene expression in human adipose tissue. J Biol Chem 1993; 268:19463-19470.
9. Bulun S. Aromatase deficiency and estrogen resistance: from molecular genetics to clinic. Semin Reprod Med 2000; 2000:31-39.
10. Zhao Y NJ, Bulun SE, Mendelson CR et al. Aromatase P450 gene expression in human adipose tissue: Role of a Jak/STAT pathway in regulation of the adiposespecific promoter. J Biol Chem 1995; 270:16449-16457.
11. Kamat A, Alcorn J, Kunczt C et al. Characterization of the regulatory regions of the human aromatase (P450arom) gene involved in placentaspecific expression. Mol Endocrinol 1998; 12:1764-1777.
12. Jiang B, Kamat A, Mendelson C. Hypoxia prevents induction of aromatase expression in human trophoblast cells in culture: potential inhibitory role of the hypoxia-inducible transcription factor Mash-2 (mammalian achaetescute homologous protein-2). Mol Endocrinol 2000; 14:1661-1673.
13. Zhao Y, Agarwal VR, Mendelson CR et al. Estrogen biosynthesis proximal to a breast tumor is stimulated by PGE2 via cyclic AMP, leading to activation of promoter II of the CYP19 (aromatase) gene. Endocrinology 1996; 137(12):5739-5742.
14. Bulun SE, Noble LS, Takayama K et al. Endocrine disorders associated with inappropriately high aromatase expression. J Steroid Biochem Mol Biol 1997; 61:133-139.
15. Bulun SE, Lin Z, Imir G et al. Regulation of aromatase expression in estrogen-responsive breast and uterine disease: from bench to treatment. Pharmacol Rev 2005; 57(3):359-383.
16. Bulun SE, Economos K, Miller D et al. CYP19 (aromatase cytochrome P450) gene expression in human malignant endometrial tumors. J Clin Endocrinol Metab 1994; 79:1831-1834.
17. Burnett AF BA, Amezcua C. Anastrozole, an aromatase inhibitor and medroxyprogesterone acetate therapy in premenopausal obese women with endometrial cancer: a report of two cases successfully treated without hysterectomy. Gynecol Oncol 2004; 94:832-834.
18. Rose PG BV, VanLe L, Bell J et al. A phase II trial of anastrozole in advanced recurrent or persistent endometrial carcinoma: a Gynecologic Oncology Group Study. Gynecol Oncol 2000; 78(2):212-216.
19. Somigliana E, Vigano P, Parazzini F et al. Association between endometriosis and cancer: a comprehensive review and a critical analysis of clinical and epidemiological evidence. Gynecol Oncol 2006; 101(2):331-341.
20. Vercellini P, Scarfone G, Bolis G et al. Site of origin of epithelial ovarian cancer: the endometriosis connection. Br J Obst Gynec 2000; 107(9):1155-1157.
21. Schildkraut JM, Calingaert B, Marchbanks PA et al. Impact of progestin and estrogen potency in oral contraceptives on ovarian cancer risk. J Natl Cancer Inst 2002; 94(1):32-38.
22. Rodriguez GC, Nagarsheth NP, Lee KL et al. Progestininduced apoptosis in the Macaque ovarian epithelium: differential regulation of transforming growth factorbeta. J Natl Cancer Inst 2002; 94(1):50-60.
23. Ho SM. Estrogen, progesterone and epithelial ovarian cancer. Reprod Biol Endocrinol 2003; 1:73.
24. Papadimitriou CA, Markaki S, Siapkaras J et al. Hormonal therapy with letrozole for relapsed epithelial ovarian cancer. Longterm results of a phase II study. Oncology 2004; 66(2):112-117.
25. Bowman A, Gabra H, Langdon SP et al. CA125 response is associated with estrogen receptor expression in a phase II trial of letrozole in ovarian cancer: identification of an endocrine-sensitive subgroup. Clin Cancer Res 2002; 8(7):2233-2239.
26. del Carmen MG, Fuller AF, Matulonis U et al. Phase II trial of anastrozole in women with asymptomatic mullerian cancer. Gynecol Oncol 2003; 91(3):596-602.
27. Lee EJ DM, Hughes JL, Lee JH et al. Metastasis to sigmoid colon mucosa and submucosa from serous borderline ovarian tumor: response to hormone therapy. Int J Gynecol Cancer 2006; 16(Suppl 1):295-299.
28. Meng L, Zhou J, Hironobu S et al. TNFalpha and IL-11 secreted by malignant breast epithelial cells inhibit adipocyte differentiation by selectively downregulating C/EBPalpha and PPARgamma: mechanism of desmoplastic reaction. Cancer Res 2001; 61:2250-2255.

29. Zhou J, Gurates B, Yang S et al. Malignant breast epithelial cells stimulate aromatase expression via promoter II in human adipose fibroblasts: an epithelial-stromal interaction in breast tumors mediated by C/EBPbeta. Cancer Res 2001; 61:2328-2334.

30. Haagensen CD. Diseases of the breast. Vol 3rd. Philadelphia: W.B. Saunders Company; 1986.

31. Agarwal VR, Bulun SE, Leitch M et al. Use of alternative promoters to express the aromatase cytochrome P450 (CYP19) gene in breast adipose tissues of cancer-free and breast cancer patients. J Clin Endocrinol Metab 1996; 81:3843-3849.

32. Harada N, Utsumi T, Takagi Y. Tissuespecific expression of the human aromatase cytochrome P450 gene by alternative use of multiple exons I and promoters and switching of tissue-specific exons I in carcinogenesis. Proc Natl Acad Sci U S A (USA) 1993; 90:11312-11316.

33. Utsumi T, Harada N, Maruta M et al. Presence of alternatively spliced transcripts of aromatase gene in human breast cancer. J Clin Endocrinol Metab 1996; 81:2344-2349.

34. Zhou C, Zhou D, Esteban J et al. Aromatase gene expression and its exon I usage in human breast tumors. Detection of aromatase messenger RNA by reverse transcription-polymerase chain reaction. J Steroid Biochem Mol Biol 1996; 59:163-171.

35. Sebastian S, Takayama K, Shozu M et al. Cloning and characterization of a novel endothelial promoter of the human CYP19 (aromatase P450) gene that is upregulated in breast cancer tissue. Mol Endocrinol 2002; 16:2243-2254.

36. MacDonald PC, Grodin JM, Siiteri PK. The utilization of plasma androstenedione for estrone production in women. In: Ebling CGc-eFJG, ed. Excerpta Medica Int. Congr Series No. 184, Progress in Endocrinology, Proceedings of the Third International Congress of Endocrinology 1968 (Mexico). Amsterdam: Excerpta Medica Foundation; 1968:770-776.

37. Hemsell DL GJ, Brenner PF, Siiteri PK et al. Plasma precursors of estrogen. II. Correlation of the extent of conversion of plasma androstenedione to estrone with age. J Clin Endocrin Metab 1974; 38:476-479.

38. MacDonald PC, Edman CD, Hemsell DL et al. Effect of obesity on conversion of plasma androstenedione to estrone in postmenopausal women with and without endometrial cancer. Am J Obstet Gynecol 1978; 130:448-455.

39. Hankinson S, Willett W, Manson J et al. Plasma sex steroid hormone levels and risk of breast cancer in postmenopausal women. J Natl Cancer Inst 1999; 90:1292-1299.

40. Huang Z, Hankinson SE, Colditz GA et al. Dual effects of weight and weight gain on breast cancer risk. JAMA 1997; 278:1407-1411.

41. Brodie A, Lu Q, Liu Y et al. Aromatase inhibitors and their antitumor effects in model systems. Endocr Relat Cancer 1999; 6:205-210.

42. Brodie A, Lu Q, Long B. Aromatase and its inhibitors. J Steroid Biochem and Mol Biol 1999; 69:205-210.

43. Chetrite G, Cortes-Prieto J, Philippe J et al. Comparison of estrogen concentrations, estrone sulfatase and aromatase activities in normal and in cancerous, human breast tissues. J Steroid Biochemistry and Molecular Biology 2000; 72:23-27.

44. Geisler J, Berntsen H, Lonning P. A novel HPLCRIA method for the simultaneous detection of estrone, estradiol and estrone sulphate levels in breast cancear tissue. J Steroid Biochemistry & Molecular Biology 2000; 72:259-264.

45. Van Landeghem AAJ, Poortman J, Nabuurs M et al. Endogenous concentration and subcellular distribution of estrogens in normal and malignant human breast tissue. Cancer Res 1985; 45:2907-2912.

46. O'Neill JS, Elton RA, Miller WR. Aromatase activity in adipose tissue from breast quadrants: a link with tumor site. British Medical Journal 1988; 296:741-743.

47. Bulun SE, Price TM, Mahendroo MS et al. A link between breast cancer and local estrogen biosynthesis suggested by quantification of breast adipose tissue aromatase cytochrome P450 transcripts using competitive polymerase chain reaction after reverse transcription. J Clin Endocrinol Metab 1993; 77:1622-1628.

48. Sasano H, Nagura H, Harada N et al. Immunolocalization of aromatase and other steroidogenic enzymes in human breast disorders. Hum Pathol 1994; 25:530-535.

49. Reed MJ, Topping L, Coldham NG et al. Control of aromatase activity in breast cancer cells: the role of cytokines and growth factors. J Steroid Biochem Mol Biol 1993; 44:589-596.

50. Agarwal VR, Ashanullah CI, Simpson ER et al. Alternatively spliced transcripts of the aromatase cytochrome P450 (CYP19) gene in adipose tissue of women. J Clin Endocrinol Metab 1997; 82:70-74.

51. Agarwal VR, Bulun SE, Simpson ER. Quantitative detection of alternatively spliced transcripts of the aromatase cytochrome P450 (CYP19) gene in aromataseexpressing human cells by competitive RT-PCR. Mol Cellular Probes 1995; 9:453-464.

52. Yue W, Zhou D, Chen S et al. A new nude mouse model for postmenopausal breast cancer using MCF-7 cells transfected with the human aromatase gene. Cancer Res 1994; 54:5092-5095.

53. Tekmal R, N K, Gill K et al. Aromatase overexpression and breast hyperplasia, an in vivo model—continued overexpression of aromatase is sufficient to maintain hyperplasia without circulating estrogens and aromatase inhibitors abrogate these preneoplasatic changes in mammary glands. Endocr Relat Cancer 1999; 6:307-314.

54. Kovacic A. SC, Simpson ER, Clyne CD. Inhibition of aromatase transcription via promoter II by short heterodimer partner in human preadipocytes. Mol Endocrinol 2004; 18:252-259.

55. Price T, Aitken J, Head J et al. Determination of aromatase cytochrome P450 messenger RNA in human breast tissues by competitive polymerase chain reaction (PCR) amplification. J Clin Endocrinol Metab 1992; 74:1247-1252.

56. Ackerman GE, Smith ME, Mendelson CR et al. Aromatization of androstenedione by human adipose tissue stromal cells in monolayer culture. J Clin Endocrinol Metab 1981; 53:412-417.

57. Santen RJ, Martel J, Hoagland M et al. Stromal spindle cells contain aromatase in human breast tumors. J Clin Endocrinol Metab 1994; 79:627-632.

58. Sasano H, Frost A, Saitoh R et al. Aromatase and 17beta-hydroxysteroid dehydrogenase type 1 in human breast carcinoma. J Clin Endocrinol Metab 1996; 81:4042-4046.

59. Brodie A, Long B, Lu Q. Aromatase expression in the human breast. Breast Cancer Res Treat 1998; 49:S85-91.

60. Sasano H, Edwards DP, Anderson TJ et al. Validation of new aromatase monoclonal antibodies for immunohistochemistry: progress report. J Steroid Biochem Mol Biol 2003; 86:239-244.

61. Pauley R, Santner S, Tait L et al. Regulation of CYP19 aromatase transcription in breast stromal fibroblasts. J Clin Endocrin and Metabo 2000; 85:837-846.

62. Crichton MB, Nichols JE, Zhao Y et al. Expression of transcripts of interleukin-6 and related cytokines by human breast tumors, breast cancer cells and adipose stromal cells. Mol Cell Endocrinol 1996; 118:215-220.

63. Hube F, Hauner H. The two tumor necrosis factor receptors mediate opposite effects on differentiation and glucose metabolism in human adipocytes in primary culture. Endocrinology 2000; 141:2582-2588.

64. Deb S AS, Imir AG, Yilmaz MB et al. Estrogen regulates expression of tumor necrosis factor receptors in breast adipose fibroblasts. J Clin Endocrinol Metab 2004; 89:4018-4024.

65. Clyne CD, Speed CJ, Zhou J et al. Liver receptor homologue-1 (LRH-1) regulates expression of aromatase in preadipocytes. J Biol Chem 2002; 277:20591-20597.

66. Karuppu D, Kalus A, Simpson Er et al. Aromatase and prostaglandin inter-relationships in breast adipose tissue: significance for breast cancer development. Breast Cancer Res Treat 2002; 76:103-109.

67. Brueggemeier RW, Quinn AL, Parrett ML et al. Correlation of aromatase and cyclooxygenase gene expression in human breast cancer specimens. Cancer Lett 1999(140):27-35.

68. Richards JA, Petrel TA, Brueggemeier RW. Signaling pathways regulating aromatase and cyclooxygenases in normal and malignant breast cells. J Steroid Biochem 2002; 80:203-212.

69. Deb S, Jianfeng Z, Amin SA et al. A novel role of sodium butyrate in the regulation of cancer-associated aromatase promoters I.3 and II by disrupting a transcriptional complex in breast adipose fibroblasts. J Biol Chem 2006; 281(5):2585-2597.

70. Chen S, Itoh T, Wu K et al. Transcriptional regulation of aromatase expression in human breast tissue. J Steroid Biochem Mol Biol 2002; 83:93-99.

71. Ruohola J, Valve E, Karkkainen M et al. Vascular endothelial growth factors are differentially regulated by steroid hormones and antiestrogens in breast cancer cells. Mol Cell Endocrinol 1999; 149:29-40.

72. Nakamura J, Lu Q, Aberdeen G et al. The effect of estrogen on aromatase and vascular endothelial growth factor messenger ribonucleic acid in the normal nonhuman primate mammary gland. J Clin Endocrinol Metab 1999; 84:1432-1437.

73. Nakamura J, Savinov A, Lu Q et al. Estrogen regulates vascular endothelial growth/permeability factor expression in 7,12-dimethylbenz(a)anthracene-induced rat mammary tumors. Endocrinology 1996; 137:5589-5596.

74. Shekhar M, Werdell J, Tait L. Interaction with endothelial cells is a prerequisite for branching ducta-lalveolar morphogenesis and hyperplasia of preneoplastic human breast epithelial cells: regulation by estrogen. Cancer Res 2000; 60:439-449.

75. Santen R. To block estrogen's synthesis or action: that is the question. J Clin Endocrinol Metab 2002; 87:3007-3012.

76. Baum M, Budzar AU, Cuzick J et al. Anastrozole alone or in combination with tamoxifen versus tamoxifen alone for adjuvant treatment of postmenopausal women with early breast cancer: first results of the ATAC randomised trial. Lancet 2002; 359:2131-2139.

77. Baum M, Buzdar A, Cuzick J et al. Anastrozole alone or in combination with tamoxifen versus tamoxifen alone for adjuvant treatment of postmenopausal women with early-stage breast cancer: results of the ATAC (Arimidex, Tamoxifen Alone or in Combination) trial efficacy and safety update analyses. Cancer 2003; 98(9):1802-1810.

78. Buzdar AU VI, Sainsbury R. The impact of hormone receptor status on the clinical efficacy of the newgeneration aromatase inhibitors: a review of data from first-line metastatic disease trials in postmenopausal women. Breast J 2004; 10:211-217.

79. Bonneterre J, Thurlimann B, Robertson JF et al. Anastrozole versus tamoxifen as firstline therapy for advanced breast cancer in 668 postmenopausal women: results of the tamoxifen or Arimidex randomized group efficacy and tolerability study. J Clin Oncol 2000; 18:3748-3757.

80. Goss PE, Ingle JN, Martino S et al. A randomized trial of letrozole in postmenopausal women after five years of tamoxifen therapy for early-stage breast cancer. N Engl J Med 2003; 349(19):1793-1802.

81. Mouridsen H, Gershanovich M, Sun Y et al. Superior efficacy of letrozole versus tamoxifen as first-line therapy for postmenopausal women with advanced breast cancer: results of a phase III study of the International Letrozole Breast Cancer Group. J Clin Oncol 2001; 19:2596-2606.

82. Milla-Santos A, Milla L, Portella J et al. Anastrozole versus tamoxifen as first-line therapy in postmenopausal patients with hormone-dependent advanced breast cancer: a prospective, randomized, phase III study. Am J Clin Onc 2003; 26:317-322.

83. Paridaens R, Dirix L, Lohrisch C et al. Mature results of a randomized phase II multicenter study of exemestane versus tamoxifen as first-line hormone therapy for postmenopausal women with metastatic breast cancer. Ann Oncol 2003; 14:1391-1398.

84. Lu Q, Yue W, Wang J et al. The effects of aromatase inhibitors and antiestrogens in the nude mouse model. Breast Cancer Res Treat 1998; 50:63-71.

85. Dixon J, Renshaw L, Bellamy C et al. The effects of neoadjuvant anastrozole (Arimidex) on tumor volume in postmenopausal women with breast cancer: a randomized, double-blind, single-center study. Clin Cancer Res 2000; 6:2229-2235.

86. Bulun SE, Yang S, Fang Z et al. Role of aromatase in endometrial disease. J Steroid Biochem Mol Biol 2001; 79:19-25.

87. Inoue M, Kyo S, Fujita M et al. Coexpression of the ckit receptor and the stem cell factor in gynecological tumors. Cancer Res 1994; 54(11):3049-3053.

88. Nagasako S, Asanuma N, Nagata Y. [Plasma concentration of estrogens and androgens in postmenopausal women with or without endometrial cancer]. Nippon Sanka Fujinka Gakkai Zasshi 1988; 40(6):707-713.

89. Potischman N, Swanson CA, Siiteri P et al. Reversal of relation between body mass and endogenous estrogen concentrations with menopausal status. J Natl Cancer Inst 1996; 88(11):756-758.

90. Sherman ME, Sturgeon S, Brinton LA et al. Risk factors and hormone levels in patients with serous and endometrioid uterine carcinomas. Mod Pathol 1997; 10(10):963-968.

91. Vermeulen-Meiners C, Poortman J, Haspels AA et al. The endogenous concentration of estradiol and estrone in pathological human postmenopausal endometrium. J Steroid Biochem 1986; 24(5):1073-1078.

92. Berstein LM, Tchernobrovkina AE, Gamajunova VB et al. Tumor estrogen content and clinico-morphological and endocrine features of endometrial cancer. J Cancer Res Clin Oncol 2003; 129(4):245-249.

93. Yamamoto T, Kitawaki J, Urabe M et al. Estrogen production of endometrium and endometrial cancer tissue; influence of aromatase on proliferation of endometrial cancer cells. J Steroid Biochem Mol Biol 1993; 44:463-468.

94. Watanabe K, Sasano H, Harada N et al. Aromatase in human endometrial carcinoma and hyperplasia. Immunohistochemical, in situ hybridization and biochemical studies. American Journal of Pathology 1995; 146:491-500.

95. Berstein L, Maximov S, Gershfeld E et al. Neoadjuvant therapy of endometrial cancer with the aromatase inhibitor letrozole: endocrine and clinical effects. Eur J Obstet Gynecol Reprod Biol 2002; 105(2):161-165.

96. Sasano H, Sato S, Ito K et al. Effects of aromatase inhibitors on the pathobiology of the human breast, endometrial and ovarian carcinoma. Endocr Relat Cancer 1999; 6(2):197-204.

97. Yamamoto T, Fukuoka M, Fujimoto Y et al. Inhibitory effect of a new androstenedione derivative, 14 alpha-hydroxy-4-androstene-3,6,17-trione (14 alpha-OHAT) on aromatase activity of human uterine tumors. J Steroid Biochem 1990; 36:517-521.

98. Duffy S, Jackson TL, Lansdown M et al. The ATAC adjuvant breast cancer trial in postmenopausal women: baseline endometrial subprotocol data. Bjog 2003; 110(12):1099-1106.

99. Lacey JV Jr, Mink PJ, Lubin JH et al. Menopausal hormone replacement therapy and risk of ovarian cancer. JAMA 2002; 288(3):334-341.

100. Anderson GL, Limacher M, Assaf AR et al. Effects of conjugated equine estrogen in postmenopausal women with hysterectomy: the Women's Health Initiative randomized controlled trial. JAMA 2004; 291(14):1701-1712.
101. Giudice L, Kao L. Endometriosis. Lancet 2004; 364:1789-1799.
102. Zeitoun K, Takayama K, Michael MD et al. Stimulation of aromatase P450 promoter (II) activity in endometriosis and its inhibition in endometrium are regulated by competitive binding of SF-1 and COUP-TF to the same cis-acting element. J Mol Endocrinol 1999; 13:239-253.
103. Yang S, Fang Z, Takashi S et al. Regulation of aromatase P450 expression in endometriotic and endometrial stromal cells by CCAT/enhancer binding proteins: decreased C/EBPbeta in endometriosis is associated with overexpression of aromatase. J Clin Endocrinol Metab 2002; 87:2336-2345.
104. Gurates B, Sebastian S, Yang S et al. WT1 and DAX-1 inhibit aromatase P450 expression in human endometrial and endometriotic stromal cells. J Clin Endocrinol Metab 2002; 87:4369-4377.
105. Fang ZJ, Yang S, Gurates G et al. Genetic or enzymatic disruption of aromatase inhibits the growth of ectopic uterine tissue. J Clin Endocrinol Metab 2002; 87:3460-3466.
106. Kitawaki J, Noguchi T, Amatsu T et al. Expression of aromatase cytochrome P450 protein and messenger ribonucleic acid in human endometriotic and adenomyotic tissues but not in normal endometrium. Biol Reprod 1997; 57:514-519.
107. Noble LS, Takayama K, Putman JM et al. Prostaglandin E2 stimulates aromatase expression in endometriosis-derived stromal cells. J Clin Endocrinol Metab 1997; 82:600-606.
108. Tsai SJ, Wu MH, Lin CC et al. Regulation of steroidogenic acute regulatory protein expression and progesterone production in endometriotic stromal cells. J Clin Endocrinol Metab 2001; 86:5765-5773.
109. Sun HS, Hsiao KY, Hsu CC et al. Transactivation of steroidogenic acute regulatory protein in human endometriotic stromalcells is mediated by the prostaglandin EP2 receptor. Endocrinology 2003; 144:3934-3942.
110. Langdon SP, Hawkes MM, Lawrie SS et al. Oestrogen receptor expression and the effects of oestrogen and tamoxifen on the growth of human ovarian carcinoma cell lines. Br J Cancer 1990; 62(2):213-216.
111. Langdon SP, Ritchie A, Young K et al. Contrasting effects of 17 beta-estradiol on the growth of human ovarian carcinoma cells in vitro and in vivo. Int J Cancer 1993; 55(3):459-464.
112. Langdon SP, Crew AJ, Ritchie AA et al. Growth inhibition of oestrogen receptor-positive human ovarian carcinoma by anti-oestrogens in vitro and in a xenograft model. Eur J Cancer 1994; 30A(5):682-686.
113. Langdon SP, Hirst GL, Miller EP et al. The regulation of growth and protein expression by estrogen in vitro: a study of 8 human ovarian carcinoma cell lines. J Steroid Biochem Mol Biol 1994; 50(3-4):131-135.
114. Langdon SP, Gabra H, Bartlett JM et al. Functionality of the progesterone receptor in ovarian cancer and its regulation by estrogen. Clin Cancer Res 1998; 4(9):2245-2251.
115. Simpson BJ, Langdon SP, Rabiasz GJ et al. Estrogen regulation of transforming growth factor-alpha in ovarian cancer. J Steroid Biochem Mol Biol 1998; 64(3-4):137-145.
116. Langdon SP, Rabiasz GJ, Hirst GL et al. Expression of the heat shock protein HSP27 in human ovarian cancer. Clin Cancer Res 1995; 1(12):1603-1609.
117. Hatch KD, Beecham JB, Blessing JA et al. Responsiveness of patients with advanced ovarian carcinoma to tamoxifen. A Gynecologic Oncology Group study of secondline therapy in 105 patients. Cancer 1991; 68(2):269-271.
118. Markman M, Iseminger KA, Hatch KD et al. Tamoxifen in platinum-refractory ovarian cancer: a Gynecologic Oncology Group Ancillary Report. Gynecol Oncol 1996; 62(1):4-6.
119. Ahlgren JD, Ellison NM, Gottlieb RJ et al. Hormonal palliation of chemoresistant ovarian cancer: three consecutive phase II trials of the Mid-Atlantic Oncology Program. J Clin Oncol 1993; 11(10):1957-1968.

Proteomics of Cancer of Hormone-Dependent Tissues

Darren R. Tyson* and David K. Ornstein

Abstract

Serum and tissue biomarkers have begun to play an increasingly important role in the detection and management of many cancers of hormone-sensitive tissues. Specifically, the introduction of serum PSA measurements into clinical practice has dramatically altered detection and treatment of prostate cancer and serum tumor markers play a critical role in the management of testicular cancer. Serum biomarkers are used for ovarian and pancreatic cancers, but their usefulness is limited by poor specificity. Tissue biomarkers are used to help guide breast cancer treatment but are not widely used in other cancers. Even the "best" biomarkers such as PSA have substantial limitations. The discovery of new biomarkers for both early detection and prognosis of cancer is critical to the hope of better clinical outcomes. Recently there has been an expanding understanding of the underlying molecular etiology of cancer and molecular targeted therapies for some particularly aggressive cancers such as renal cell carcinoma have been developed. Better understanding of the molecular etiology of cancer and identification of additional therapeutic targets remain important research goals. Currently, there are very few patient-tailored therapies and there is a great need to better understand the molecular alterations associated with cancer and to use this information to design need cancer therapies and prevention strategies.

Advances in proteomic technologies have created tremendous opportunities for biomarker discovery and biological studies of cancer. The potential that proteomics will impact clinical practice is currently greater than ever, but there main several obstacles in making this a reality. A major hurdle to overcome continues to be the proper acquisition of patient tissues and body fluids for investigation and clinical diagnostics. Each cancer has specific issues in this regard and it is incumbent upon investigators and collaborating clinicians to understand the various nuances of tissue and biofluid procurement. This chapter not only reviews the clinical need and potential impact of proteomic studies of hormone-sensitive cancers, but details specific technologies and discusses the issues surrounding tissue/biofluid procurement.

Introduction and Overview

Clinical Perspective

In the United States, cancer of hormone-sensitive tissues represent a majority of solid tumors, with prostate and breast cancers being the most common types of noncutaneous malignancies in men and women, respectively. Ovarian and pancreatic cancers are less common but usually lethal when they do occur. Pancreatic cancer is responsible for 6% of cancer deaths in both men

*Corresponding Author: Darren R. Tyson—Departments of Urology and Physiology and Biophysics, University of California Irvine Medical Center, 101 The City Dr. South, Bldg 55, Rm. 300, Orange, CA 92868, USA. Email: darren@uci.edu

Innovative Endocrinology of Cancer, edited by Lev M. Berstein and Richard J. Santen.
©2008 Landes Bioscience and Springer Science+Business Media.

and women and ovarian cancer for 6% of cancer deaths in women.[1] In contemporary practice, serum biomarkers have the greatest role in prostate cancer management. Prostate specific antigen (PSA) is widely accepted as a serum biomarker for prostate cancer (CaP) and is used extensively for screening, staging and monitoring patients after treatment.[2] CA-125 is considered the best biomarker for ovarian cancer, although it is not recommended for widespread screening due to a lack of specificity.[3] Similarly, CA19-9 is a widely used marker of pancreatic cancer, but it lacks sufficient specificity and sensitivity to be used for screening purposes.[4] Biomarkers play an important role in staging and monitoring patient with testicular cancer. Alpha-fetoprotein (AFP) is highly specific for nonseminomatous germ cell tumors and human chorionic gonadotropin (bHCG) is elevated in more than 50% of nonseminomatous germ cell tumors and approximately 10% of pure seminomas.[5] There are currently no useful serum biomarkers for the detection of breast or adrenal cancers. In most cases, early detection improves the outcome for cancer treatment. Although biomarkers have begun to play a role in detection and management of some cancers, for most there is either no useful serum biomarkers or the available biomarker lacks sufficient specificity and sensitivity for use as a screening tool.

Although serum (or potentially another body fluid) is the most useful source to measure biomarkers for early detection, tissue biomarkers are now being used more often to help determine the most appropriate treatment for a specific patient or follow response to therapy. For example, tissue biomarkers such as HER-2 and estrogen and progesterone receptor levels are used for prognostication and to direct treatment in breast cancer. Unfortunately, targeting these molecules has not proven to be a sufficient means to completely eradicate these cancers as they tend to develop resistance to uni-targeted therapies.[6] CA-125 is often used to monitor treatment of ovarian cancer, but is not always helpful since many of these tumors do not express this protein.[3] For testicular cancer, AFP and bHCG are used to monitor response to chemotherapy and are used to direct further therapy.[7] The molecular determinants of prostate, ovarian, endometrial and pancreatic carcinogenesis remain ill-defined; therefore, no molecular based prognostic tools are commonly used for these cancers.

The Cancer Phenotype

It is a widely held belief that in most cases the malignant phenotype originates from inherited germline genetic alterations, acquired somatic mutations, or by epigenetic phenomena. Examination of the changes occurring in cancer at the nucleic acid level has resulted in invaluable information about disease development and progression. More recently, advances in gene expression profiling technologies have allowed for global analysis of expression levels of thousands of mRNA transcripts simultaneously. This information has begun to be used for disease classification to help clinicians with prognosis and treatment. Malignant transforming genetic alterations are typically manifested as either a loss or a gain of function of a specific regulatory protein. These tumor suppressors or oncogenes are commonly responsible for how a cell responds to its environment and may cause inappropriate proliferation, migration, survival or other cancer-defining responses.

Although many biomarker discovery studies have focused on RNA expression analysis, there are, however, distinct advantages of proteomic studies; above all, proteins are ultimately responsible for the disease phenotype. In addition, proteomics can identify alterations in posttranslational modifications, subcellular localization and proteolytic cleavage events, and protein levels are not necessarily reflective of RNA-based expression studies. Furthermore, since most FDA-approved diagnostic tests are protein based, directly studying proteins and their variants should expedite the development of clinically useful tests. Traditionally, proteomic studies have focused on biomarker discovery and clinical tests are typically antibody-based and directed at individual biomarkers. Technological advances, however, have increased the throughput and accuracy of protein analysis and it is possible that some of these analytical instruments will be usable for proteomic-based clinical assays rather than relying on the development of antibodies, a laborious and time-consuming process that is not guaranteed to succeed.[8]

Many different scientific strategies have utilized a variety of biospecimens to identify novel cancer biomarkers. Some studies have focused on the molecular alterations occurring in cancerous tissue as well as the surrounding stroma; others have concentrated on circulating blood, other body fluids, or distant tissues that may be affected by the developing tumor. The study of these tissues and fluids at the protein level is broadly referred to as proteomics.

Proteomics Defined

Proteomics can be defined in many ways depending on the desired scope and complexity of the analysis. In the main, proteomic analyses aim to characterize all the proteins present within a particular cell, tissue or organ. However, since a single gene can encode multiple proteins via different exon usage or splicing events and proteins are invariably modified posttranslationally (e.g., phosphorylation and acetylation), a single gene can produce tens to hundreds and possibly thousands of unique proteins within a single cell. In addition, proteins are constantly being modified and any single analysis only represents a snapshot of the ongoing milieu. Not surprisingly, variability is a considerable problem in the field of proteomics. In spite of these difficulties, proteomic analyses have provided substantial new insight into our understanding of cancer as well as powerful new techniques for finding biological markers to detect and analyze cancer development, progression and response to treatment. The goal of this chapter is to summarize some of the recent studies using proteomic analyses on endocrine-regulated cancers, to describe advantages and limitations of these approaches, to discuss potential clinical applications of these findings and to provide insight into the future directions that proteomics will take cancer biology and clinical management of these common cancers. Proteomic techniques that have been used to identify biomarkers in different sample sources (e.g., blood or tumor tissue) will also be discussed.

Biomarkers versus Biology

Numerous tools have been developed to provide both quantitative and qualitative information about protein composition in tumor tissue and biofluids. Application of these tools to the study of cancer has generally focused on two distinct yet complementary goals: (1) understanding how cancer develops and progresses and (2) cataloguing new biomarkers associated with a particular tumor type. In each case, the application of proteomics is primarily discovery-driven and does not have a specific hypothesis as a prerequisite. Regardless, validation of results generated using discovery-based approaches are critical.[9] To date, most of the efforts in this arena have been put toward the discovery phase with very little follow through on the validation. Few, if any, biomarkers identified with proteomic technologies have been validated by clinical trials and approved by regulatory agencies.[8]

In the past, studies designed to understand the biological basis of cancer have involved a reductionist approach aimed to reduce the complexity of analysis.[10] However, with recent major advances in the fields of bioinformatics and computational technology the inherent complexity can now be examined en masse in what is referred to as systems biology.[10-12] Thus, the use of highly sensitive and quantitative proteomic techniques coupled with the new computational capabilities permit an unbiased cataloging of molecular changes associated with cancer initiation and progression. This provides an unprecedented opportunity for discovering new clinically useful biomarkers and gaining new insight into tumor biology.

Cancer Proteomics: Sample Sources and Methodological Approaches

Cancerous Human Tissue

Typically, cancerous tissue is the most fertile source to procure relevant molecular information. However, for many human cancers an invasive procedure is required to obtain tissue samples for analysis. For example, in order to procure prostate cancer specimens a transrectal needle biopsy of the prostate or a radical prostatectomy is required. In addition, due to widespread screening and better detection modalities for cancers of the breast and prostate, most of these cancers are detected as low-volume disease; there is often only a limited amount of cancerous tissue present even within a radical prostatectomy specimen. Furthermore, the infiltrative nature of prostatic adenocarcinomas makes isolation of pure cell populations of cancer cells difficult. This is also true for pancreatic ductal adenocarcinoma in which the tumor is comprised of 30-90% tumor cells with a large amount of fibroblastic infiltration.[13] While it is becoming much more appreciated that the surrounding stroma is a major contributor to tumor biology,[14] the primary focus of most studies of the tumor involve the cancerous epithelial cells themselves (the vast majority of cancers are adenocarcinomas).

In order to minimize the contribution of contaminated stroma and inflammatory cells in the proteomic analyses, different methods have been developed for procuring pure populations of cells from human tissues. Laser capture microdissection is a relatively new technique that allows researchers to visualize a tissue section via light microscopy and procure the desired cells by activating a 7.5 to 30 μm diameter infrared laser beam to "weld" the tissue to a plastic cap. Intact DNA, RNA and protein can then be extracted from the "welded" tissue and analyzed by conventional methods.[15,16] Proteomic studies utilizing two-dimensional gel electrophoresis (2DGE) analysis of LCM procured benign and cancerous prostate cells have been successfully performed. Through this approach annexin I was found to be under-expressed in early stage CaP,[17,18] and subsequent studies have confirmed that annexin I and annexin II are commonly reduced in CaP and that these molecules may be useful tissue biomarkers.[19] LCM has been used extensively to isolate tumor cells from breast cancer for subsequent proteomic analyses,[20-29] and at least two groups have used LCM to aid in the isolation of pure populations of tumor cells from ovarian tumors that are frequently highly infiltrative at initial detection.[30,31] Similarly, studies on pancreatic,[32] and renal cancers[33] have also relied on LCM to enrich the tumor cell population for proteomic-based studies. The major limitations of LCM are: 1) it is extremely labor intensive (although new systems that provide automated cell selection and cutting have at least partially alleviated this) and 2) for optimal extraction of macromolecules the input tissue should be cryopreserved rather than formalin-fixed.

Although LCM is the most frequently employed tool for separating tumor cells from benign cells and stroma, other techniques have also been employed. These include short-term culture of enzymatically disaggregated cells[34-36] or immunomagnetic bead separation of individual cells.[37,38] Short-term culture is useful to provide a cellular amplification step to increase sample size when available tissue is limiting. However, even short-term culture of cells may induce changes in response to nonnative growth conditions that may mask relevant markers of malignancy. The use of immunocapture beads to isolate cells from disaggregated tumors allows tumor cell enrichment without requiring the cells to proliferate and would therefore alleviate the risk of cellular changes induced by culture but would eliminate the amplification step.

Historically, the stalwart platform for proteomics has been two dimensional gel electrophoresis (2DGE).[39] Although the technique has been in use for over three decades, recent modifications to the technique have enhanced the dynamic range and resolution of protein discrimination enabling this technique to remain as a common platform for proteomic analyses. Despite these advances, 2DGE is still limited by a relatively small dynamic range (two to three orders of magnitude), difficulty separating highly basic or acidic proteins or those of low molecular mass and the relatively low throughput. Advances in separation technologies and bioinformatics have greatly enhanced the use of mass spectrometry (MS)-based approaches and have begun to replace 2DGE as the proteomic analytic technique of choice.

Determining the cellular source of protein production is of critical importance for the proper identification of molecular alterations occur during the transition from benign to malignant tissue. For 2DGE, relative expression levels can now be determined much more accurately using differentially labeled samples that are run simultaneously on the same gel.[39] Gel-to-gel variability, a well-known problem of 2DGE, is also mitigated by the use of dually labeled samples run simultaneously. The identification of individual spots on 2D gels is generally accomplished using liquid chromatographic separation of trypsin-digested fragments subjected to tandem mass spectrometry (LC-MS/MS) or matrix-assisted laser desorption/ionization time-of-flight (MALDI-TOF) mass spectrometry.

As outlined in Table 1, many other techniques have been employed to examine the proteome of clinical cancer specimens from hormone-regulated organs, but mass spectrometry (MS) has become the preferred technology. The description and use of MS for proteomic studies has been extensively reviewed.[40-45] However, several innovative MS technologies are worth describing further. Relevant to the analysis of tumor tissue, the elegant work conducted by Caprioli and colleagues has provided a new dimension to MS spectra, specifically tissue localization.[46-48] This is accomplished by directly adding micron-sized matrix droplets onto whole tissue sections and subjecting the tissue to direct MALDI-TOF analysis.[49] This technique has been used to analyze normal mammary epithelium, ductal carcinoma in situ, invasive breast adenocarcinoma and surrounding stroma from sectioned human breast cancer samples.[50] Although no specific peaks were identified, this approach demonstrated definite alterations of spectral patterns from tissue sections containing the various histological phenotypes easily allowing their discrimination on the spectral data alone.[50] The use of spectral data alone has previously been suggested as a diagnostic tool for analyzing serum constituents as described below.

Body Fluids

In clinical practice, most useful biomarkers are measured in serum or plasma. There is an emerging body of data suggesting that for most cancers the assessment of a pattern of multiple biomarkers provides more robust diagnostic and prognostic information than the measurement of a single biomarker. Advances in proteomic technologies have made it possible to rapidly assess complex protein expression patterns in a large number of clinical samples. Surface-enhanced laser desorption ionization time-of-flight (SELDI-TOF) mass spectrometry is a relatively new technology that can profile low molecular weight peptides. SELDI-TOF is a proprietary modification of MALDI-TOF that incorporates an affinity resin on the MALDI plate to facilitate protein capture and purification in a single step prior to subsequent MALDI-TOF analysis.[51-53] This technology produces crude but rapid protein purification and signal amplification with very high throughput and provides a strong platform for cancer biomarker screening by generating a reproducible low molecular protein fingerprint from a miniscule amount of sample (i.e., 1 μl of blood). In addition, no a priori knowledge of specific protein components is required. SELDI-TOF has been used extensively to profile cancer of hormone-sensitive tissues. For example, it has been used to identify protein signatures from nipple aspirates for the discrimination of women with breast cancer from healthy women,[54-56] to discriminate between microdissected benign and malignant cells from prostate tissue[57,58] and to screen for presence of kidney cancer in serum[59] and urine.[60] SELDI-TOF has also been used to detect alterations in serum profiles of men undergoing androgen ablation therapy[61] or radiation[62] for prostate cancer and to screen for diagnostic markers in thyroid cancer[63] and renal cancer.[64]

Because of its ability to rapidly analyze a large number of samples, SELDI-TOF is particularly well suited to generate informative proteomic patterns from serum. Because visual analysis only detects gross changes in protein expression, bioinformatics tools are required to detect subtle differences in patterns of protein expression. Importantly, because of the huge dimensionality of the data, advanced pattern recognition algorithms are required to find the hidden, non-apparent signatures in a background of noise and chaos. Bioinformatics tools, some of which have utilized artificial intelligence based pattern recognition algorithms that evolve and learn, can facilitate the analysis of complex data sets and have been applied to the detection of ovarian and prostate cancer. Using this approach, a diagnostic algorithm was generated that yielded an overall positive predictive value (PPV) of 94% for the diagnosis of ovarian cancer and all 18 women with stage I ovarian cancer were correctly classified by the algorithm.[65] Although these preliminary studies generated highly promising data and demonstrated feasibility of a new diagnostic paradigm, a lack of reproducibility and the inability to identify the proteins and peptides comprising the spectra drew significant criticism of the approach. The use of high-end mass spectrometers like the API QSTAR Pulsar LC/MS/MS System (Applied Biosystems Inc.) has increased mass accuracy that reduces machine-to-machine difference in mass drift. Moreover, the QSTAR can perform direct

Table 1. Examples of proteomic analyses performed on cancers of hormone-regulated organs

Cancer Type	Sample Source	Prefractionation	Analysis Technology	Quantitation	Study Goal	Ref.
Prostate	urine	reverse phase	LC-MS/MS	protein coverage	diagnostic	72
	urine	none	2DGE	spot intensity	diagnostic	73
	serum	none	SELDI-TOF	peak height	diagnostic	68
	serum	cation X	LC-MS/MS	protein coverage	diagnostic	67
	serum	none	antigen array	spot intensity	diagnostic	85
	serum	none	SELDI-TOF	peak height	prognostic	61
	serum	none	Autoantibody array	spot intensity	diagnostic	86
	tumors	LCM	SELDI-TOF	peak height	diagnostic	58
	tumors	manual dissection	high-throughput IB	band intensity	diagnostic	87
	tumor	LCM	SELDI-TOF	peak height	diagnostic	57
	tumor	manual dissection	2DGE	radioiodine	diagnostic	88
	tumor	manual dissection	2DGE	spot intensity	diagnostic	89
	tumor	LCM	2DGE	spot intensity	diagnostic	90
	tumor biopsies	none	LC-MS/MS	none	diagnostic	91
	FFPE tumors	LCM	LC-MS/MS	O^{16}/O^{18}	diagnostic	92
	tumor, LNCaP	LCM	2DGE	spot intensity	diagnostic	93
	LNCaP	microsomal prep	LC-MS/MS	ICAT	diagnostic	94
	LNCaP	secretome	LC-MS/MS	ICAT	diagnostic	95
	LNCaP	none	2DGE	spot intensity	prognostic	96
	LNCaP	none	2DGE	ICAT	diagnostic	97
Breast	nipple aspirate	none	2DGE	spot intensity	diagnostic	75
	nipple aspirate	none	SELDI-TOF	peak height	diagnostic	54
	nipple aspirate	metal affinity cation X	SELDI-TOF	peak height	diagnostic	55
	nipple aspirate	1D-PAGE	LC-MS/MS	ICAT	diagnostic	76
	nipple aspirate	hydrophobic anion X	SELDI-TOF	peak height	diagnostic	56
	serum	none	immunobead array	fluorescence	diagnostic	83
	adipose tissue/fluid	none	2DGE and antibody array	spot intensity	diagnostic	80
	tumor	LCM	reverse-phase array	spot intensity	diagnostic	29
	tumor (HER-2$^{-/+}$)	metal affinity	SELDI	peak height	prognostic	25
	tumor (PR$^{-/+}$)	LCM	2DGE	radioiodine	prognostic	26
	tumor	LCM	2DGE	spot intensity	diagnostic	21
	tumor	LCM	MALDI-TOF	peak height	diagnostic	22
	tumor	LCM	2DGE	O^{16}/O^{18}	diagnostic	23
	tumor(HER-2$^{-/+}$)	LCM	2DGE	spot intensity	prognostic	98

continued on next page

Table 1. Continued

Cancer Type	Sample Source	Prefractionation	Analysis Technology	Quantitation	Study Goal	Ref.
Ovaries	serum	albumin-bound	1D-PAGE/ LC-MS/MS	none	diagnostic	69
	serum	albumin-bound	MALDI-TOF	none	diagnostic	99
	serum	hydrophobic	SELDI-TOF	peak height	diagnostic	65
	tumor	LCM	2DGE	spot intensity	diagnostic	31
	tumor	LCM	reverse-phase array	spot intensity	diagnostic	100
Pancreas	serum	anion X	SELD-TOF	peak height	diagnostic	101
	serum	none	2DGE	fluorescence	diagnostic	102
	plasma	anion X	SELDI-TOF	peak height	diagnostic	103
	plasma	none	2DGE	fluorescence	diagnostic	104
	plasma	none	2DGE	spot intensity	diagnostic	105
	pancreatic juice	1D-PAGE	LC-MS/MS	protein coverage	diagnostic	77
	tumor	LCM	2DGE	spot intensity	diagnostic	32
	tumor	none	high-throughput IB	band intensity	diagnostic	106
	tumor	cation X	LC-MS/MS	ICAT	diagnostic	37
	tumor	LCM	2DGE	fluorescence	diagnostic	107
	cell line	secretome	LC-MS/MS	ICAT	diagnostic	108
	cell line (–/+ Tx)	none	2DGE	spot intensity	prognostic	109
	cell line (–/+ Tx)	none	2DGE	spot intensity	prognostic	110
Kidney	serum	anion X	SELDI-TOF	peak height	diagnostic	59
	urine	cation X	SELDI-TOF	peak height	diagnostic	60
	urine	none	2DGE	spot intensity	diagnostic	74
	tumor	none	2DGE	spot intensity	diagnostic	111
	tumor	LCM	2DGE	radioiodine	diagnostic	112
	tumor	manual dissection	2DGE	spot intensity	diagnostic	33
	tumor	LCM	2DGE	spot intensity	diagnostic	113
	primary cells	none	2DGE	spot intensity	diagnostic	36
	primary cells	none	2DGE	spot intensity	diagnostic	114
	tumor	cation X/metal affinity	SELDI-TOF	peak height	diagnostic	63
Thyroid	serum	C8 reverse phase	MALDI-TOF	peak height	diagnostic	115
	tumor	none	2DGE	fluorescence	diagnostic	116
	tumor	manual dissection	2DGE	spot intensity	diagnostic	117
Endometrium	serum	none	immunobead array	fluorescence	diagnostic	84

continued on next page

Table 1 Abbreviations: LC-MS/MS, liquid chromatography—tandem mass spectrometry; 2DGE, two dimensional gel electrophoresis; SELDI-TOF, surface-enhanced laser desorption/ionization—time of flight mass spectrometry; MALDI-TOF, matrix-assisted laser desorption/ionization—time of flight mass spectrometry; LCM, laser capture microdissection; X, exchange; ICAT, isotope-coded affinity tag; FFPE, formalin-fixed, paraffin-embedded; Tx, treatment

---

MS/MS protein identification, alleviating a major drawback to the use of SELDI, the lack of peak identification.[66]

This concept is not limited to just one type of cancer. An algorithm capable of predicting the presence of prostate cancer with 41% sensitivity has been generated. The artificial intelligence-type pattern recognition algorithm identified correctly 36 of 38 men with prostate cancer (i.e., 95% sensitivity) and 177 of 228 men with benign biopsies (i.e., specificity of 76%). For men with total PSA levels between 4.0 and 10.0 ng/ml, 97 of 137 (71%) were correctly classified as having benign prostates. Thus, if serum proteomic analysis had been used to determine the need for prostate biopsy, 70% of "unnecessary" biopsies could have been prevented while only 5% of cancers would have been missed. Importantly, the algorithm correctly classified all of these men with prostate cancer.[67] Another analytical strategy utilizes a decision tree algorithm that relies on binomial decisions based on heights of a predefined set of specific protein peaks. Using this approach in a blinded test set of 60 men (30 with prostate cancer and 30 with benign prostates) yielded a sensitivity of 83% and a specificity of 97%.[68]

Although body fluids are fertile sources for biomarker discovery they pose several challenges that complicate biomarker discovery. A major difficulty in the direct identification of serum or plasma biomarkers is the high abundance of albumin and other larger carrier molecules, which has historically made it impossible to identify small molecule biomarkers directly from serum or plasma. Traditionally, serum-based biomarker studies have utilized strategies to deplete albumin and immunoglobulins to increase the sensitivity for the lesser abundant proteins. Recent data challenges this experimental paradigm as it has become increasingly apparent that an immense archive of potentially relevant clinical biomarkers exists bound to albumin. In fact, it has been demonstrated that depletion strategies for high-abundant carrier proteins can be exploited as a means to amplify low abundant serum proteins and peptide fragments.[69] This approach and other examples of innovative solutions to technical challenges in clinical proteomics are listed in Table 2.

Blood likely contains only minute quantities of tumor-specific biomarkers due to its presence throughout the body. Hence, organ-proximal fluids (e.g., pancreatic juice and nipple aspirate fluid) may be more useful as source materials, albeit with a loss of ease of acquisition. For urogenital malignancies, urine provides an easily obtainable source material that is likely enriched in tumor-specific molecules. However, urine is also known to vary significantly in protein content even from the same individual, making its analysis more challenging.[70,71] Urine has been screened for markers of prostate[72,73] and kidney[60,74] cancer and has provided several potential markers for each. Nipple aspirate fluid has been studied extensively for the presence of tumor markers and may be a particularly useful sample source for diagnosis of breast cancer.[54-56,75,76] Several potential markers of breast cancer found in nipple aspirate fluid include vitamin D binding protein, lipophilin B, hemopexin, alpha1-acid glycoprotein and GCDFP-15.[75,76] Likewise, human pancreatic juice has also been analyzed for the presence of cancer-specific biomarkers.[77] This extensive study produced a very large list of proteins present in pancreatic juice from patients undergoing pancreatectomy for pancreatic cancer and many of the proteins identified have previously been shown to be markers of pancreatic cancer.[77]

There is an emerging body of evidence supporting the role of adipose tissue as an endocrine organ and fat has recently garnered attention as a source of biomarkers for breast and other cancers. Adipose tissue is a major component of mammary glands and has been shown to contribute to the development of the glands[78,79] and several studies have suggested a direct role of mammary adipose tissue in the progression of breast tumors. Initial studies of mammary adipose tissue and

Table 2. *Examples of limitations and challenges of clinical proteomics and recent innovative solutions*

Limitations/Challenges	Needs	Recent Innovative Solutions
Lack of sensitivity during discovery phase	Signal amplification, removal of abundant proteins, more sensitive discovery methods	Carrier-protein amplification (e.g., characterization of LMW peptides bound to albumin[99]) Use of antibodies during discovery stage (e.g., multiplex formats of antibody-bound beads[83,84] or arrays;[86] reverse-phase lysate arrays[82]) Computer model of protein abundance distributions to assist experimental design[118]
Enormous datasets with different levels of quantitation and unknown associations	Bioinformatic and computational tools to handle multidimensional data	Development of software for examining multi-dimensional datasets using interval estimation[119] Development of software for analyzing potential interacting molecules[120-123] Development of a computer algorithm that uses neural network processing to discern discriminatory patterns from mass spectrometry data[68]
Limited supply of clinical specimens with long-term clinical annotation to better determine risk of recurrence or death	Tissue procurement programs incorporating annotated databases, alternative source materials in more abundance	Use of archived formalin-fixed paraffin-embedded tissue as source material[92]
Cells in low abundance within tumors (e.g., cancer stem cells) are not well represented	Direct analysis or prior isolation of low protein abundance cells in complex tissues	Microdissection of cells based on expression[124,125]

its interstitial fluid from human patients undergoing mastectomy for breast cancer were analyzed by 2DGE and an antibody array to detect signaling proteins in tissue lysates.[80] This extensive characterization provides a substantial list of proteins (359 identifiable proteins) found within and around the adipose tissue, including numerous growth factors and cytokines well documented as mediators of cancer progression.[80] These studies suggest that mammary adipose tissue should be considered as part of the tumor stroma since it contributes significantly to the secreted factors surrounding the tumor cells. This may also be the case for other malignancies. Adipose tissue surrounding organs likely provide organ-specific functions and can be expected to actively participate in organ homeostasis. Therefore, organ-proximal adipose tissue may interact bi-directionally with developing tumors.

Cultured Cells

The use of clinical samples provides the most relevant tissue for discovery-based approaches to cancer. However, the limiting supply of tissue and the extreme heterogeneity of samples provide substantial hurdles to these studies. Model systems by design are reductive approaches to understanding a particular system and are limited in the global applicability, but cultured cells can be extremely useful in alleviating the problems of sample supply and heterogeneity. For these reasons, cultured cells have been used extensively to study many human diseases, especially cancer and comprise the main source material for molecular analyses. Primary cell lines are isolated directly from tissue and grown in culture. Sufficient cell separation techniques are required to assure a high enrichment of cancer cells, otherwise the benign cells within the culture can mask any cancer-specific alterations. Short-term cultures generally have a short life span (often under five passages) but have been shown to maintain many of their phenotypic properties over this time.[34] A potential problem with short-term cultures is that the growth medium may be selective for a particular cell population, thereby misrepresenting the true cellular population of the initial tumor.[81]

Recent Innovations and Technological Advances

Aside from 2DGE and MS-based techniques there are a wide variety of protein arrays that can provide alternative modalities for detecting cancer-specific factors, such as reverse phase lysate arrays, antibody arrays, kinase substrate arrays and others.[82] Numerous techniques have been developed that aim to reduce the complexity of the samples by focusing on specific subsets of proteins (e.g., kinases by measuring activity with peptide substrate arrays) and the use of array-based proteomics for clinical management of cancer has been excellently reviewed by Gulmann et al.[82] In addition to solid phase arrays, a new quantitative platform based on flow cytometric separation of fluorescently labeled beads (xMAP™) is becoming more widely used. The technology allows for linkage of many types of molecules, including antibodies, peptides, carbohydrates, etc. to beads with different fluorescent properties that can then be used as affinity capture reagents. As many as 100 different beads can be discriminated in a single tube, which allows for a highly multiplexed analysis of samples. This technology has already been used to examine several components in blood of patients with prostate cancer[83] or endometrial cancer.[84] A limitation of this technology is that knowledge is required a priori to determine which types of molecules to detect. Major advantages of this approach are that the beads are small enough to provide binding kinetics similar to those in solution, the results are quantitative over approximately five orders of magnitude and only very small sample sizes are required.

The Future of Clinical Proteomics

The utilization of proteomics for discovery-based studies has generated extensive lists of proteins and peptides that may be clinically useful biomarkers. Although the generation of these lists has been the focus of the majority of clinical proteomic studies, discerning the true relevance of these biomarkers to a particular disease state is much more important and presents a much greater challenge. The evaluation of clinical biomarkers is an arduous process and will likely lead to the removal of many of the candidates from the list. However, it is imperative that these studies are performed so that the truly relevant and useful biomarkers can be applied toward minimizing pain and suffering from endocrine-related cancers. There are several critical factors that are of utmost importance for achieving this goal: (1) the development of data and sample repositories with accurate and thorough clinical annotation, (2) the continual development of new technologies to address the deficiencies of current approaches, (3) standardized protocols and data management procedures to ensure that results from multiple groups can be directly compared, (4) the development of new computational and informatic systems that can integrate the multidimensional data from multiple investigators into unifying theories relevant to disease development and progression, (5) incorporation of other data sets (e.g., genomic, transcriptomic and metabolomic information) into these models and (6) continual basic research at the cellular and molecular level to aid in our understanding of carcinogenesis and tumor progression.

The application of proteomics to patient-tailored diagnosis and treatment has not yet come to fruition, but with vigilant efforts this goal may still be achieved. Until such time that cancer is no longer a major cause of morbidity and mortality, such efforts remain imperative.

References

1. Jemal A, Siegel R, Ward E et al. Cancer statistics. CA Cancer J Clin 2007; 57(1):43-66.
2. Thompson IM, Ankerst DP. Prostate-specific antigen in the early detection of prostate cancer. CMAJ 2007; 176(13):1853-1858.
3. Bast RC Jr, Badgwell D, Lu Z et al. New tumor markers: CA125 and beyond. Int J Gynecol Cancer 2005; 15 Suppl 3:274-281.
4. Goggins M. Molecular markers of early pancreatic cancer. J Clin Oncol 2005; 23(20):4524-4531.
5. Neill M, Warde P, Fleshner N. Management of low-stage testicular seminoma. Urol Clin North Am 2007; 34(2):127-136; abstract vii-viii.
6. Ocana A, Cruz JJ, Pandiella A. Trastuzumab and antiestrogen therapy: focus on mechanisms of action and resistance. Am J Clin Oncol 2006; 29(1):90-95.
7. Sim HG, Lange PH, Lin DW. Role of post-chemotherapy surgery in germ cell tumors. Urol Clin North Am 2007; 34(2):199-217; abstract ix.
8. Zolg W. The proteomic search for diagnostic biomarkers: lost in translation? Mol Cell Proteomics 2006; 5(10):1720-1726.
9. Ransohoff DF. Rules of evidence for cancer molecular-marker discovery and validation. Nat Rev Cancer 2004; 4(4):309-314.
10. Strange K. The end of "naive reductionism": rise of systems biology or renaissance of physiology? Am J Physiol Cell Physiol 2005; 288(5):C968-974.
11. Weston AD, Hood L. Systems biology, proteomics and the future of health care: toward predictive, preventative and personalized medicine. J Proteome Res 2004; 3(2):179-196.
12. Huang S, Wikswo J. Dimensions of systems biology. Rev Physiol Biochem Pharmacol 2006; 157:81-104.
13. Chen R, Yi EC, Donohoe S et al. Pancreatic cancer proteome: the proteins that underlie invasion, metastasis and immunologic escape. Gastroenterology 2005; 129(4):1187-1197.
14. Liotta LA, Kohn EC. The microenvironment of the tumour-host interface. Nature 2001; 411(6835):375-379.
15. Bonner RF, Emmert-Buck M, Cole K et al. Laser capture microdissection: molecular analysis of tissue. Science 1997; 278(5342):1481,1483.
16. Emmert-Buck MR, Bonner RF, Smith PD et al. Laser capture microdissection. Science 1996; 274(5289):998-1001.
17. Kang JS, Calvo BF, Maygarden SJ et al. Dysregulation of annexin I protein expression in high-grade prostatic intraepithelial neoplasia and prostate cancer. Clin Cancer Res 2002; 8(1):117-123.
18. Paweletz CP, Ornstein DK, Roth MJ et al. Loss of annexin 1 correlates with early onset of tumorigenesis in esophageal and prostate carcinoma. Cancer Res 2000; 60(22):6293-6297.
19. Yee DS, Narula N, Ramzy I et al. Reduced annexin II protein expression in high-grade prostatic intraepithelial neoplasia and prostate cancer. Arch Pathol Lab Med 2007; 131(6):902-908.
20. Burgemeister R. New aspects of laser microdissection in research and routine. J Histochem Cytochem 2005; 53(3):409-412.
21. Wulfkuhle JD, Sgroi DC, Krutzsch H et al. Proteomics of human breast ductal carcinoma in situ. Cancer Res 2002; 62(22):6740-6749.
22. Xu BJ, Caprioli RM, Sanders ME et al. Direct analysis of laser capture microdissected cells by MALDI mass spectrometry. J Am Soc Mass Spectrom 2002; 13(11):1292-1297.
23. Zang L, Palmer Toy D, Hancock WS et al. Proteomic analysis of ductal carcinoma of the breast using laser capture microdissection, LC-MS and 16O/18O isotopic labeling. J Proteome Res 2004; 3(3):604-612.
24. Zhang DH, Tai LK, Wong LL et al. Proteomics of breast cancer: enhanced expression of cytokeratin19 in human epidermal growth factor receptor type 2 positive breast tumors. Proteomics 2005; 5(7):1797-1805.
25. Nakagawa T, Huang SK, Martinez SR et al. Proteomic profiling of primary breast cancer predicts axillary lymph node metastasis. Cancer Res 2006; 66(24):11825-11830.
26. Neubauer H, Clare SE, Kurek R et al. Breast cancer proteomics by laser capture microdissection, sample pooling, 54-cm IPG IEF and differential iodine radioisotope detection. Electrophoresis 2006; 27(9):1840-1852.
27. Yang F, Foekens JA, Yu J et al. Laser microdissection and microarray analysis of breast tumors reveal ER-alpha related genes and pathways. Oncogene 2006; 25(9):1413-1419.

28. Umar A, Luider TM, Foekens JA et al. NanoLC-FT-ICR MS improves proteome coverage attainable for approximately 3000 laser-microdissected breast carcinoma cells. Proteomics 2007; 7(2):323-329.
29. Cowherd SM, Espina VA, Petricoin EF 3rd, Liotta LA. Proteomic analysis of human breast cancer tissue with laser-capture microdissection and reverse-phase protein microarrays. Clin Breast Cancer 2004; 5(5):385-392.
30. Takeshima Y, Amatya VJ, Daimaru Y et al. Heterogeneous genetic alterations in ovarian mucinous tumors: application and usefulness of laser capture microdissection. Hum Pathol 2001; 32(11):1203-1208.
31. Jones MB, Krutzsch H, Shu H et al. Proteomic analysis and identification of new biomarkers and therapeutic targets for invasive ovarian cancer. Proteomics 2002; 2(1):76-84.
32. Shekouh AR, Thompson CC, Prime W et al. Application of laser capture microdissection combined with two-dimensional electrophoresis for the discovery of differentially regulated proteins in pancreatic ductal adenocarcinoma. Proteomics 2003; 3(10):1988-2001.
33. Unwin RD, Craven RA, Harnden P et al. Proteomic changes in renal cancer and co-ordinate demonstration of both the glycolytic and mitochondrial aspects of the Warburg effect. Proteomics 2003; 3(8):1620-1632.
34. Peehl DM. Primary cell cultures as models of prostate cancer development. Endocr Relat Cancer 2005; 12(1):19-47.
35. Everley PA, Bakalarski CE, Elias JE et al. Enhanced analysis of metastatic prostate cancer using stable isotopes and high mass accuracy instrumentation. J Proteome Res 2006; 5(5):1224-1231.
36. Craven RA, Stanley AJ, Hanrahan S et al. Proteomic analysis of primary cell lines identifies protein changes present in renal cell carcinoma. Proteomics 2006; 6(9):2853-2864.
37. Chen R, Pan S, Brentnall TA et al. Proteomic profiling of pancreatic cancer for biomarker discovery. Mol Cell Proteomics 2005; 4(4):523-533.
38. Sarto C, Valsecchi C, Mocarelli P. Renal cell carcinoma: handling and treatment. Proteomics 2002; 2(11):1627-1629.
39. Issaq HJ, Veenstra TD. The role of electrophoresis in disease biomarker discovery. Electrophoresis 2007; 28(12):1980-1988.
40. Diamandis EP. Mass spectrometry as a diagnostic and a cancer biomarker discovery tool: opportunities and potential limitations. Mol Cell Proteomics 2004; 3(4):367-378.
41. Domon B, Broder S. Implications of new proteomics strategies for biology and medicine. J Proteome Res 2004; 3(2):253-260.
42. Hortin GL. The MALDI-TOF mass spectrometric view of the plasma proteome and peptidome. Clin Chem 2006; 52(7):1223-1237.
43. Schiffer E, Mischak H, Novak J. High resolution proteome/peptidome analysis of body fluids by capillary electrophoresis coupled with MS. Proteomics 2006; 6(20):5615-5627.
44. van der Merwe DE, Oikonomopoulou K, Marshall J et al. Mass spectrometry: uncovering the cancer proteome for diagnostics. Adv Cancer Res 2007; 96:23-50.
45. Semmes OJ, Malik G, Ward M. Application of mass spectrometry to the discovery of biomarkers for detection of prostate cancer. J Cell Biochem 2006; 98(3):496-503.
46. McLean JA, Ridenour WB, Caprioli RM. Profiling and imaging of tissues by imaging ion mobility-mass spectrometry. J Mass Spectrom 2007; 42(8):1099-1105.
47. Chaurand P, Sanders ME, Jensen RA et al. Proteomics in diagnostic pathology: profiling and imaging proteins directly in tissue sections. Am J Pathol 2004; 165(4):1057-1068.
48. Schwartz SA, Reyzer ML, Caprioli RM. Direct tissue analysis using matrix-assisted laser desorption/ionization mass spectrometry: practical aspects of sample preparation. J Mass Spectrom 2003; 38(7):699-708.
49. Chaurand P, Schwartz SA, Caprioli RM. Assessing protein patterns in disease using imaging mass spectrometry. J Proteome Res 2004; 3(2):245-252.
50. Cornett DS, Mobley JA, Dias EC et al. A novel histology-directed strategy for MALDI-MS tissue profiling that improves throughput and cellular specificity in human breast cancer. Mol Cell Proteomics 2006; 5(10):1975-1983.
51. Merchant M, Weinberger SR. Recent advancements in surface-enhanced laser desorption/ionization-time of flight-mass spectrometry. Electrophoresis 2000; 21(6):1164-1177.
52. Verma M, Wright GL Jr, Hanash SM et al. Proteomic approaches within the NCI early detection research network for the discovery and identification of cancer biomarkers. Ann N Y Acad Sci 2001; 945:103-115.
53. von Eggeling F, Junker K, Fiedle W et al. Mass spectrometry meets chip technology: a new proteomic tool in cancer research? Electrophoresis 2001; 22(14):2898-2902.

54. Paweletz CP, Trock B, Pennanen M et al. Proteomic patterns of nipple aspirate fluids obtained by SELDI-TOF: potential for new biomarkers to aid in the diagnosis of breast cancer. Dis Markers 2001; 17(4):301-307.
55. Pawlik TM, Fritsche H, Coombes KR et al. Significant differences in nipple aspirate fluid protein expression between healthy women and those with breast cancer demonstrated by time-of-flight mass spectrometry. Breast Cancer Res Treat 2005; 89(2):149-157.
56. Sauter ER, Zhu W, Fan XJ et al. Proteomic analysis of nipple aspirate fluid to detect biologic markers of breast cancer. Br J Cancer 2002; 86(9):1440-1443.
57. Cazares LH, Adam BL, Ward MD et al. Normal, benign, preneoplastic and malignant prostate cells have distinct protein expression profiles resolved by surface enhanced laser desorption/ionization mass spectrometry. Clin Cancer Res 2002; 8(8):2541-2552.
58. Cheung PK, Woolcock B, Adomat H et al. Protein profiling of microdissected prostate tissue links growth differentiation factor 15 to prostate carcinogenesis. Cancer Res 2004; 64(17):5929-5933.
59. Hara T, Honda K, Ono M et al. Identification of 2 serum biomarkers of renal cell carcinoma by surface enhanced laser desorption/ionization mass spectrometry. J Urol 2005; 174(4 Pt 1):1213-1217.
60. Rogers MA, Clarke P, Noble J et al. Proteomic profiling of urinary proteins in renal cancer by surface enhanced laser desorption ionization and neural-network analysis: identification of key issues affecting potential clinical utility. Cancer Res 2003; 63(20):6971-6983.
61. Kohli M, Siegel E, Bhattacharya S et al. Surface-enhanced laser desorption/ionization time-of-flight mass spectrometry (SELDI-TOF MS) for determining prognosis in advanced stage hormone relapsing prostate cancer. Cancer Biomark 2006; 2(6):249-258.
62. Menard C, Johann D, Lowenthal M et al. Discovering clinical biomarkers of ionizing radiation exposure with serum proteomic analysis. Cancer Res 2006; 66(3):1844-1850.
63. Suriano R, Lin Y, Ashok BT et al. Pilot study using SELDI-TOF-MS based proteomic profile for the identification of diagnostic biomarkers of thyroid proliferative diseases. J Proteome Res 2006; 5(4):856-861.
64. Nakamura K, Yoshikawa K, Yamada Y et al. Differential profiling analysis of proteins involved in anti-proliferative effect of interferon-alpha on renal cell carcinoma cell lines by protein biochip technology. Int J Oncol 2006; 28(4):965-970.
65. Petricoin EF, Ardekani AM, Hitt BA et al. Use of proteomic patterns in serum to identify ovarian cancer. Lancet 2002; 359(9306):572-577.
66. Conrads TP, Zhou M, Petricoin EF et al. Cancer diagnosis using proteomic patterns. Expert Rev Mol Diagn 2003; 3(4):411-420.
67. Ornstein DK, Rayford W, Fusaro VA et al. Serum proteomic profiling can discriminate prostate cancer from benign prostates in men with total prostate specific antigen levels between 2.5 and 15.0 ng/ml. J Urol 2004; 172(4 Pt 1):1302-1305.
68. Petricoin EF 3rd, Ornstein DK, Paweletz CP et al. Serum proteomic patterns for detection of prostate cancer. J Natl Cancer Inst 2002; 94(20):1576-1578.
69. Lowenthal MS, Mehta AI, Frogale K et al. Analysis of albumin-associated peptides and proteins from ovarian cancer patients. Clin Chem 2005; 51(10):1933-1945.
70. Pieper R, Gatlin CL, McGrath AM et al. Characterization of the human urinary proteome: a method for high-resolution display of urinary proteins on two-dimensional electrophoresis gels with a yield of nearly 1400 distinct protein spots. Proteomics 2004; 4(4):1159-1174.
71. Pisitkun T, Johnstone R, Knepper MA. Discovery of urinary biomarkers. Mol Cell Proteomics 2006; 5(10):1760-1771.
72. M'Koma AE, Blum DL, Norris JL et al. Detection of preneoplastic and neoplastic prostate disease by MALDI profiling of urine. Biochem Biophys Res Commun 2007; 353(3):829-834.
73. Rehman I, Azzouzi AR, Catto JW et al. Proteomic analysis of voided urine after prostatic massage from patients with prostate cancer: a pilot study Urology 2004; 64(6):1238-1243.
74. Perroud B, Lee J, Valkova N et al. Pathway analysis of kidney cancer using proteomics and metabolic profiling. Mol Cancer 2006; 5:64.
75. Alexander H, Stegner AL, Wagner-Mann C et al. Proteomic analysis to identify breast cancer biomarkers in nipple aspirate fluid. Clin Cancer Res 2004; 10(22):7500-7510.
76. Pawlik TM, Hawke DH, Liu Y et al. Proteomic analysis of nipple aspirate fluid from women with early-stage breast cancer using isotope-coded affinity tags and tandem mass spectrometry reveals differential expression of vitamin D binding protein. BMC Cancer 2006; 6:68.
77. Gronborg M, Bunkenborg J, Kristiansen TZ et al. Comprehensive proteomic analysis of human pancreatic juice. J Proteome Res 2004; 3(5):1042-1055.
78. Stingl J, Eirew P, Ricketson I et al. Purification and unique properties of mammary epithelial stem cells. Nature 2006; 439(7079):993-997.

79. Fata JE, Werb Z, Bissell MJ. Regulation of mammary gland branching morphogenesis by the extracellular matrix and its remodeling enzymes. Breast Cancer Res 2004; 6(1):1-11.

80. Celis JE, Moreira JM, Cabezon T et al. Identification of extracellular and intracellular signaling components of the mammary adipose tissue and its interstitial fluid in high risk breast cancer patients: toward dissecting the molecular circuitry of epithelial-adipocyte stromal cell interactions. Mol Cell Proteomics 2005; 4(4):492-522.

81. Litvinov IV, Vander Griend DJ, Xu Y et al. Low-calcium serum-free defined medium selects for growth of normal prostatic epithelial stem cells. Cancer Res 2006; 66(17):8598-8607.

82. Gulmann C, Sheehan KM, Kay EW et al. Array-based proteomics: mapping of protein circuitries for diagnostics, prognostics and therapy guidance in cancer. J Pathol 2006; 208(5):595-606.

83. Drukier AK, Ossetrova N, Schors E et al. High-sensitivity blood-based detection of breast cancer by multi photon detection diagnostic proteomics. J Proteome Res 2006; 5(8):1906-1915.

84. Yurkovetsky Z, Ta'asan S, Skates S et al. Development of multimarker panel for early detection of endometrial cancer. High diagnostic power of prolactin. Gynecol Oncol 2007; 107(1):58-65.

85. Casiano CA, Mediavilla-Varela M, Tan EM. Tumor-associated antigen arrays for the serological diagnosis of cancer. Mol Cell Proteomics 2006; 5(10):1745-1759.

86. Qin S, Qiu W, Ehrlich JR et al. Development of a "reverse capture" autoantibody microarray for studies of antigen-autoantibody profiling. Proteomics 2006; 6(10):3199-3209.

87. Varambally S, Yu J, Laxman B et al. Integrative genomic and proteomic analysis of prostate cancer reveals signatures of metastatic progression. Cancer Cell 2005; 8(5):393-406.

88. Wozny W, Schroer K, Schwall GP et al. Differential radioactive quantification of protein abundance ratios between benign and malignant prostate tissues: cancer association of annexin A3. Proteomics 2007; 7(2):313-322.

89. Lexander H, Palmberg C, Hellman U et al. Correlation of protein expression, Gleason score and DNA ploidy in prostate cancer. Proteomics 2006; 6(15):4370-4380.

90. Ahram M, Best CJ, Flaig MJ et al. Proteomic analysis of human prostate cancer. Mol Carcinog 2002; 33(1):9-15.

91. Hwang SI, Thumar J, Lundgren DH et al. Direct cancer tissue proteomics: a method to identify candidate cancer biomarkers from formalin-fixed paraffin-embedded archival tissues. Oncogene 2007; 26(1):65-76.

92. Hood BL, Darfler MM, Guiel TG et al. Proteomic analysis of formalin-fixed prostate cancer tissue. Mol Cell Proteomics 2005; 4(11):1741-1753.

93. Ornstein DK, Gillespie JW, Paweletz CP et al. Proteomic analysis of laser capture microdissected human prostate cancer and in vitro prostate cell lines. Electrophoresis 2000; 21(11):2235-2242.

94. Wright ME, Tsai MJ, Aebersold R. Androgen receptor represses the neuroendocrine transdifferentiation process in prostate cancer cells. Mol Endocrinol 2003; 17(9):1726-1737.

95. Martin DB, Gifford DR, Wright ME et al. Quantitative proteomic analysis of proteins released by neoplastic prostate epithelium. Cancer Res 2004; 64(1):347-355.

96. Rowland JG, Robson JL, Simon WJ et al. Evaluation of an in vitro model of androgen ablation and identification of the androgen responsive proteome in LNCaP cells. Proteomics 2007; 7(1):47-63.

97. Meehan KL, Sadar MD. Quantitative profiling of LNCaP prostate cancer cells using isotope-coded affinity tags and mass spectrometry. Proteomics 2004; 4(4):1116-1134.

98. Zhang D, Tai LK, Wong LL et al. Proteomic study reveals that proteins involved in metabolic and detoxification pathways are highly expressed in HER-2/neu-positive breast cancer. Mol Cell Proteomics 2005; 4(11):1686-1696.

99. Lopez MF, Mikulskis A, Kuzdzal S et al. A novel, high-throughput workflow for discovery and identification of serum carrier protein-bound peptide biomarker candidates in ovarian cancer samples. Clin Chem 2007; 53(6):1067-1074.

100. Wulfkuhle JD, Aquino JA, Calvert VS et al. Signal pathway profiling of ovarian cancer from human tissue specimens using reverse-phase protein microarrays. Proteomics 2003; 3(11):2085-2090.

101. Bhattacharyya S, Siegel ER, Petersen GM et al. Diagnosis of pancreatic cancer using serum proteomic profiling. Neoplasia 2004; 6(5):674-686.

102. Yu KH, Rustgi AK, Blair IA. Characterization of proteins in human pancreatic cancer serum using differential gel electrophoresis and tandem mass spectrometry. J Proteome Res 2005; 4(5):1742-1751.

103. Honda K, Hayashida Y, Umaki T et al. Possible detection of pancreatic cancer by plasma protein profiling. Cancer Res 2005; 65(22):10613-10622.

104. Lin Y, Goedegebuure PS, Tan MC et al. Proteins associated with disease and clinical course in pancreas cancer: a proteomic analysis of plasma in surgical patients. J Proteome Res 2006; 5(9):2169-2176.

105. Deng R, Lu Z, Chen Y et al. Plasma proteomic analysis of pancreatic cancer by 2-dimensional gel electrophoresis. Pancreas 2007; 34(3):310-317.

106. Crnogorac-Jurcevic T, Gangeswaran R, Bhakta V et al. Proteomic analysis of chronic pancreatitis and pancreatic adenocarcinoma. Gastroenterology 2005; 129(5):1454-1463.
107. Sitek B, Luttges J, Marcus K et al. Application of fluorescence difference gel electrophoresis saturation labelling for the analysis of microdissected precursor lesions of pancreatic ductal adenocarcinoma. Proteomics 2005; 5(10):2665-2679.
108. Gronborg M, Kristiansen TZ, Iwahori A et al. Biomarker discovery from pancreatic cancer secretome using a differential proteomic approach. Mol Cell Proteomics 2006; 5(1):157-171.
109. Marengo E, Robotti E, Cecconi D et al. Identification of the regulatory proteins in human pancreatic cancers treated with Trichostatin A by 2D-PAGE maps and multivariate statistical analysis. Anal Bioanal Chem 2004; 379(7-8):992-1003.
110. Cecconi D, Donadelli M, Scarpa A et al. Proteomic analysis of pancreatic ductal carcinoma cells after combined treatment with gemcitabine and trichostatin A. J Proteome Res 2005; 4(6):1909-1916.
111. Hwa JS, Park HJ, Jung JH et al. Identification of proteins differentially expressed in the conventional renal cell carcinoma by proteomic analysis. J Korean Med Sci 2005; 20(3):450-455.
112. Poznanovic S, Wozny W, Schwall GP et al. Differential radioactive proteomic analysis of microdissected renal cell carcinoma tissue by 54 cm isoelectric focusing in serial immobilized pH gradient gels. J Proteome Res 2005; 4(6):2117-2125.
113. Zhuang Z, Huang S, Kowalak JA et al. From tissue phenotype to proteotype: sensitive protein identification in microdissected tumor tissue. Int J Oncol 2006; 28(1):103-110.
114. Perego RA, Bianchi C, Corizzato M et al. Primary cell cultures arising from normal kidney and renal cell carcinoma retain the proteomic profile of corresponding tissues. J Proteome Res 2005; 4(5):1503-1510.
115. Villanueva J, Martorella AJ, Lawlor K et al. Serum peptidome patterns that distinguish metastatic thyroid carcinoma from cancer-free controls are unbiased by gender and age. Mol Cell Proteomics 2006; 5(10):1840-1852.
116. Brown LM, Helmke SM, Hunsucker SW et al. Quantitative and qualitative differences in protein expression between papillary thyroid carcinoma and normal thyroid tissue. Mol Carcinog 2006; 45(8):613-626.
117. Torres-Cabala C, Bibbo M, Panizo-Santos A et al. Proteomic identification of new biomarkers and application in thyroid cytology. Acta Cytol 2006; 50(5):518-528.
118. Eriksson J, Fenyo D. Improving the success rate of proteome analysis by modeling protein-abundance distributions and experimental designs. Nat Biotechnol 2007; 25(6):651-655.
119. Park Y, Downing SR, Kim D et al. Simultaneous and exact interval estimates for the contrast of two groups based on an extremely high dimensional variable: application to mass spec data. Bioinformatics 2007; 23(12):1451-1458.
120. Lubovac Z, Gamalielsson J, Olsson B. Combining functional and topological properties to identify core modules in protein interaction networks. Proteins 2006; 64(4):948-959.
121. Bernaschi M, Castiglione F, Ferranti A et al. ProtNet: a tool for stochastic simulations of protein interaction networks dynamics. BMC Bioinformatics 2007; 8 Suppl 1:S4.
122. Wolf-Yadlin A, Hautaniemi S, Lauffenburger DA et al. Multiple reaction monitoring for robust quantitative proteomic analysis of cellular signaling networks. Proc Natl Acad Sci USA 2007; 104(14):5860-5865.
123. Shannon P, Markiel A, Ozier O et al. Cytoscape: a software environment for integrated models of biomolecular interaction networks. Genome Res 2003; 13(11):2498-2504.
124. Tangrea MA, Chuaqui RF, Gillespie JW et al. Expression microdissection: operator-independent retrieval of cells for molecular profiling. Diagn Mol Pathol 2004; 13(4):207-212.
125. Buckanovich RJ, Sasaroli D, O'Brien-Jenkins A et al. Use of immuno-LCM to identify the in situ expression profile of cellular constituents of the tumor microenvironment. Cancer Biol Ther 2006; 5(6):635-642.

CHAPTER 10

Endogenous Hormone Levels and Risk of Breast, Endometrial and Ovarian Cancers:
Prospective Studies

A. Heather Eliassen* and Susan E. Hankinson

Abstract

Multiple lines of evidence support a central role of hormones in the etiology of breast, endometrial and ovarian cancers. Evidence of an association between circulating hormones and these cancers varies by both hormone and cancer site, with the most consistent associations observed for sex steroid hormones and breast cancer risk among postmenopausal women. Recently, evidence has begun to accumulate suggesting an important role for endogenous hormones in premenopausal breast cancer, endometrial cancer and possibly ovarian cancer. In this chapter, prospective epidemiologic studies, where endogenous hormones are measured in study subjects prior to disease diagnosis, are summarized. Overall, a strong positive association between breast cancer risk and circulating levels of both estrogens and testosterone has now been well confirmed among postmenopausal women; women with hormone levels in the top 20% of the distribution (versus bottom 20%) have a two-to-three-fold higher risk of breast cancer. Evidence among premenopausal women is more limited, though increased risk associated with higher levels of testosterone is consistent. Evidence to date of hormonal associations for endometrial cancer is limited, though a strong association with sex steroid hormones is suggested. Studies of ovarian cancer have been few and small with no consistent associations observed with endogenous hormones. Clearly more evaluation is needed to confirm the role of endogenous hormones in premenopausal breast cancer, endometrial cancer and ovarian cancer.

Introduction

A hormonal etiology has long been suspected for breast, endometrial and ovarian cancers as several risk factors for each cancer are hormonally related. Early age at menarche, nulliparity and late age at menopause, increase the risk of breast cancer.[1] In addition, after menopause, adipose tissue is the major source of estrogen and obese postmenopausal women have both higher levels of endogenous estrogen and a higher risk of breast and endometrial cancer.[2,3] In addition to body mass index, early menarche, late age at menopause, nulliparity and postmenopausal hormone use increase the risk and oral contraceptive use decreases the risk of endometrial cancer.[3] Finally, ovarian cancer risk is reduced with increasing parity, oral contraceptive use and risk is increased by postmenopausal hormone use.[4,5] More recently, evidence has begun to accumulate of a direct

*Corresponding Author: Heather Eliassen—Channing Laboratory, Department of Medicine, Brigham and Women's Hospital, 181 Longwood Avenue, Boston, MA 02115, USA. Email: heather.eliassen@channing.harvard.edu

Innovative Endocrinology of Cancer, edited by Lev M. Berstein and Richard J. Santen. ©2008 Landes Bioscience and Springer Science+Business Media.

involvement of hormone concentrations in each of these cancers. Although there are limited data for ovarian and endometrial cancers, as well as for premenopausal breast cancer, direct evidence of a hormonal etiology of breast cancer is quite strong among postmenopausal women. This chapter reviews the current literature on endogenous hormones and breast, endometrial and ovarian cancer. The hormones included are estrogens, androgens, insulin-like growth factor I and its binding proteins, prolactin (breast cancer) and gonadotropins (ovarian cancer). Because of the potential for these tumors to affect circulating levels of hormones, only data from prospective studies (i.e., "nested" case-control studies), in which hormone levels are measured prior to cancer diagnosis, will be reviewed.

Mechanistically, estrogens contribute to tumor growth by promoting the proliferation of cells with existing mutations or perhaps by increasing the opportunity for mutations.[6] Androgens have been hypothesized to increase cancer risk either directly, by increasing cellular growth and prolif-eration, or indirectly, by their conversion to estrogen.[7-9] Insulin-like growth factor I (IGF-I) may increase cell proliferation and decrease apoptosis while the IGF binding proteins (IGFBPs) limit the bioavailability of IGF-I.[10-12] Prolactin also may increase breast cell proliferation and inhibit apoptosis.[13] Progesterone has been hypothesized to both decrease and increase breast cancer risk and evidence from animal and in vitro studies supports each hypothesis.[14,15] While postmenopausal estrogen use alone increases breast cancer risk, the association is stronger with the combination of estrogen and progestin.[1] Progesterone is hypothesized to decrease endometrial and ovarian cancer risk,[16,17] although to our knowledge no prospective studies have evaluated progesterone levels with respect to these cancers. Gonadotropins have been hypothesized to increase ovarian cancer risk directly or indirectly by stimulating the production of steroid hormones.[18]

Methodologic Considerations

Evaluating the association of circulating hormones with cancer risk is complicated in epide-miologic studies. Because of logistic and financial restraints, most studies only have a single blood sample for each study subject. However, a single blood sample has been found to reflect long-term hormone levels fairly well. For example, over a two-to-three year period, the correlations for IGF-I, the IGFBPs and postmenopausal gonadotropin and steroid hormones, ranged from 0.5 to 0.9.[19-25] In premenopausal women androgens are similarly well correlated over time[19,24,25] but estrogens (evaluated separately in the follicular and luteal phase) and progesterone (evaluated in the luteal phase) are more modestly correlated.[19,26] Thus, the use of a single blood measure likely causes some attenuation of relative risk (RR) estimates. However, this reproducibility is similar to that of blood pressure or serum cholesterol, parameters that are reasonably measured and consistent predictors of disease in epidemiologic studies.[27]

Although circulating hormone levels are most often measured in epidemiologic studies, relatively little is known about how these levels correlate with exposure in breast, endometrial or ovarian tissue. Levels of 17β-estradiol within the breast tissue are higher than circulating levels,[28] due to its conversion from steroid precursors.[29] The correlation between local nonmalignant tissue levels and circulating levels is not known because most studies evaluated the correlation between circulating levels and tumor tissue hormone levels or did not present correlations between circu-lating levels and nonmalignant tissue.[30-32] However, the consistent positive associations between circulating hormone levels and risk in postmenopausal women (described below) indicate these levels may be an important marker of tissue exposure. Although few studies have assessed the association between circulating and endometrial tissue hormone levels, evidence suggests the cor-relation is high and circulating levels of some hormones have been associated with endometrial hyperplasia.[3,33] Given the avascular nature of ovarian epithelium, it is possible that paracrine and autocrine hormonal activity is more important than endocrine activity within the ovaries.[34] In addition, evidence of an association between circulating hormones and ovarian cancer (described below) is more limited.

Breast Cancer

Postmenopausal Women

Estrogens

Substantial prospective data have accrued over the last several years on estrogen concentrations and breast cancer risk in postmenopausal women. In 2002, a pooled analysis was published consisting of all nine prospective studies available at that time.[35] None of the women were using exogenous hormones at blood collection and the analysis included 663 breast cancer cases and 1765 controls. Median time between blood collection and cancer diagnosis ranged from 2 to 12 years. Circulating estrogen levels were positively associated with breast cancer risk. The RRs (95% confidence interval (CI)) for increasing quintiles of estradiol level, relative to the lowest quintile, were 1.4, 1.2, 1.8 and 2.0 (1.5-2.7) (Table 1). Estrone, estrone sulfate and free estradiol were similarly related to risk. The variation in RRs between studies was not statistically significant for any of the hormones and the associations did not vary significantly according to the type of laboratory assay used. Subsequent to the pooled analysis, a Swedish prospective study with 173 cases reported similar positive associations between circulating estrogens and postmenopausal breast cancer.[36] In addition, urinary estrogen levels also were positively associated with breast cancer risk in two prospective studies.[37,38]

More recently, findings from the large multi-country European Prospective Investigation into Cancer and Nutrition (EPIC) study were reported.[39] In EPIC, 677 incident breast cancer cases and 1309 age and recruitment center matched controls were accrued among postmenopausal women over six years of follow-up; findings confirmed those of the pooled analysis of nine studies. For example, for circulating estradiol, the RRs (95% CI) for increasing quintile of levels were 1.0, 1.1, 1.4, 1.7, 2.3 (1.6-3.2) (Table 1). Other estrogens again were similarly related to risk.

Updated analyses from two cohorts included in the pooled analysis have expanded upon the observed associations in important ways. With 13 years of follow-up after blood collection in the New York University Women's Health Study (NYUWHS), the associations with circulating hormones remained unchanged with the exclusion of the first five years of follow-up.[40] In addition, the authors assessed if the change in levels over time varied between cases and controls with two blood samples collected from a large number of women (for cases, one within five years of diagnosis and a second at least five years post diagnosis). Changes in estrogens and testosterone were comparable between the two groups. Thus, this study provides strong evidence that circulating hormones are truly a marker of increased risk in postmenopausal women and not simply a result of tumor-related hormone production.

Only a single detailed assessment of the association between plasma hormones and breast cancer risk by estrogen and progesterone receptor (ER/PR) status of the tumor has been published.[41] While strong positive associations were observed for ER+/PR+ tumors, weak or no associations were noted for ER+/PR− and ER−/PR− tumor types (too few ER−/PR+ tumors were available to evaluate separately). For example, for estradiol, the top versus bottom quartile RR (95% CI) was 3.3 (2.0-5.4) for ER+/PR+ tumors (p-trend<0.001), 1.0 (0.4-2.6; p-trend = 0.82) for ER+/PR- tumors and 1.0 (0.4-2.4; p-trend = 0.46) for ER−/PR− tumors (p for heterogeneity<0.001).

In two recent studies, whether the association between plasma estrogens and postmenopausal breast cancer is similar in women at varying levels of breast cancer risk has been evaluated. No association between plasma estradiol and breast cancer risk was observed among 89 cases and 141 non-cases in the high risk population of the National Surgical Adjuvant Breast and Bowel Project Cancer Prevention Trial (P-1) (top versus bottom quartile RR = 0.96, 95% CI (0.5-2.0)).[42] Within the Nurses' Health Study (NHS) cohort, with 418 cases and 817 controls,[43] the associations of plasma estradiol and estrone sulfate with breast cancer were robust across risk categories regardless of which metric was used to define risk (e.g., 5-year modified Gail score or by family history of breast cancer). For example, estradiol appeared as or more strongly associated with breast cancer in women with higher predicted risk by the Gail risk score (modified Gail score >2.25%: RR = 4.5, 95% CI (2.1-9.5)), compared to lower risk (modified Gail score <1.66%: RR = 2.1, 95% CI

Table 1. *Circulating hormone levels and breast cancer risk in postmenopausal women*

	Study	Cases/Controls	Category Unit	RR (95% CI)
Estradiol				
	EHBCCG*, 2002	663/1765	Quintiles	2.0 (1.5-2.7)
	Zeleniuch-Jacquotte, 2004**	297/563	Quintiles	2.5 (1.5-4.2)
	Kaaks, 2005	677/1309	Quintiles	2.3 (1.6-3.2)
	Missmer, 2004***	322/643	Quartiles	2.1 (1.5-3.2)
	Manjer, 2003	173/438	Top 20% vs. bottom 80%	1.7 (0.7-1.7)
Testosterone				
	EHBCCG, 2002	585/1574	Quintiles	2.2 (1.6-3.1)
	Zeleniuch-Jacquotte, 2004**	297/562	Quintiles	2.4 (1.4-4.0)
	Kaaks, 2005	668/1280	Quintiles	1.9 (1.3-2.6)
	Missmer, 2004***	312/628	Quartiles	1.6 (1.0-2.4)
	Manjer, 2003	154/417	Quartiles	1.9 (1.1-3.3)
Progesterone				
	Missmer, 2004***	270/530	Quartiles	0.9 (0.6-1.5)
IGF-I				
	Hankinson, 1998	305/483	Quartiles	0.9 (0.5-1.4)
	Toniolo, 2000	115/220	Quartiles	1.0 (0.5-1.9)
	Kaaks, 2002	274/519	Quartiles	1.3 (0.8-2.1)
	Krajcik, 2002	60/60	Quartiles	0.8 (0.2-2.6)
	Muti, 2002	64/238	Quartiles	0.6 (0.2-1.4)
	Keinan-Boker, 2003	149/333	Quartiles	1.1 (0.6-2.1)
	Gronbaek, 2004	411/397	25 unit increase	1.0 (1.0-1.1)
	Schernhammer, 2005	514/754	Quintiles	1.0 (0.7-1.4)
	Allen, 2005	47/141	Tertiles	0.8 (0.3-1.7)
	Rollison, 2006	152/152#	Tertiles	1.4 (0.8-2.4)
		91/91##	Tertiles	1.7 (0.8-3.6)
	Rinaldi, 2006	808/1560###	Quintiles	1.4 (1.0-1.9)
	Baglietto, 2007	220/8885	Quartiles	1.6 (1.0-2.4)
Prolactin				
	Wang, 1992	40/1180	Quintiles	1.6 (0.6-4.7)
	Hankinson, 1999	306/448	Quartiles	2.0 (1.3-3.3)
	Kabuto, 2000	26/56	Log_{10} unit increase	6.5 (0.0-43.9)
	Manjer, 2000	173/438	Quartiles	1.3 (0.8-2.2)
	Tworoger, 2004	851/1275	Quartiles	1.3 (1.0-1.8)
	Tworoger, 2007	916/1410	Quartiles	1.3 (1.1-1.7)

*Endogenous Hormone and Breast Cancer Collaborative Group. **Extension of study included in EHBCCG analysis; 168 new cases and 316 new controls included here. ***Extension of study included in EHBCCG analysis; 167 new cases and 333 new controls included here. #Premenopausal at blood collection, postmenopausal at diagnosis. ##Postmenopausal at blood collection and diagnosis. ###Age at diagnosis >50 years.

(1.2-3.6)), but these differences in relative risk were not statistically significant. The association between plasma estrone sulfate and breast cancer also was similar in the two groups. Thus evidence from this larger cohort suggests that circulating estrogens are predictive of risk in women across both low and high predicted risk of breast cancer, however confirmation in other studies is needed.

Only one prospective study has addressed whether estradiol levels are associated with breast cancer risk in women using postmenopausal hormones.[44] Modest positive associations were observed (top versus bottom quartile RR (95% CI) for estradiol = 1.3 (0.9-2.0) p-trend = 0.20) which were stronger and statistically significant among women who were older, leaner and who had the longest duration of non-use of hormones since menopause. Thus, even in postmenopausal hormone users, plasma estradiol levels appear to be at least modestly associated with risk.

Androgens

Although androstenedione, DHEA and DHEAS have been investigated with respect to breast cancer risk in postmenopausal women, this chapter will focus on associations with testosterone specifically given the amount of data available and limited space. The pooled analysis of nine prospective studies described above[35] and the recently published report from the EPIC study[39] provide a comprehensive summary of evidence on circulating testosterone levels and breast cancer risk in postmenopausal women (Table 1). In the pooled analysis, breast cancer risk increased with increasing testosterone levels: the RRs (95% CI) for increasing quintile (relative to the lowest quintile) were 1.3, 1.6, 1.6 and 2.2 (1.6-3.1). Results were similar in analyses excluding cases diagnosed within two years of blood collection. Extensions of these findings, with up to 13 years of follow-up after the initial blood collection, have been published for 2 of the studies included in the pooled analysis and the observed associations were very similar.[40,43] In the EPIC cohort, similar associations were observed.[39] In addition, the association of plasma testosterone levels and subsequent breast cancer risk was generally similar in women using postmenopausal hormones.[44]

In each of these analyses, adjustment for estradiol in the statistical models only modestly attenuated relative risks for testosterone, suggesting some independent association of testosterone levels with breast cancer.[35,39] However, possible differences between estradiol and testosterone in assay precision, stability of levels 'within woman' over time and intracellular conversion of androgens to estrogens complicate the interpretation of these epidemiologic analyses.

In the NHS, the association between testosterone and breast cancer was stronger for ER+/PR+ tumors (p for heterogeneity = 0.03).[41] Specifically, the top versus bottom quartile RR (95% CI) was 2.0 (1.2-3.4; p-trend<0.001) for ER+/PR+ tumors, 1.9 (0.7-5.0; p-trend = 0.12) for ER+/PR– tumors and 0.7 (0.3-1.6; p-trend = 0.35) for ER–/PR– tumors.

In the two studies previously described, the association between circulating testosterone and breast cancer risk across categories of predicted risk has been addressed. No association was observed between testosterone levels and breast cancer risk in the P-1 trial with 89 cases and 141 non-cases (RR (95% CI) for top versus bottom quartile: 0.5 (0.2-1.1)),[42] although the association was noted to be quite robust in the larger NHS cohort.[43]

Progesterone

Only one large prospective study, with 270 cases, has evaluated the association of postmenopausal circulating progesterone and breast cancer risk. No association was observed either overall (top versus bottom quartile of levels: RR = 0.9; 95% CI = 0.6-1.5; p-trend = 0.90) (Table 1), when evaluated by tumor hormone receptor status or stratified by circulating estradiol levels.[41]

Insulin-Like Growth Factor I and IGF Binding Proteins

The association between IGF-I and IGFBP-3 levels and breast cancer risk has been investigated in 11 prospective studies to date, with a weak positive or no association observed (Table 1).[45-55] In the two largest studies to date, no association was observed in the NHS with 514 cases (top versus bottom quintile RR = 1.0, 95% CI (0.7-1.4)) and a weak positive association was observed in EPIC with 808 cases (top versus bottom quintile RR = 1.4, 95% CI (1.0-1.9)).[51,54] The association between IGFBP-3 and breast cancer risk is more ambiguous, with studies suggesting positive, inverse and null associations.[20,46-48,51]

Prolactin

Prolactin levels and risk of breast cancer among postmenopausal women has been evaluated in several studies to date.[36,56-60] Most, though not all,[36] studies have observed a significant positive association, with case numbers ranging from 26[56] to 915[60] (Table 1). In the largest to date, an updated analysis within the NHS and NHSII cohorts with 915 postmenopausal women, a marginally significant trend was observed across quartiles of prolactin level, (top versus bottom quartile RR = 1.4, 95% CI (1.0-1.9), p-trend = 0.05).[60] In this two-cohort analysis, the association of prolactin with breast cancer did not differ by menopausal status (p = 0.95). Among premenopausal and postmenopausal women combined (1539 cases), the association was stronger for invasive cases (top versus bottom quartile RR = 1.4, 95% CI (1.1-1.7), p-trend = 0.001) than in situ cases (comparable RR = 1.2, 95% CI (0.8-1.6), p-trend = 0.43). In addition, the association was significantly different by ER/PR status of the tumor (p-heterogeneity = 0.03) with RRs (95% CI) for top versus bottom quartiles of 1.6, (1.3-2.0), p-trend<0.001 for ER+/PR+, 1.7, (1.0-2.7), p-trend = 0.06 for ER+/PR– and 0.9, (0.6-1.3), p-trend = 0.70 for ER–/PR–. There were too few ER–/PR+ cases to evaluate separately.

Conclusion

The positive association between circulating estrogens and testosterone in postmenopausal women and subsequent risk of breast cancer is now well established. For both estradiol and testosterone, women in the top, versus bottom, 20% of estrogen levels have a two- to three-fold higher breast cancer risk. Although confirmation is needed, the association appears strongest for ER+ breast tumors and seems robust across groups of women at varying risk of breast cancer. Whether the association observed with testosterone is direct or indirect (through its conversion to estradiol) is unclear; both may be true. Although recent results are mixed for an association between IGFBP-3 and breast cancer, accumulated evidence suggests no strong association between IGF-I and breast cancer risk among postmenopausal women. Prolactin levels appear to be a modest risk factor for both premenopausal and postmenopausal breast cancer with a stronger association among invasive and ER+ breast tumors.

Studies are now needed to determine if circulating hormone measurements add substantially to existing breast cancer risk prediction models. Several statistical models have been developed for use as an entry criterion into breast cancer chemoprevention trials (e.g., NSABP P-1 trial), in counseling women on the potential use of chemopreventives (e.g., tamoxifen or aromatase inhibitors) and to provide general insight into a woman's individual breast cancer risk[61-64] but none of them include circulating hormone levels. Similarly, whether circulating sex steroid levels can be used to identify women who would most benefit from anti-estrogens is as yet unknown; baseline estradiol levels predicted the subsequent reduction in breast cancer risk associated with raloxifene use in the MORE trial[65] but not with tamoxifen use in the P-1 trial.[42]

Premenopausal Women

In contrast to the rapidly accumulating data on postmenopausal women, relatively few studies on circulating hormone levels and breast cancer have been conducted in premenopausal women. This is largely due to the variation in sex steroid hormone levels, particularly estrogen levels, over the menstrual cycle thus making epidemiologic studies with a single blood sample from each study subject particularly complex.

Estrogens

Seven prospective studies in premenopausal women have been published to date, although five of the seven had fewer than 80 cases (range 14-79 cases).[56,66-69] In none of the five smaller studies were significant associations between estrogen levels and breast cancer risk noted, although as expected given their size, precision of the estimates was uniformly low. Two much larger studies have recently been published. In the largest study to date, conducted in the EPIC cohort, with 285 invasive breast cancer cases and 555 controls, a single blood sample was collected per woman and the day of collection within the menstrual cycle was recorded.[70] Controls were matched to cases on age, study center and time of day of collection and phase of the menstrual cycle at blood collection (in five categories). Comparisons between case and control hormone levels were based on residuals from spline regression models; the residuals indicated how much an individual's hormone level deviated from the predicted hormone levels on that day. Overall, no association was observed for either estradiol or estrone (e.g., top to bottom quartile comparison RR = 1.0, 95% CI (0.7-1.5) for estradiol) (Table 2). Of note, because blood samples were collected across the menstrual cycle, the investigators had relatively limited ability to evaluate associations within specific parts of the cycle.

In the second large prospective study, conducted within the NHSII, both early follicular (day three to five) and mid-luteal (seven to nine days prior to next cycle) samples were collected from each woman.[71] Timing of the luteal sample collection was by backward dating from the onset of the next menstrual cycle. The analysis included 197 cases (in situ and invasive combined) with 394 controls matched on age, luteal day, date and time of blood draw and fasting status. Follicular, but not luteal, total and free estradiol were significantly associated with breast cancer risk (top to bottom quartile comparison RR = 2.1, 95% CI (1.1-4.1) for follicular total estradiol) (Table 2). Associations were stronger among the 89 ER+/PR+ cases (comparable RR = 2.7, 95% CI (1.2-6.0) for follicular total estradiol). No association was observed with either estrone or estrone sulfate (in either phase of the cycle).

Testosterone

As with estrogens, few prospective studies have evaluated the association between circulating testosterone and breast cancer. Of the five prospective studies published to date, three had 65 or fewer cases; in these studies significant positive[72] or null[66,69] associations with testosterone were reported. Again, confidence intervals were wide.

In the large EPIC cohort, with 370 invasive breast cancer cases and 726 controls, significant positive associations were observed between circulating levels of testosterone and risk of breast cancer.[70] The RRs (95% CI) with increasing testosterone level (in quartile categories) were 1.0, 1.4, 1.4 and 1.7 (1.2-2.6) (p-trend = 0.01) (Table 2).

In the NHSII, with 197 cases (including both in situ and invasive disease) and 394 controls, modest, but not statistically significant, positive associations were observed for testosterone (in both the follicular and luteal phase); the associations, particularly for follicular testosterone, did not appear entirely linear.[71] The associations were stronger and statistically significant when restricting to invasive (comparable case group to the EPIC study) or ER+/PR+ tumors. For example, in the luteal phase, women in the top (versus bottom) 25% of testosterone levels had a twofold increased risk of invasive cancer (RR = 2.0, 95% CI (1.1-3.6), p-trend = 0.05) and a threefold higher risk of an ER+/PR+ tumor (RR = 2.9, 95% CI (1.4-6.0), p-trend = 0.02). Findings for free testosterone generally mirrored those for total testosterone.

Progesterone

To date, only six prospective studies have examined progesterone levels and breast cancer risk in premenopausal women, with four of the six studies including 65 or fewer cases.[66,67,72,73] Nonsignificant inverse associations were observed in three of the smaller studies,[66,69,72] and a nonsignificant positive association was observed in the fourth.[67]

In the large EPIC cohort study, with 285 cases and 555 controls, a significant inverse association was observed between progesterone levels (residuals from spline regression model) and breast cancer risk (top to bottom quartile comparison RR = 0.6, 95% CI (0.4-1.0)) (Table 2).[70] This association was driven by women with samples drawn in the luteal phase and was only apparent among cases and controls matched by forward dating, not among those matched by the more accurate backward dating approach. In the second large study, utilizing backward dating with 197 cases and 394 controls, no association was observed between luteal progesterone levels and risk.[71]

Insulin-Like Growth Factor I and IGF Binding Proteins

Eleven analyses within nine cohort studies have examined IGF-I levels and breast cancer risk in premenopausal women.[20,45-48,51,52,54,55,74,75] Among earlier studies, with a range of 66[48] to 121[47] cases, most but not all[47] studies observed an increased risk of breast cancer with higher levels of IGF-I (Table 2). For instance, in both the NHS and NYUWHS studies, women in the top 20-25%

Table 2. *Circulating hormone levels and breast cancer risk in premenopausal women*

	Study	Cases/Controls	Category Unit	RR (95% CI)
Estradiol				
	Kaaks, 2005	285/555	Quartiles	1.0 (0.7-1.5)
	Eliassen, 2006	185/368	Quartiles	2.1 (1.1-4.1)
	Follicular			
	Luteal	175/349	Quartiles	1.0 (0.5-1.9)
Testosterone				
	Micheli, 2004	40/108	Tertiles	2.2 (0.6-7.6)
	Kaaks, 2005	370/726	Quartiles	1.7 (1.2-2.6)
	Eliassen, 2006	190/374	Quartiles	1.3 (0.8-2.4)
	Follicular			
	Luteal	192/390	Quartiles	1.6 (0.9-2.8)
Progesterone				
	Micheli, 2004	40/108	Tertiles	0.1 (0.0-0.5)
	Kaaks, 2005	277/524	Quartiles	0.6 (0.4-1.0)
	Eliassen, 2006	195/391	Quartiles	0.9 (0.5-1.7)
	Luteal			
IGF-I				
	Hankinson, 1998	76/105	Quintiles	2.3 (1.1-5.2)
	Toniolo, 2000	172/486	Quartiles	2.3 (1.1-4.9)
	Kaaks, 2002	116/330*	Quartiles	0.6 (0.3-1.4)
	Krajcik, 2002	66/66	Quartiles	3.5 (0.7-18.7)
	Muti, 2002	69/265	Quartiles	3.1 (1.1-8.6)
	Allen, 2005	70/209	Tertiles	1.2 (0.6-2.5)
	Rinaldi, 2005	138/259	Quartiles	1.9 (1.0-3.7)
	Schernhammer, 2005	218/281	Tertiles	1.6 (1.0-2.5)
	Schernhammer, 2006	239/478	Quartiles	1.0 (0.7-1.5)
	Rinaldi, 2006	270/528**	Quintiles	1.0 (0.6-1.8)
	Baglietto, 2007	151/6352	Quartiles	0.8 (0.5-1.4)
Prolactin				
	Wang, 1992	71/2596	Quintile	1.1 (0.5-2.2)
	Helzlsouer, 1994	21/42	Tertile	1.1 (0.3-4.1)
	Kabuto, 2000	46/94	Log_{10} unit increase	1.0 (0.0-47.4)
	Tworoger, 2006	239/478	Quartile	1.5 (1.0-2.5)
	Tworoger, 2007	492/1001	Quartile	1.4 (1.0-1.9)

*Age <50 years at blood collection. **Age at diagnosis ≤50.

of IGF-I levels had a significant 2.3-fold higher risk of breast cancer compared to women in the lowest category.[45,46] However, in an analysis of two Swedish cohorts combined, no increased risk was observed (top vs. bottom quartile RR = 0.6, 95% CI (0.3-1.4)).[47] In more recent studies, estimates have been more modest[51,74] or null[54,55,75] (Table 2). In an extended analysis within the NHS, with 218 cases, a modest increased risk was observed (top versus bottom tertile RR = 1.6, 95% CI (1.0-2.5)).[51] In the largest analysis of premenopausal women to date, in EPIC with 270 cases, no overall association was observed between IGF-I levels and breast cancer risk (top versus bottom quintile RR = 1.0, 95% CI (0.6-1.8)).[54]

Analyses of IGFBP-3 levels and breast cancer risk in premenopausal women have been, as with postmenopausal women, quite inconsistent, with suggested positive,[20,46,48,74] null[47,51,75] and suggested inverse[52] associations observed. To date, four studies have examined IGFBP-1 levels and breast cancer risk in premenopausal women, with no association observed in any of the four.[47,48,51,75]

Prolactin

To date there have been only five prospective studies of prolactin levels and breast cancer risk among premenopausal women (Table 2). In three small studies, with 21-71 cases each,[56,57,67] no association was observed, but a significant positive association was observed among 239 cases in the NHSII.[76] As noted above, in the combined analysis of NHS and NHSII no significant difference was observed by menopausal status and prolactin levels were modestly associated with breast cancer risk in premenopausal women.[60] With 492 premenopausal cases, the top versus bottom quartile RR was 1.4, 95% CI (1.0-1.9), p-trend = 0.05.

Conclusion

Although there are few prospective studies of premenopausal testosterone and breast cancer risk, a positive association has been observed consistently with approximate twofold increases in invasive breast cancer risk among women with high levels. The associations between estrogen and progesterone levels in premenopausal women and breast cancer risk have not been consistent and further assessments are needed. In the only study to detect a significant association with estrogen, follicular, but not luteal, estradiol levels were associated with risk. It is possible that follicular levels better reflect breast tissue estrogen exposure[77-79] or that estradiol has a greater impact in the low-progesterone environment of the follicular phase.[80-84] This finding was not consistent across estrogens, as no associations were observed with estrone or estrone sulfate. The stronger associations observed with ER+/PR+ tumors is consistent with findings among postmenopausal women, although again this needs to be replicated in future studies. The two largest studies also had conflicting findings for progesterone. The importance of timing within the menstrual cycle needs to be resolved since the association was only apparent in the EPIC study when the less accurate form of menstrual cycle timing was utilized. Thus, while evidence is beginning to accumulate supporting an association between premenopausal sex steroid hormones and breast cancer risk, the nature and magnitude of the associations require further study.

Earlier evidence suggested a positive association between IGF-I and breast cancer risk among premenopausal women, but more recent evidence from larger studies has been null. Whether the differences in results are attributable to differences in study populations or assay methods needs to be examined to determine the source of these substantial inconsistencies. Assessments of IGFs and breast cancer survival are also needed. While there are still few studies of prolactin levels and breast cancer risk in premenopausal women, accumulated evidence suggests that prolactin is a modest, independent risk factor for breast cancer in premenopausal women.

Endometrial Cancer

Estrogens

To date, the association between estrogen levels and endometrial cancer risk has been investigated in only two prospective studies, both among postmenopausal women not using postmenopausal hormones. Cases (n = 57) from the first study from NYUWHS,[85] were then included in a combined analysis of the NYUWHS, Umea Sweden and Hormones and Diet in the Etiology of Breast Cancer Risk (ORDET) cohorts[86] among postmenopausal women (124 cases). Estradiol and estrone were both strongly and significantly associated with endometrial cancer risk (top versus bottom quartile RR = 5.4, 95% CI (2.5-11.6), p-trend = 0.0001 for estradiol and RR = 4.6, 95% CI (2.3-9.1), p-trend = 0.0001 for estrone). Adjustment for BMI, SHBG levels, or androgen levels slightly attenuated these associations but they remained strong and statistically significant (Table 3).

SHBG was inversely associated with endometrial cancer risk in the combined analysis (top versus bottom quartile RR = 0.4, 95% CI (0.2-0.7), p-trend = 0.0006), as expected given the strong inverse association between BMI and SHBG.[86]

Androgens

The association between circulating androgens and endometrial cancer risk has only been investigated in the combined analysis of postmenopausal women (124 cases),[86] with significant direct associations observed for androstenedione (top versus bottom quartile RR = 2.1, 95% CI (1.1-4.0), p-trend = 0.03), testosterone (comparable RR = 2.1, 95% CI (1.1-4.0), p-trend = 0.02) and DHEAS (comparable RR = 3.1, 95% CI (1.5-6.0), p-trend = 0.0001). After adjustment for BMI, the associations were attenuated but remained strong and all but the testosterone association remained statistically significant (Table 3). Adjusting for estradiol and estrone significantly attenuated the associations and the effects of androstenedione and testosterone were no longer significant, but DHEAS, though attenuated, remained significant after adjustment for estrone and was marginally significant after adjustment for estradiol.

Insulin-Like Growth Factor I and IGF Binding Proteins

Only one study, combining the NYUWHS, Umea and ORDET cohorts with 166 cases in total, has investigated circulating IGF-I and endometrial cancer risk and no association was observed.[87] Similarly, no association was observed with IGFBP-3. IGFBP-1 and -2 have been investigated in the combined analysis[87] as well as within EPIC,[88] with conflicting findings. In the combined analysis, IGFBP-2 was unrelated to endometrial cancer risk but IGFBP-1 was inversely associated with risk (top versus bottom quintile RR = 0.3, 95% CI (0.2-0.6), p-trend = 0.002); the association with IGFBP-1 was substantially weakened after adjusting for BMI (p-trend = 0.06).[87] In contrast, in the EPIC investigation, no association was observed with IGFBP-1 levels, but a significant inverse association was observed with IGFBP-2 levels (top versus bottom quartile RR = 0.6, 95% CI (0.4-0.9), p-trend = 0.03).[88]

Conclusion

Although few studies have been conducted to date, evidence suggests strong positive associations between circulating androgens, estrogens and endometrial cancer. These findings should be confirmed and better quantified in future, larger prospective studies. Evidence for an association with IGF-I and its binding proteins is limited and more mixed, with null and inverse associations observed. While the question remains of whether there is a correlation between circulating and tissue levels of hormones, the strong positive associations with estrogens and androgens suggest that circulating levels are an indirect marker of tissue exposure.

Ovarian Cancer

Gonadotropins

Although gonadotropins have been hypothesized to contribute to a hormonal etiology of ovarian cancer,[18] the few studies that have investigated FSH and LH levels have found either null or inverse associations (Table 4). In the NYUWHS study with 58 cases (22 premenopausal and 36 postmenopausal), the point estimate for the highest tertile of LH levels, compared with the lowest, was below one but was not statistically significant (RR = 0.4, 95% CI (0.1-2.1)).[89] Similarly, in a small study by Helzlsouer et al, with 31 cases, a nonsignificant inverse association was observed among premenopausal and postmenopausal women combined (RR = 0.4, 95% CI (0.1-2.0)).[90] FSH levels were statistically significantly inversely associated with ovarian cancer in this study (top versus bottom tertile RR = 0.1, 95% CI (0.0-1.0), p-trend = 0.02), with the association most apparent among postmenopausal women (p = 0.05). However, in a combined analysis of the NYUWHS, Umea and ORDET cohorts, with 88 postmenopausal cases, no association was observed (top versus bottom tertile RR = 0.9, 95% CI (0.4-2.0)).[91] Thus, the limited data available to date do not support a positive relation between gonadotropins and ovarian cancer as originally hypothesized.

Table 3. Circulating hormone levels and endometrial cancer risk

	Study	Menopausal Status	Hormone	Cases/Controls	Category Unit	RR (95% CI)
Estrogens						
	Lukanova, 2004(a)	Postmenopausal	Estradiol	122/230	Quartiles	4.1 (1.8-9.7)
			Estrone	122/230	Quartiles	3.7 (1.7-7.9)
Androgens						
	Lukanova, 2004(a)	Postmenopausal	Androstenedione	124/236	Quartiles	2.2 (1.1-4.4)
			Testosterone	124/236	Quartiles	1.7 (0.9-3.5)
			DHEAS	124/236	Quartiles	2.9 (1.4-5.9)
IGF-I						
	Lukanova, 2004(b)	Pre and Postmenopausal	IGF-I	166/314	Quintiles	0.9 (0.4-1.8)

Estrogens

Estrone levels have been examined in two studies (119 cases in total), with no significant associations observed in premenopausal and postmenopausal women combined,[90] or in postmenopausal women alone (Table 4).[92] In a small study of both premenopausal and postmenopausal women estradiol levels were not significantly different between cases and controls.[90]

Androgens

Several studies have investigated the associations between both ovarian and adrenal androgens, including androstenedione, testosterone, DHEA and DHEAS, and the risk of ovarian cancer. In an early small (31 cases) study androstenedione levels were significantly positively associated with ovarian cancer risk (Table 4).[90] However, in two subsequent, larger studies (132 and 192 cases) results generally were null,[92,93] although in one study a positive association among premenopausal women was suggested (44 cases) (RR = 2.4, 95% CI (0.8-6.8)).[92] Testosterone levels have been investigated in two studies, with no associations observed; however a significant inverse association was observed between free testosterone and ovarian cancer risk among postmenopausal, but not premenopausal, cases (n = 136) (Table 4).[93] DHEA levels were significantly higher in cases compared with controls in one small study;[90] to our knowledge plasma DHEA levels have not been examined in any other study. DHEAS levels were suggestive positively associated with ovarian cancer risk in a small study,[90] but no association was observed among premenopausal or postmenopausal women in two subsequent, larger studies (Table 4).[92,93]

Insulin-like Growth Factor I and IGF Binding Proteins

Only four analyses have examined the association between IGF-I, its binding proteins and ovarian cancer risk. In a combined analysis of three cohorts (NYUWHS, Umea Sweden and ORDET), with 132 cases, no overall association was observed with IGF-I (Table 4), but an increased risk was observed among 41 cases who were diagnosed at ages <55 years (top versus bottom tertile RR = 5.0, 95% CI (1.2-20.2)).[94] A similar pattern was observed in the EPIC cohort, with 214 cases, with no overall association (Table 4) but a suggested increased risk among those diagnosed at ages <55 years (66 cases) (top versus bottom tertile RR = 2.4, 95% CI (0.9-6.4)).[95] In a combined analysis within the NHS, NHSII and Women's Health Study (WHS) cohorts, with 179 cases, a modest inverse association was observed (top versus bottom quartile RR = 0.6, 95% CI (0.3-1.0)), but the trend was not significant (p-trend = 0.14).[96] In contrast to the two previous studies, no significant association was observed among the 59 cases diagnosed at ages <55 years. In all three studies, the association with IGFBP-3 was null among all cases and among those diagnosed at ages <55 years. In the only study to date to investigate IGFBP-1 no association was observed for levels of the binding protein overall or among cases diagnosed at ages <55 years.[97] Two studies have investigated IGFBP-2, with no associations observed overall or among younger women.[96,97]

Conclusions

While ovarian cancer has a hormonal etiology, at least in part, studies to date of circulating hormone levels and risk have not consistently shown the hypothesized associations. Data on estrogens and ovarian cancer are limited and one of the prior studies combined premenopausal and postmenopausal women, which is likely not appropriate for estrogen levels that differ so substantially by menopausal status. To date, circulating androgen levels do not appear important in predicting risk. IGF-I levels may be directly related to ovarian cancer in younger women, although the data again are limited and not entirely consistent; associations with IGF binding proteins have thus far been null. Future larger prospective studies are needed and separate examination by menopausal status would be important for estrogens and gonadotropins. A potential explanation for the lack of associations observed could be that circulating levels of hormones do not reflect hormone exposure at the ovarian epithelial cell. In addition, most epidemiologic studies include a combination of subtypes of epithelial ovarian cancer. While it is possible that these subtypes have different etiologies, the limited case numbers in prospective analyses of ovarian cancer currently preclude any subtype specific assessments.

Table 4. Circulating hormone levels and ovarian cancer risk

	Study	Menopausal Status	Hormone	Cases/Controls	Category Unit	RR (95% CI)
Estrogens	Helzlsouer, 1995	Pre and Postmenopausal	Estradiol	31/62	Tertiles	3.0 (0.6–14.9)
			Estrone	31/62	Tertiles	1.7 (0.4–7.6)
	Lukanova, 2003	Postmenopausal	Estrone	88/171	Quartiles	1.2 (0.5–2.8)
Androgens	Helzlsouer, 1995	Pre and Postmenopausal	Androstenedione	31/62	Tertiles	7.6 (1.2–48.7)
			DHEA	31/62	Tertiles	2.3 (0.7–7.6)
			DHEAS	31/62	Tertiles	2.7 (0.7–10.0)
	Lukanova, 2003	Premenopausal	Androstenedione	44/84	Tertiles	2.4 (0.8–6.8)
			Testosterone	44/83	Tertiles	1.4 (0.5–4.1)
			DHEAS	44/84	Tertiles	1.5 (0.5–4.3)
		Postmenopausal	Androstenedione	86/173	Quartiles	0.6 (0.3–1.3)
			Testosterone	88/169	Quartiles	1.3 (0.6–3.1)
			DHEAS	87/172	Quartiles	1.0 (0.4–2.3)
	Rinaldi, 2007	Premenopausal	Androstenedione	54/104	Above vs. below median	1.1 (0.6–2.3)
			Testosterone	52/97	Above vs. below median	1.2 (0.5–2.7)
			DHEAS	56/109	Above vs. below median	1.2 (0.6–2.5)
			Free testosterone	50/92	Above vs. below median	1.3 (0.6–2.9)
		Postmenopausal	Androstenedione	128/222	Tertiles	0.7 (0.4–1.2)
			Testosterone	125/203	Tertiles	0.7 (0.4–1.3)
			DHEAS	134/232	Tertiles	0.8 (0.5–1.4)
			Free testosterone	118/186	Tertiles	0.5 (0.2–0.9)
IGF-I	Lukanova, 2002	Pre and Postmenopausal	IGF-I	132/263	Quartiles	1.4 (0.7–2.8)
	Peeters, 2007	Pre and Postmenopausal	IGF-I	214/388	Tertiles	1.1 (0.7–1.7)
	Tworoger, 2007	Pre and Postmenopausal	IGF-I	179/599	Quartiles	0.6 (0.3–1.0)
Gonadotropins	Akhmedkhanov, 2001	Pre and Postmenopausal	LH	58/116	Tertiles	0.4 (0.1–2.1)
	Helzlsouer, 1995	Pre and Postmenopausal	LH	31/62	Tertiles	0.4 (0.1–2.0)
			FSH	31/62	Tertiles	0.1 (0.0–1.0)
	Arslan, 2003	Postmenopausal	FSH	88/168	Tertiles	0.9 (0.4–2.0)

Summary

As cumulative indirect evidence has suggested, sex steroid hormones are important in the etiology of breast cancer. Among postmenopausal women, the associations between estrogens, testosterone and breast cancer risk are consistent and well established. IGF-I and its binding proteins have not been consistently associated with an increased risk, but prolactin levels appear to be a modest relatively well confirmed risk factor for breast cancer. Recent work has helped identify subgroups of women in whom hormone levels appear particularly important (e.g., those with ER+/PR+ tumors) and hormone levels may improve current models used to predict a woman's risk of breast cancer. Premenopausal sex steroid hormones also appear to play an important role in breast cancer although evidence is not as plentiful nor as consistent hence further research is necessary to elucidate these relationships. IGF-I results have been puzzlingly inconsistent, with more recent studies not confirming the positive association observed among premenopausal women in earlier studies. Accumulating evidence suggests that prolactin levels in premenopausal women are predictive of breast cancer risk, with a similar magnitude observed for both premenopausal and postmenopausal women.

In contrast to breast cancer, fewer studies have investigated circulating hormone levels and risk of endometrial and ovarian cancer. Sex steroid hormones appear to be an important and strong predictor of endometrial cancer risk, but results from studies of ovarian cancer do not suggest a strong association. From the current literature, it is unclear whether IGF-I is an important risk factor for either endometrial or ovarian cancer. Several studies have investigated the role of circulating gonadotropins and ovarian cancer risk, but thus far none has supported the gonadotropin hypothesis of the etiology of ovarian cancer.

Further study is required to continue to elucidate the hormonal etiology of these three cancers. With strong evidence to date of a role of sex steroid hormones in the etiology of postmenopausal breast cancer, the next step is to consider the roles of these hormones in existing prediction models to help determine a woman's risk of breast cancer. Among premenopausal women, further prospective studies with careful attention paid to menstrual cycle timing are necessary to confirm the magnitude and direction of estimates. Although all of the studies summarized are prospective, it is possible that blood collected shortly before diagnosis may be affected by a subclinical tumor. However, evidence to date suggests that hormone concentrations are associated with breast cancer risk in postmenopausal women at least 10 years after blood collection; with more follow-up the importance of timing can be confirmed in both premenopausal and postmenopausal women. Larger prospective studies are required to confirm the sex steroid hormone association with endometrial cancer and further investigation into growth factors and the associations with obesity are necessary. The continuing investigation of the role of circulating hormones in the etiology of ovarian cancer in larger prospective studies is necessary, with separate analysis of premenopausal and postmenopausal women and attention to menstrual cycle timing among premenopausal women. In addition, larger studies may allow a separation of subtypes, which may have different etiologies.

Acknowlegement

This work was supported by Research Grant CA49449 and CA67262 from the National Cancer Institute. Dr. Eliassen was supported by Cancer Education and Career Development Grant R25 CA098566-02 from the National Cancer Institute.

References

1. Hankinson SE, Colditz GA, Willett WC. Towards an integrated model for breast cancer etiology: the lifelong interplay of genes, lifestyle and hormones. Breast Cancer Res 2004; 6:213-218.
2. van den Brandt PA, Spiegelman D, Yaun SS et al. Pooled analysis of prospective cohort studies on height, weight and breast cancer risk. Am J Epidemiol 2000; 152:514-527.
3. Kaaks R, Lukanova A, Kurzer MS. Obesity, endogenous hormones and endometrial cancer risk: a synthetic review. Cancer Epidemiol Biomarkers Prev 2002; 11:1531-1543.
4. Lukanova A, Kaaks R. Endogenous hormones and ovarian cancer: epidemiology and current hypotheses. Cancer Epidemiol Biomarkers Prev 2005; 14:98-107.

5. Danforth KN, Tworoger SS, Hecht JL et al. A prospective study of postmenopausal hormone use and ovarian cancer risk. Br J Cancer 2007; 96:151-156.
6. Henderson BE, Feigelson HS. Hormonal carcinogenesis. Carcinogenesis 2000; 21:427-433.
7. Liao DJ, Dickson RB. Roles of androgens in the development, growth and carcinogenesis of the mammary gland. J Steroid Biochem Mol Biol 2002; 80:175-189.
8. Syed V, Ulinski G, Mok SC et al. Expression of gonadotropin receptor and growth responses to key reproductive hormones in normal and malignant human ovarian surface epithelial cells. Cancer Res 2001; 61:6768-6776.
9. Legro RS, Kunselman AR, Miller SA et al. Role of androgens in the growth of endometrial carcinoma: an in vivo animal model. Am J Obstet Gynecol 2001; 184:303-308.
10. Khandwala HM, McCutcheon IE, Flyvbjerg A et al. The effects of insulin-like growth factors on tumorigenesis and neoplastic growth. Endocr Rev 2000; 21:215-244.
11. Rajaram S, Baylink DJ, Mohan S. Insulin-like growth factor-binding proteins in serum and other biological fluids: regulation and functions. Endocr Rev 1997; 18:801-831.
12. Yu H, Rohan T. Role of the insulin-like growth factor family in cancer development and progression. J Natl Cancer Inst 2000; 92:1472-1489.
13. Clevenger CV, Furth PA, Hankinson SE et al. The role of prolactin in mammary carcinoma. Endocr Rev 2003; 24:1-27.
14. Lanari C, Molinolo AA. Progesterone receptors—animal models and cell signalling in breast cancer. Diverse activation pathways for the progesterone receptor: possible implications for breast biology and cancer. Breast Cancer Res 2002; 4:240-243.
15. Campagnoli C, Clavel-Chapelon F, Kaaks R et al. Progestins and progesterone in hormone replacement therapy and the risk of breast cancer. J Steroid Biochem Mol Biol 2005;96:95-108.
16. Siiteri PK. Steroid hormones and endometrial cancer. Cancer Res 1978; 38:4360-4366.
17. Risch HA. Hormonal etiology of epithelial ovarian cancer, with a hypothesis concerning the role of androgens and progesterone. J Natl Cancer Inst 1998; 90:1774-1786.
18. Cramer DW, Welch WR. Determinants of ovarian cancer risk. II. Inferences regarding pathogenesis. J Natl Cancer Inst 1983; 71:717-721.
19. Missmer SA, Spiegelman D, Bertone-Johnson ER et al. Reproducibility of plasma steroid hormones, prolactin and insulin-like growth factor levels among premenopausal women over a 2-3 year period. Cancer Epidemiol Biomarkers Prev 2006; 15:972-978.
20. Muti P, Quattrin T, Grant BJ et al. Fasting glucose is a risk factor for breast cancer: a prospective study. Cancer Epidemiol Biomarkers Prev 2002; 11:1361-1368.
21. Arslan AA, Zeleniuch-Jacquotte A, Lukanova A et al. Reliability of follicle-stimulating hormone measurements in serum. Reprod Biol Endocrinol 2003; 1:49.
22. Toniolo P, Koenig KL, Pasternack BS et al. Reliability of measurements of total, protein-bound and unbound estradiol in serum. Cancer Epidemiol Biomarkers Prev 1994; 3:47-50.
23. Hankinson SE, Manson JE, Spiegelman D et al. Reproducibility of plasma hormone levels in postmenopausal women over a 2-3-year period. Cancer Epidemiol Biomarkers Prev 1995; 4:649-654.
24. Micheli A, Muti P, Pisani P et al. Repeated serum and urinary androgen measurements in premenopausal and postmenopausal women. J Clin Epidemiol 1991; 44:1055-1061.
25. Muti P, Trevisan M, Micheli A et al. Reliability of serum hormones in premenopausal and postmenopausal women over a one-year period. Cancer Epidemiol Biomarkers Prev 1996; 5:917-922.
26. Michaud DS, Manson JE, Spiegelman D et al. Reproducibility of plasma and urinary sex hormone levels in premenopausal women over a one-year period. Cancer Epidemiol Biomarkers Prev 1999; 8:1059-1064.
27. Willett WC. Nutritional Epidemiology. 2nd ed. New York: Oxford University Press 1998.
28. van Landeghem AA, Poortman J, Nabuurs M et al. Endogenous concentration and subcellular distribution of estrogens in normal and malignant human breast tissue. Cancer Res 1985; 45:2900-2906.
29. Thijssen JH, Blankenstein MA, Miller WR et al. Estrogens in tissues: uptake from the peripheral circulation or local production. Steroids 1987; 50:297-306.
30. Vermeulen A, Deslypere JP, Paridaens R et al. Aromatase, 17 beta-hydroxysteroid dehydrogenase and intratissular sex hormone concentrations in cancerous and normal glandular breast tissue in postmenopausal women. Eur J Cancer Clin Oncol 1986; 22:515-525.
31. Recchione C, Venturelli E, Manzari A et al. Testosterone, dihydrotestosterone and oestradiol levels in postmenopausal breast cancer tissues. J Steroid Biochem Mol Biol 1995; 52:541-546.
32. Mady EA, Ramadan EE, Ossman AA. Sex steroid hormones in serum and tissue of benign and malignant breast tumor patients. Disease Markers 2000; 16:151-157.
33. Porias H, Sojo I, Carranco A et al. A simultaneous assay to quantitate plasma and endometrial hormone concentrations. Fertil Steril 1978; 30:66-69.

34. Godwin AK, Perez RP, Johnson SW et al. Growth regulation of ovarian cancer. Hematol Oncol Clin North Am 1992; 6:829-841.

35. Endogenous Hormones and Breast Cancer Collaborative Group. Endogenous sex hormones and breast cancer in postmenopausal women: reanalysis of nine prospective studies. J Natl Cancer Inst 2002; 94:606-616.

36. Manjer J, Johansson R, Berglund G et al. Postmenopausal breast cancer risk in relation to sex steroid hormones, prolactin and SHBG (Sweden). Cancer Causes Control 2003; 14:599-607.

37. Key TJ, Wang DY, Brown JB et al. A prospective study of urinary oestrogen excretion and breast cancer risk. Br J Cancer 1996; 73:1615-1619.

38. Onland-Moret NC, Kaaks R, van Noord PA et al. Urinary endogenous sex hormone levels and the risk of postmenopausal breast cancer. Br J Cancer 2003; 88:1394-1399.

39. Kaaks R, Rinaldi S, Key TJ et al. Postmenopausal serum androgens, oestrogens and breast cancer risk: the European prospective investigation into cancer and nutrition. Endocr Relat Cancer 2005; 12:1071-1082.

40. Zeleniuch-Jacquotte A, Shore RE, Koenig KL et al. Postmenopausal levels of oestrogen androgen and SHBG and breast cancer: long-term results of a prospective study. Br J Cancer 2004; 90:153-159.

41. Missmer SA, Eliassen AH, Barbieri RL et al. Endogenous estrogen androgen and progesterone concentrations and breast cancer risk among postmenopausal women. J Natl Cancer Inst 2004; 96:1856-1865.

42. Beattie MS, Costantino JP, Cummings SR et al. Endogenous sex hormones, breast cancer risk and tamoxifen response: an ancillary study in the NSABP Breast Cancer Prevention Trial (P1). J Natl Cancer Inst 2006; 98:110-115.

43. Eliassen AH, Missmer SA, Tworoger SS et al. Endogenous steroid hormone concentrations and risk of breast cancer: does the association vary by a woman's predicted breast cancer risk? J Clin Oncol 2006; 24:1823-1830.

44. Tworoger SS, Missmer SA, Barbieri RL et al. Plasma sex hormone concentrations and subsequent risk of breast cancer among women using postmenopausal hormones. J Natl Cancer Inst 2005; 97:595-602.

45. Hankinson SE, Willett WC, Colditz GA et al. Circulating concentrations of insulin-like growth factor-I and risk of breast cancer. Lancet 1998; 351:1393-1396.

46. Toniolo P, Bruning PF, Akhmedkhanov A et al. Serum insulin-like growth factor-I and breast cancer. Int J Cancer 2000; 88:828-832.

47. Kaaks R, Lundin E, Rinaldi S et al. Prospective study of IGF-I, IGF-binding proteins and breast cancer risk, in northern and southern Sweden. Cancer Causes Control 2002; 13:307-316.

48. Krajcik RA, Borofsky ND, Massaro S et al. Insulin-like growth factor I (IGF-I), IGF-binding proteins and breast cancer. Cancer Epidemiol Biomarkers Prev 2002; 11:1566-1573.

49. Keinan-Boker L, Bueno De Mesquita HB, Kaaks R et al. Circulating levels of insulin-like growth factor I, its binding proteins -1,-2, -3, C-peptide and risk of postmenopausal breast cancer. Int J Cancer 2003; 106:90-95.

50. Gronbaek H, Flyvbjerg A, Mellemkjaer L et al. Serum insulin-like growth factors, insulin-like growth factor binding proteins and breast cancer risk in postmenopausal women. Cancer Epidemiol Biomarkers Prev 2004; 13:1759-1764.

51. Schernhammer ES, Holly JM, Pollak MN et al. Circulating levels of insulin-like growth factors, their binding proteins and breast cancer risk. Cancer Epidemiol Biomarkers Prev 2005; 14:699-704.

52. Allen NE, Roddam AW, Allen DS et al. A prospective study of serum insulin-like growth factor-I (IGF-I), IGF-II, IGF-binding protein-3 and breast cancer risk. Br J Cancer 2005; 92:1283-1287.

53. Rollison DE, Newschaffer CJ, Tao Y et al. Premenopausal levels of circulating insulin-like growth factor I and the risk of postmenopausal breast cancer. Int J Cancer 2006; 118:1279-1284.

54. Rinaldi S, Peeters PH, Berrino F et al. IGF-I, IGFBP-3 and breast cancer risk in women: The European Prospective Investigation into Cancer and Nutrition (EPIC). Endocr Relat Cancer 2006; 13:593-605.

55. Baglietto L, English DR, Hopper JL et al. Circulating insulin-like growth factor-I and binding protein-3 and the risk of breast cancer. Cancer Epidemiol Biomarkers Prev 2007; 16:763-768.

56. Kabuto M, Akiba S, Stevens RG et al. A prospective study of estradiol and breast cancer in Japanese women. Cancer Epidemiol Biomarkers Prev 2000; 9:575-579.

57. Wang DY, De Stavola BL, Bulbrook RD et al. Relationship of blood prolactin levels and the risk of subsequent breast cancer. Int J Epidemiol 1992; 21:214-221.

58. Hankinson SE, Willett WC, Michaud DS et al. Plasma prolactin levels and subsequent risk of breast cancer in postmenopausal women. J Natl Cancer Inst 1999; 91:629-634.

59. Tworoger SS, Eliassen AH, Rosner B et al. Plasma prolactin concentrations and risk of postmenopausal breast cancer. Cancer Res 2004; 64:6814-6819.

60. Tworoger SS, Eliassen AH, Sluss P et al. A prospective study of plasma prolactin concentrations and risk of premenopausal and postmenopausal breast cancer. J Clin Oncol 2007; 25:1482-1488.

61. Fisher B, Costantino JP, Wickerham DL et al. Tamoxifen for prevention of breast cancer: report of the National Surgical Adjuvant Breast and Bowel Project P-1 Study. J Natl Cancer Inst 1998; 90:1371-1388.
62. Colditz GA, Rosner B. Cumulative risk of breast cancer to age 70 years according to risk factor status: data from the Nurses' Health Study. Am J Epidemiol 2000; 152:950-964.
63. Tyrer J, Duffy SW, Cuzick J. A breast cancer prediction model incorporating familial and personal risk factors. Stat Med 2004; 23:1111-1130.
64. Freedman AN, Seminara D, Gail MH et al. Cancer risk prediction models: a workshop on development, evaluation and application. J Natl Cancer Inst 2005; 97:715-723.
65. Cummings SR, Duong T, Kenyon E et al. Serum estradiol level and risk of breast cancer during treatment with raloxifene. JAMA 2002; 287:216-220.
66. Wysowski DK, Comstock GW, Helsing KJ et al. Sex hormone levels in serum in relation to the development of breast cancer. Am J Epidemiol 1987; 125:791-799.
67. Helzlsouer KJ, Alberg AJ, Bush TL et al. A prospective study of endogenous hormones and breast cancer. Cancer Detect Prev 1994; 18:79-85.
68. Rosenberg CR, Pasternack BS, Shore RE et al. Premenopausal estradiol levels and the risk of breast cancer: a new method of controlling for day of the menstrual cycle. Am J Epidemiol 1994; 140:518-525.
69. Thomas HV, Key TJ, Allen DS et al. A prospective study of endogenous serum hormone concentrations and breast cancer risk in premenopausal women on the island of Guernsey. Br J Cancer 1997; 75:1075-1079.
70. Kaaks R, Berrino F, Key T et al. Serum sex steroids in premenopausal women and breast cancer risk within the European Prospective Investigation into Cancer and Nutrition (EPIC). J Natl Cancer Inst 2005; 97:755-765.
71. Eliassen AH, Missmer SA, Tworoger SS et al. Endogenous steroid hormone concentrations and risk of breast cancer among premenopausal women. J Natl Cancer Inst 2006; 98:1406-1415.
72. Micheli A, Muti P, Secreto G et al. Endogenous sex hormones and subsequent breast cancer in premenopausal women. Int J Cancer 2004; 112:312-318.
73. Thomas HV, Key TJ, Allen DS et al. A prospective study of endogenous serum hormone concentrations and breast cancer risk in postmenopausal women on the island of Guernsey. Br J Cancer 1997; 76:401-405.
74. Rinaldi S, Kaaks R, Zeleniuch-Jacquotte A et al. Insulin-like growth factor-I, IGF binding protein-3 and breast cancer in young women: a comparison of risk estimates using different peptide assays. Cancer Epidemiol Biomarkers Prev 2005; 14:48-52.
75. Schernhammer ES, Holly JM, Hunter DJ et al. Insulin-like growth factor-I, its binding proteins (IGFBP-1 and IGFBP-3) and growth hormone and breast cancer risk in The Nurses Health Study II. Endocr Relat Cancer 2006; 13:583-592.
76. Tworoger SS, Sluss P, Hankinson SE. Association between plasma prolactin concentrations and risk of breast cancer among predominately premenopausal women. Cancer Res 2006; 66:2476-2482.
77. Siiteri PK, Schwarz BE, Moriyama I et al. Estrogen binding in the rat and human. Adv Exp Med Biol 1973; 36:97-112.
78. Siiteri PK. Extraglandular oestrogen formation and serum binding of oestradiol: relationship to cancer. J Endocrinol 1981;89 Suppl:119P-129P.
79. Bulun SE, Price TM, Aitken J et al. A link between breast cancer and local estrogen biosynthesis suggested by quantification of breast adipose tissue aromatase cytochrome P450 transcripts using competitive polymerase chain reaction after reverse transcription. J Clin Endocrinol Metab 1993; 77:1622-1628.
80. Ricketts D, Turnbull L, Ryall G et al. Estrogen and progesterone receptors in the normal female breast. Cancer Res 1991; 51:1817-1822.
81. Markopoulos C, Berger U, Wilson P et al. Oestrogen receptor content of normal breast cells and breast carcinomas throughout the menstrual cycle. Br Med J (Clin Res Ed) 1988; 296:1349-1351.
82. Yue W, Santner SJ, Masamura S et al. Determinants of tissue estradiol levels and biologic responsiveness in breast tumors. Breast Cancer Res Treat. 1998;49 Suppl. 1:S1-7; discussion S33-37.
83. Gompel A, Somai S, Chaouat M et al. Hormonal regulation of apoptosis in breast cells and tissues. Steroids 2000; 65:593-598.
84. Sabourin JC, Martin A, Baruch J et al. bcl-2 expression in normal breast tissue during the menstrual cycle. Int J Cancer 1994; 59:1-6.
85. Zeleniuch-Jacquotte A, Akhmedkhanov A, Kato I et al. Postmenopausal endogenous oestrogens and risk of endometrial cancer: results of a prospective study. Br J Cancer 2001; 84:975-981.
86. Lukanova A, Lundin E, Micheli A et al. Circulating levels of sex steroid hormones and risk of endometrial cancer in postmenopausal women. Int J Cancer 2004; 108:425-432.

87. Lukanova A, Zeleniuch-Jacquotte A, Lundin E et al. Prediagnostic levels of C-peptide, IGF-I, IGFBP-1, -2 and -3 and risk of endometrial cancer. Int J Cancer 2004; 108:262-268.

88. Cust AE, Allen NE, Rinaldi S et al. Serum levels of C-peptide, IGFBP-1 and IGFBP-2 and endometrial cancer risk; results from the European prospective investigation into cancer and nutrition. Int J Cancer 2007; 120:2656-2664.

89. Akhmedkhanov A, Toniolo P, Zeleniuch-Jacquotte A et al. Luteinizing hormone, its beta-subunit variant and epithelial ovarian cancer: the gonadotropin hypothesis revisited. Am J Epidemiol 2001; 154:43-49.

90. Helzlsouer KJ, Alberg AJ, Gordon GB et al. Serum gonadotropins and steroid hormones and the development of ovarian cancer. JAMA 1995; 274:1926-1930.

91. Arslan AA, Zeleniuch-Jacquotte A, Lundin E et al. Serum follicle-stimulating hormone and risk of epithelial ovarian cancer in postmenopausal women. Cancer Epidemiol Biomarkers Prev 2003; 12:1531-1535.

92. Lukanova A, Lundin E, Akhmedkhanov A et al. Circulating levels of sex steroid hormones and risk of ovarian cancer. Int J Cancer 2003; 104:636-642.

93. Rinaldi S, Dossus L, Lukanova A et al. Endogenous androgens and risk of epithelial ovarian cancer: results from the European Prospective Investigation into Cancer and Nutrition (EPIC). Cancer Epidemiol Biomarkers Prev 2007; 16:23-29.

94. Lukanova A, Lundin E, Toniolo P et al. Circulating levels of insulin-like growth factor-I and risk of ovarian cancer. Int J Cancer 2002; 101:549-554.

95. Peeters PH, Lukanova A, Allen N et al. Serum IGF-I, its major binding protein (IGFBP-3) and epithelial ovarian cancer risk: the European Prospective Investigation into Cancer and Nutrition (EPIC). Endocr Relat Cancer 2007; 14:81-90.

96. Tworoger SS, Lee IM, Buring JE et al. Insulin-like growth factors and ovarian cancer risk: a nested case-control study in three cohorts. Cancer Epidemiol Biomarkers Prev 2007 (In press).

97. Lukanova A, Lundin E, Micheli A et al. Risk of ovarian cancer in relation to prediagnostic levels of C-peptide, insulin-like growth factor binding proteins-1 and -2 (USA, Sweden, Italy). Cancer Causes Control 2003; 14:285-292.

CHAPTER 11

Hormonal Heterogeneity of Endometrial Cancer

Carsten Gründker, Andreas R. Günthert and Günter Emons*

Abstract

Endometrial cancer is the most common malignant tumor of the female genital tract in the developed world. Increasing evidence suggests that the majority of cases can be divided into two different types of endometrial cancer based on clinico-pathological and molecular characteristics. Type I is associated with an endocrine milieu of estrogen predominance. These tumors are of endometroid histology and develop from endometrial hyperplasia. They have good prognosis and are sensitive to endocrine treatment. Type II endometrial cancers are not associated with a history of unopposed estrogens and develop from the atrophic endometrium of elderly women. Mainly, they are of serous papillary or clear cell morphology, have a poor prognosis and do not react to endocrine treatment. Both types of endometrial cancer probably differ markedly with regard to the molecular mechanisms of transformation. The transition from normal endometrium to a malignant tumor is thought to involve a stepwise accumulation of alterations in cellular mechanisms leading to dysfunctional cell growth. This chapter reviews the current knowledge of the molecular mechanisms commonly associated with development of type I and type II endometrial cancer.

Introduction

With 142,000 new cases every year, endometrial cancer (EC) is worldwide the seventh most frequent carcinoma of women. About 42,000 women die of this malignancy every year. In the developed world EC is the most common malignancy of the female genital tract and the fourth most common malignancy in women. In the Western industrialized countries, annual incidence rates between 10 per 100,000 women (U.K, Spain, France) and 25 per 100,000 women (U.S.A, Canada) are observed.[1,2] Though the curability of EC is high, tumors with particular morphological variants, adverse histopathological features and /or advanced stage are characterized by aggressive behavior and poor prognosis.

Increasing evidence suggests that at least two different types of EC exist. Type I is associated with an endocrine milieu of estrogen predominance. It frequently develops via a characteristic sequence of hyperplastic lesions of the endometrium with increasing premalignant potential. These tumors have a favorable prognosis.[3] On the molecular level mutations of the *ras*-oncogene, loss of *PTEN* tumor suppressor gene expression and dysfunction of DNA-mismatch repair genes are involved.[4,5] Additional mutations (e.g., in the *p53* tumor suppressor gene, loss of estrogen and/or progesterone receptor expression) are typical features of a further malignant transformation to aggressive, dedifferentiated endometrioid endometrial carcinomas with poor prognosis.[4,5]

*Corresponding Author: Günter Emons—Department of Gynecology and Obstetrics, Georg-August-University, Robert-Koch-Street 40, 37075 Göttingen, Germany.
Email: emons@med.uni-goettingen.de

Innovative Endocrinology of Cancer, edited by Lev M. Berstein and Richard J. Santen.
©2008 Landes Bioscience and Springer Science+Business Media.

About 10% of endometrial cancers are type II lesions. Type II EC is not associated with systemic hyperestrogenism and typically develops from the atrophic endometrium of elderly women. The histological type is either poorly differentiated endometrioid or non-endometrioid. The initial molecular event for the development of type II EC is probably a mutation of *p53* resulting in intraepithelial endometrial cancer which rapidly progresses to invasive serous-papillary carcinoma or other high-risk types of endometrial cancer. Sex steroid hormones are probably not involved in the tumorogenesis of these highly aggressive EC.[4,5]

However, the molecular mechanisms involved in development of EC remain poorly understood. This chapter reviews the current knowledge of the molecular mechanisms commonly associated with development of type I and type II EC.

Etiology

Type I and type II EC differ substantially with respect to etiology, pathogenesis and clinical behavior. For details see Table 1.[2,5]

Type I EC is driven by continuous exposure to estrogens in the absence of sufficient levels of progestogens. Typical risk factors are obesity, anovulatory states, early menarche and late menopause, nulliparity and unopposed exogenous estrogens. Multiparity, physically fitness and use of oral contraceptives decreases the risk to develop these cancers.[2,5,6] A continuous combined estrogen-progestagen therapy in the peri- and postmenopause possibly also reduces the risk to develop type I EC while the effects of a therapy with Tibolone on the endometrium are still controversial.[7] Type I EC develops via a characteristic sequence of hyperplastic changes of the endometrium with increasing premalignant potential.[3,4,8-11] Histologically, these estrogen-related ECs are accompanied by endometrial hyperplasia. They are well-to-intermediately differentiated, are normally diagnosed at an early stage and have an excellent prognosis. They strongly express estrogen and progestin receptors and have high response rates to progestin treatment of advanced stages.[3,4,8-13]

Type II EC has an aggressive clinical course and mostly non-endometrioid histology (usually papillary serous or clear cell) and is not associated with hyperestrogenic states.[3,8,9] It develops from the atrophic endometrium of elderly women, who do not have the classical risk factors for EC. These patients tend to be slim, are physically fit and as a rule have never used estrogen-replacement therapy. On diagnosis, type II EC is characterized by deep myometrial invasion and early lymph node or distant metastases. These cancers rarely express functional estrogen and/or progestin

Table 1. Differential aspects of type I and type II EC

Parameter	Type I EC	Type II EC
Cycle	Anovulatory	No disturbance
Fertility	Reduced	No disturbance
Age at menopause	>50 years	<50 years
Menopausal stage	Perimenopausal	Late postmenopausal
Endometrium adjacent to EC	Hyperplastic	Atrophic
Obesity	Mostly present	Mostly absent
Metabolic syndrome	Mostly present	Mostly absent
Tumor differentiation	>80% G1/G2	>60% G3 or upgraded
Histologic subtype	Endometroid carcinoma	Serous-papillary, clear-cell or adenosquamous carcinoma
Myometrial invasion	Superficial myometrial invasion	Deep myometrial invasion
Lymph space invasion	Rare	Frequent
Expression of PR	High	Low/ absent
Prognosis	favorable	poor

Reproduced from Emons G et al. 2000; 7(4):227-242;[5] with copyright permission from the Society for Endocrinology (2007).

Table 2.   Genetic differences between type I and type II EC

Parameter	Type I EC	Type II EC
K-ras	Mutational activation	—
C-myc, c-jun		Overexpression
hTERT		Overexpression
β-catenin	Gain of function mutations	—
PTEN	Loss of function mutations	—
p53	Inactivating mutations (late event, 5-10%)	Inactivating mutations (early event, 80-90%)
BRCA	—	Mutation -> Increase of risk
MSI	Yes	Rare
EGF-R		Overexpression
HER-2/erb-B2	Overexpression (10-30%)	Overexpression (45-70%)
IGF-R		Overexpression
ER-α	Decrease of expression to higher grade	Rarely expressed

receptors and their response rates to endocrine therapies tend to be low. The only known risk factors are the age and a radiotherapy of the uterus (e.g., because of cervical cancer).[14] In type II EC, mutations are found early in the p53 gene. Overexpression of the *HER-2/erb-B2* gene is also discussed.[2] Their prognosis is poor.

The morphologic and clinical differences between type I and type II EC are paralleled by genetic distinctions and carry mutations of independent sets of genes (Table 2).[15-20]

Estrogen-Aassociated Endometrial Cancer (Type I)

The association between the endocrine milieu of estrogen predominance, resulting in hyper-stimulation of the endometrium and an increased incidence of EC was first formally reported by Gusberg in 1947.[21] The normal endometrium is a hormonally responsive tissue. Estrogenic stimulation produces cellular growth and glandular proliferation, which is cyclically balanced by the maturational effects of progesterone.[22] Abnormal proliferation and neoplastic transformation is associated with chronic unopposed exposure to estrogenic stimulation. In a series of 170 patients who received no therapeutic intervention other than diagnostic curettage, Kurman et al[23] found that at least one-quarter of patients with atypical endometrial hyperplasia developed carcinoma compared with only 2% of patients with other types of hyperplasia. It is currently believed that estrogen-associated type I endometrial cancers (endometroid adenocarcinoma) progress through a premalignant stage of atypical adenomatous hyperplasia.[23] Type I EC's are characterized by large numbers of genetic changes in which the temporal sequence of mutation and the final combination of defects differ substantially between individual cases. Common genetic changes in type I EC include, but are not limited to, microsatellite instability (MSI),[24-27] or specific mutations of PTEN,[28-33] K-ras,[25,34-38] and β-catenin genes.[39-41] Additional mutations in the *p53* tumor suppressor gene and/or loss of estrogen and/or progesterone receptor expression are typical features of a further malignant transformation to aggressive, dedifferentiated endometrioid endometrial carcinomas with poor prognosis (Fig. 1).[4,5]

Non-Estrogen-Associated Endometrial Cancer (Type II)

Women with type II EC are at high risk of relapse and metastatic disease. Type II EC is not estrogen driven and most are associated with endometrial atrophy (Fig. 2). Serous carcinoma is the most aggressive type of type II EC.[42,43] Clear cell carcinoma is another type of type II EC.[44] About 40% of type II EC are mixed, with an endometrioid component.[43] Histopathologic studies

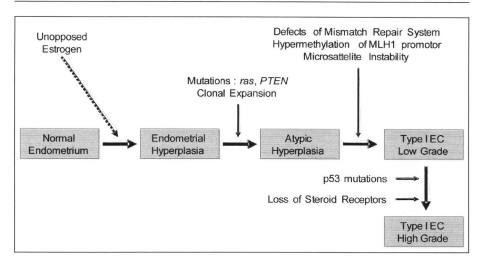

Figure 1. Carcinogenetic pathway of type I EC.

suggest that the majority of serous carcinomas develop from a distinctive lesion termed endometrial intraepithelial carcinoma (EIC), which appears to represent malignant transformation of atrophic surface endometrium.[4,45] In uteri containing serous carcinoma, the uninvolved endometrium is usually atrophic. It has been shown that when endometrial hyperplasia is identified in an uterus containing a carcinoma that is partly or exclusively serous, the hyperplasia and the carcinoma are usually topographically unrelated and appear distinct.[4] Sherman et al found that obesity and exogenous hormone use were not related to risk for serous carcinoma.[46] With advancing age, the probability of the accumulation of mutations leading to malignant transformation increases.[47]

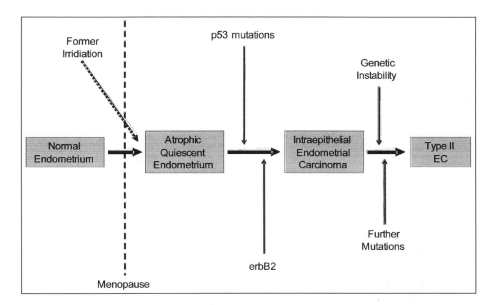

Figure 2. Carcinogenetic pathway of type II EC.

Pelvic irradiation might also add to the accumulation of mutations. The declining competence of the immune system with advancing age has been suggested as a further possible reason.[8,9,11] Mutations in the *p53* gene are well documented in type II EC and in its putative precursor EIC.[2,45] Tashiro et al found higher rates of loss of heterozygosity in serous carcinoma (100%) compared with EIC (43%) and suggested that loss of the wild-type *p53* allele can result in EIC, whereas serous carcinoma develops after the loss of the second allele.[48] Overexpression of *HER-2/erb-B2* is also discussed.[2] The timing of the appearance of *HER-2/erb-B2* mutations in the pathogenesis of type II EC is not known.

Uterine Carcinosarcomas (Malignant Mixed Müllerian Tumors)

The malignant mixed Müllerian tumor (MMMT) is a combination of carcinoma and sarcoma and is also termed uterine carcinosarcoma (UCS). MMMT's have been traditionally regarded as a subtype of type II EC. These neoplasms are rare (1-2% of all malignancies of the uterine corpus), highly aggressive and with an extremely poor prognosis. They are usually arising in elderly post-menopausal women and often presenting at an advanced stage.[49] There is an increasing evidence (clinical and molecular) suggesting that MMMT's are monoclonal malignancies, being derived from a single stem cell.[49-56] Immunological studies have suggested a common epithelial origin of MMMT's.[51] In vivo studies using nude mice have demonstrated that carcinoma cells derived from a MMMT cell line can give rise to tumors that include both epithelial and mesenchymal components whereas sarcoma cells do not.[52] In addition, the epithelial and mesenchymal components frequently share identical patterns of X-inactivation, allelic loss and p53 mutations.[53, 54] This would be highly unlikely if both components were not derived from a single stem cell. This all provides indirect evidence for the monoclonal theory of carcinogenesis in MMMT's with the carcinomatous component being the driving force and the sarcomatous component being derived from this as a result of dedifferentiation. Further molecular studies have shown that more than 25% of MMMT's have defects in their DNA mismatch repair system.[57] There is increasing evidence suggesting that MSI, a hallmark of defective DNA mismatch repair, is a common genetic change in MMMT and that defective DNA mismatch repair is a feature unique to the epithelial component of MMMT's.[58-60]

Molecular Pathogenesis of Endometrial Cancer

Oncogenes

K-ras

The *ras* (retrovirus-assiciated DNA sequences) genes are a family of proteins that have GTPase activity and are involved in signal transduction and mediate pleiotropic effects, including cell proliferation and migration. Ras genes are widely conserved among animal species. All of the genes have a similar structure and each gene encodes a 21-kDa protein. The C-terminus is necessary for full activation of downstream effectors such as Raf kinase and PI-3 kinase.[61] Point mutations in the mutational hot-spot codons 12, 13 and 61 are frequently detected in human malignancies and in different types of experimentally induced tumors in animals.[62-64] Ras mutations have been detected in different human cancers including endometrial cancer.[65,66] K-ras mutations have been identified in 19% to 46% of type I EC, but not in normal endometrium.[35,38,67-69] The frequency of K-ras mutations is higher in cancers with MSI.[69] Although both K-ras mutation and estrogen receptor (ER) are associated with type I EC, the relationship of these two factors is unclear. Tu et al could demonstrate that ER is positively regulated by Ras signaling.[70] Furthermore, the estrogen- and tamoxifen-induced transcriptional activity is enhanced by K-ras mutations.[70,71] ER seems to be one of the effectors of Ras/Raf signal transduction, involved in the tumorigenesis of type I EC.[70] Alterations of K-ras are also found in endometrial hyperplasia at a similar rate to EC suggesting that mutation in the K-ras gene is an early event in tumorigenesis of type I EC.[68] In type II EC MSI and K-ras mutations seem to be uncommon.[72-74]

C-myc and C-jun

Estrogen treatment induces immediate and transient activation of a number of nuclear oncogens in the uterus, including *c-fos, c-jun, junB, junD, N-myc* and *c-myc*.[75-78] Increased expression of these genes appears to be a direct effect of estrogen.[76] Among such estrogen-inducible oncogenes, some are considered to contribute to malignant transformation in the endometrium.[79] *C-myc* and *c-jun* are not only involved in normal growth, but may also play a role in the development of neoplasia.[79] Bai et al could demonstrate that overexpression and localization of the *c-myc* gene product may have an important role in the initiation, differentiation and progression of EC.[80] Bircan et al suggested in a study analyzing the expression of *c-myc, c-jun* and ER-alpha in cyclic endometrium, endometrial hyperplasia and EC that estrogen may induce *c-myc* expression leading to neoplastic transformation in human endometrium.[81] In addition, they found a positive correlation between *c-jun* expression and tumor grade in EC.[81] The association between ER and *c-jun* and hormone-mediated signaling pathways in EC seems to be different from that of normal endometrium. However, the involvement of *c-jun* in initiation, differentiation, or progression of EC is discussed controversially. *C-myc* is overexpressed in between 3% and 19% of EC. In addition, it was shown that nuclear and cytoplasmic immunohistochemical staining of *c-myc* is an independent prognostic factor in EC.[71,82,83] Neither *c-myc* nor *c-jun* seem to have specific prevalence in type I or type II EC.

hTERT

Telomerase is a unique ribonucleoprotein responsible for adding the telomeric repeats back onto the 3'-end of chromosome before each cell division and plays an important role in cellular immortalization and carcinogenesis.[84,85] Human telomerase reverse transcriptase (hTERT) is the catalytic part and therefore a key component of the telomerase.[86] In most normal somatic cell types, telomerase activity is usually undetectable but not in the endometrium.[87] This activity is dynamic throughout the menstrual cycle. It is high during the proliferative phase under influence of estrogen. In the secretory phase telomerase activity decreases under the influence of progesterone.[88] Overexpression of hTERT is involved in the development of cancer by causing telomere maintenance and potential cell immortalization.[89] Kyo et al have shown that estrogen activates telomerase through direct interaction of ligand-activated ER with the estrogen responsive element (ERE) in the hTERT 5' regulatory region of ER-positive endometrial cancer cells.[90] Other sex steroids also directly or indirectly regulate the hTERT promoter.[91,92] Wang et al demonstrated that the hTERT gene is a target of tamoxifen in a cell-specific manner.[93] Tamoxifen exerted E2 antagonistic effects on hTERT transcription in breast cancer cells but an agonistic effect in endometrial cancer cells. The authors could further show that tamoxifen activates the MAPK cascade in the endometrial cancer cells, but not in breast cancer cells. The activation of hTERT mRNA expression was effectively blocked by a MEK inhibitor, suggesting that the MAPK pathway is involved in the tamoxifen-induced activation of hTERT.[93] The effects of tamoxifen on abnormal endometrial proliferation are complex, but induction of hTERT and subsequent telomerase activation may be one component of these effects. Patients undergoing a prolonged adjuvant tamoxifen therapy against breast cancer should therefore be monitored for endometrial telomerase activity.[93] Recently Chen et al have shown that antisense oligonucleotides of hTERT effectively inhibit the growth of EC.[94] In a more recent study Zhou et al demonstrated that arsenic trioxide inhibits proliferation of EC cells through induction of apoptosis and by inhibition of telomerase activity and hTERT mRNA transcription.[95] Inhibition of telomerase activity might be a new strategy for therapy or prevention of EC. However, further studies are necessary to establish the exact role of hTERT in EC.

β-Catenin

Catenins are a group of cytosolic proteins which interact with the cytoplasmic domain of cadherins.[96,97] Cadherins are essential to the formation of cell-cell contacts and the stabilization of tissue architecture.[97] β- and γ-catenin bind to the catenin-binding domain of cadherins and mediate the binding of the complex to α-catenin.[96,97] Besides β- and γ-catenin are central players in the oncogenic Wnt signaling pathway.[98] They are downstream transcriptional activators in the Wnt signal transduction in which their activity is closely controlled by the APC tumor suppressor gene.[99] In this context β-catenin plays an important role in oncogenesis and is implicated in the development of EC.[41] Mutations affecting the phosphorylation sites of the β-catenin gene (CTNNB1) produce constitutively stable proteins in a variety of human cancers, including type I EC.[100,101] Consequently, increased nuclear levels of β-catenin induces a higher transcriptional activation through lymphoid enhancer factor/T cell factor (LEF/TCF).[102] LEF/TCFs normally mediate Wnt signals in the nucleus by recruiting β-catenin and its co-activators to Wnt response elements (WREs) of target genes. Overactive LEF/TCFs drive the cells to transform.[103] Gain of function mutations of CTNNB1 are found in 25% to 38% of type I EC but none were observed in type II EC.[39-41,104] CTNNB1 mutations and nuclear accumulation (activation) of β-catenin have been also demonstrated in atypical hyperplasia suggesting that β-catenin abnormalities arise early in the development of type I EC.[105] Nuclear accumulation is also induced by abnormal Wnt signaling as found in some type I EC with MSI.[106]

Tumor Suppressor Genes

PTEN

The tumor suppressor gene *PTEN* (phosphatase and tensin homolog deleted on chromosome 10) codes for a phosphatase that downregulates the phosphatidyinositol 3-kinase (PI3-K)/Akt signaling pathway of growth factor receptors.[107-109] The *PTEN* gene is localized to 10q23, a chromosomal region subject to frequent loss of heterozygosity (LOH).[107] Decreased *PTEN* activity and therefore increased activation of Akt lead to increased cell proliferation and resistance to apoptosis.[110,111] Inactivation of *PTEN* is the most common genetic defect in type I EC with rates ranging from 34% to 83%.[28,32] When analyzed according to histological type, *PTEN* mutations are found almost exclusively in type I EC. In the normal endometrium no *PTEN* mutations were found. *PTEN* mutations are found at higher rates in tumors with MSI (up to 85%) and are also seen in endometrial hyperplasia with and without atypia.[30,31] *PTEN* mutations occur at the earliest detectable stage of endometrial carcinogenesis.[112] The *PTEN* defect observed most frequently is an inactivation of both alleles resulting in a complete loss of function. Even a hemizygous inactivation leading to a protein deficient state seems to be functionally significant when combined with defects of other genes within this pathway. Oda et al demonstrated that the PI3K/Akt pathway is extensively activated in EC and that a combination of defects in the catalytic subunit alpha of PI3K (PIK3CA) and *PTEN* plays an important role in the development of these tumors.[113,114] The tumor suppressor gene *PTEN* is also involved in the regulation of telomerase activity by inhibition of Akt activation and a subsequent decrease of hTERT expression. Loss of *PTEN* may therefore allow endometrial cells to express high levels of telomerase activity, facilitating neoplastic transformation.[115] Highly mitotic cells, such as normal estrogen-stimulated proliferative endometrial glands, contain abundant *PTEN* protein. Suppression of *PTEN* expression in a mitotically active estrogenic environment (unopposed by progestins) may compromise growth control more than loss of *PTEN* protein in mitotically quiescent cells. Individual *PTEN*-negative glands in estrogen-exposed endometria represent the earliest recognizable stage of endometrial carcinogenesis, which is followed by proliferation into dense clusters that form discrete premalignant lesions.[5,28]

p53

The *p53* tumor suppressor gene is located on chromosome 17 and encodes a 53 kDa nuclear phosphoprotein that induces proliferative arrest or apoptosis through induction of p21[Wafl/Cip1] and hMdm2 to prevent propagation of cells with damaged DNA.[116] Mutations in *p53* can introduce stop codons resulting in a truncated, nonfunctional protein. Since these truncations often involve the C-terminus, hMdm2 cannot bind to the *p53* protein (TP53) and therefore nonfunctional TP53 accumulates in the cell. Almost 80% of *p53* mutations are missense mutations leading to synthesis of a TP53, lacking its specific DNA binding function and accumulation in the nucleus.[117,118] In addition, missense mutations in *p53* often affect amino acids involved in post-translational modifications affecting the stability of TP53.[119] *p53* protein overexpression in EC is associated with high grade tumors, lymph node metastasis and myometrial invasion.[67] In type I EC, TP53 overexpression is frequently observed, however, *p53* mutations are rare and, if present, not related to TP53 overexpression.[67,120] Most type I EC that harbor *p53* mutations are large high-grade tumors, which suggests that *p53* mutations in type I EC are more closely related with dedifferentiation, as in the case of other tumor systems.[4,67] Aberrant accumulation of inactivated TP53 is found in approximately 5% of type I EC.[67] A high level of inactivated TP53 is also an independent prognostic factor.[121] Pijnenborg et al demonstrated that TP53 overexpression is predictive for recurrent type I EC and mostly not correlated with *p53* mutations.[122] Concomitant low expression of hMdm2 and p21$^{Waf1/Cip1}$ in tumors with TP53 overexpression suggests a dysfunction in this signal transduction pathway.[122] In type II EC, TP53 overexpression is also frequently present but associated with truncating *p53* mutations.[48] *p53* mutations are found in 71% to 85% of the type II EC and in contrast to type I EC are early events in the development of type II EC.[123-125]

BRCA

Germline *BRCA* gene mutation carriers are found to have an increased risk of developing breast or ovarian cancer and to a lesser degree, colon cancer. Male *BRCA* mutation carriers are also inclined to an increased risk of breast, colon, or prostate cancer.[126,127] Following the paradigm of tumor suppressor genes, one mutated allele of *BRCA1* or *BRCA2* is inherited and then somatic mutation occurs to alter the second allele, such that tumors invariably contain two mutant alleles. There are limited data regarding whether or not *BRCA* mutation carriers are also at increased risk for EC. Thompson and Easton have recently reported that *BRCA1* mutation carriers have a 2.7-fold increased risk to develop EC.[128] Other studies suggest that *BRCA* mutation carriers have an increased risk of type II EC.[129,130] Other groups did not find any correlation.[131,132] In a prospective study Beiner et al did not find that *BRCA* mutations directly increase the risk of EC.[133] They suggested that the main contributor to the increased risk of EC among these women was tamoxifen treatment of previous breast cancer or the preventive use of tamoxifen.[133] Hornreich et al observed two sisters with advanced serous papillary carcinomas of endometrial and ovarian origin, carrying the same *BRCA1* mutation.[134] LOH analysis of the EC showed loss of the wild-type allele, suggesting a causal relationship between the germline *BRCA1* mutation and development of type II EC.[134] However, whether or not germline *BRCA* mutations play a role in the development of EC remains unclear.

DNA-Mismatch Repair Genes

Type I ECs are characterized by defects in DNA mismatch repair, as evidenced by the microsatellite instability (MSI) or replication error repair (RER) phenotype. Microsatellites are short segments of repetitive DNA bases that are scattered throughout the genome and found predominantly in noncoding DNA. MSI is the property to develop changes in the number of repeat elements as compared with normal tissue due to DNA repair errors made during replication. MSI is found in 17 to 25% of sporadic type I EC but is rarely (<5%) present in type II EC.[29,72,135] MSI was detected in atypical hyperplasia associated with carcinoma but not in atypical hyperplasia without associated carcinoma, suggesting that mismatch repair defects may occur in the transition between the two lesion.[4,24] Somatic mutational inactivation of known mismatch repair genes does not account for the great majority of sporadic ECs with MSI. Instead, mismatch repair genes (i.e., MLH-1) are inactivated or silenced by gene promoter hypermethylation (epigenetic effect).[136] This mechanism is not found in type II EC.[136]

Growth Factor Receptors

EGF Receptor

The role of epidermal growth factor receptor (EGF-R) in endometrial cancer is still disputable. The EGF-signaling pathways involve four known receptors (EGF-R, erbB2/HER-2/neu, erbB3 and erbB4) and various ligands, like e.g., epidermal growth factor (EGF), amphiregulin and transforming growth factor-alpha (TGF-α).[137] The members of the erb-B family belong to transmembrane receptor tyrosine kinases and activation of these receptors generally requires tyrosine phosphorylation of the cytoplasmatic tyrosine kinase domain.[138,139] Most tyrosine kinase receptors are activated by ligand-induced dimerization. EGF and TGF-α stimulate homodimerization of the EGF receptor, but, under certain conditions, heterodimerization with other family members like HER-2 also occurs. Activation of the EGF-R by its ligands induces activation of *ras* and phosphorylates further downstream substrates of the mitogen activated protein-kinase (MAP-kinase) family including extracellular signal-regulated kinases (ERK-1/2), *c-jun* N-terminal kinase (JNK) and MAP-kinase p38 and activates EREs.[137] EGF-R is expressed at comparable levels in normal and hyperplastic endometrium and may be overexpressed in invasive EC.[140] Niikura et al, however, described in advanced disease increased co-expression of EGF-R and TGF-α.[140] Overexpression of TGF-α was described in poorly differentiated EC and negatively correlates with ER expression.[140-142] Jasonni et al found low levels of EGF-R expression in type I EC and high levels in EC with benign squamous metaplasia, whereas in mucinous and serous EC EGF-R and TGF-α expression was not found.[143,144] In contrast, overexpression of EGF-R was found to be strongly correlated with tumor metastases and survival in patients with EC, independent of the histologic type.[145,146] In a more recent publication EGF-R expression was described not to be increased in endometrioid EC compared to normal endometrium, but the authors found an increased expression of HER-4 and the EGF-R ligands TGF-α and heparin-binding epidermal growth factor-like growth factor (HB-EGF).[147] EGF-R expression was also described in the majority of endometrial carcinosarcomas. Interestingly EGF-R was predominantly overexpressed in the sarcomatous components of the tumors, whereas HER-2 was predominantly overexpressed in the carcinomatous components.[148] Taken together, EGF-R expression and expression of its ligands TGF-α and HB-EGF correlate with occurrence of myometrial invasion and/or metastases and poor prognosis in patients with EC. Negative correlation of ER expression and TGF-α expression in advanced disease indicates a conversion of formerly ER dependent growth to predominantly EGF-R mediated autocrine growth-regulation by alternative ligands like TGF-α and HB-EGF. Smith et al found a strong correlation of G-protein coupled receptor 30 (GPR30), a 7-transmembrane receptor for estrogen and EGF-R expression in patients with advanced EC, high grade and biologically aggressive histologic subtypes.[149] GPR30 represents an alternative cytoplasmic estrogen-responsive receptor that is overexpressed in tumors where estrogen and progesterone receptors are down-regulated and in high-risk EC patients with lower survival rates. Activation of GPR30 by estradiol induces metalloproteinase activity, release of growth factors like HB-EGF by tumor cells and trans-activation of the EGF-R.[150] In vitro experiments with specific EGF-R tyrosine kinase inhibitor gefitinib showed equal inhibition of EGF-R autophosphorylation and MAP-kinase activity in cells representing type I and II EC. In cells representing type II EC high basal phosphorylation of numerous signaling molecules that were not inhibited by gefitinib indicated, that other growth factor pathways like PI3K/Akt/PKB signaling are active in addition to EGF-R.[151,152] Further investigations to understand cross-talk mechanisms of the EGF-R and its potential role in targeted therapy of EC are necessary.

HER-2/erb-B2

The *HER-2/erb-B2/neu* gene encodes a 185-kDa transmembrane receptor tyrosine kinase of the EGF-R/erb-B family. HER-2 functions as a preferred partner for heterodimerization with members of the erb-B family and induces ligand independent autosignaling via specific tyrosine kinase phosphorylation.[153] HER-2 overexpression was described in about 10-30% of type I EC and in 45-70% of type II EC, respectively.[83,154-157] However, more recent studies of large series of serous carcinomas found that only 18-43% of the tumors overexpressed HER-2.[158,159] EGF-R and HER-2 co-expression is inversely correlated with grade of differentiation and with ER and PR content and predicted a poor prognosis in patients with EC.[160] HER-2 overexpression and gene amplification correlate inversely with disease specific survival and progression-free survival in patients with EC.[159,161] In a retrospective analysis Saffari et al could show that among patients with HER-2 overexpression of EC, adjuvant chemotherapy or radiation therapy after surgery were associated with an improved overall survival.[162] HER-2 overexpression negatively correlates with expression of ER and PR and suggests the developmend of hormone-independent growth in a subgroup of EC patients.[160,163,164] Cross-talk mechanisms of HER-2 with other signal pathways (like PI3K/pAkt/PKB pathway) are comparable to those of the EGF-R. On the other hand, HER-2 associated tyrosine phosphorylation acts by ligand-independent autosignaling via HER-2/HER-X heterodimerization.[153] The extracellular domain of the HER-2 oncogene product p185 provides an attractive therapeutic target for treatment with the monoclonal antibody trastuzumab. In preclinical studies trastuzumab showed antiproliferative activity in ER positive and ER negative endometrial cancer cells.[165,166] Treeck et al could show, though, that in endometrial cancer cells HER-2 signaling was inhibited by trastuzumab only in the absence of estradiol. In these cells estradiol counteracted the inhibitory effects of trastuzumab by rapid phosphorylation of ERK-1/2, probably triggered by GPR30 and inhibitory effects of trastuzumab were restored by cotreatment with pure antiestrogen fulvestrant.[167] These findings suggest that there is intensive cross-talk between hormone-dependent growth regulation and signal transduction of members of the erbB family leading to rapid resistance of single agent targeted therapies. Recently, trastuzumab showed encouraging activity in a few patients with HER-2 overexpressing advanced EC.[168,169] Clinical trials to evaluate efficacy of trastuzumab with or without antiestrogen or chemotherapy combinations in patients with HER-2 overexpressing EC are currently ongoing.

IGF Receptor

The type I insulin-like growth factor receptor (IGF-R) is a transmembrane receptor tyrosine kinase composed of two α subunits and two β subunits.[170] The activation of IGF-R requires binding to either of its ligands, IGF-I or IGF-II. As a result of ligand-dependent IGF-R activation via intracellular tyrosine phosphorylation of the β subunits multiple downstream signaling pathways are activated, including the MAP-kinase pathway and the phosphatidylinositol 3-kinase (PI3K). The latter activates Akt/protein kinase B and induces proliferation.[171,172] PTEN negatively regulates PI3K activity by dephosphorylation of phosphoinositol triphosphate (PIP-3).[111] Lower levels of phosphatase activity like loss of PTEN expression, leads to hyperactivation of the PI3K/pAkt pathway. IGF-R is expressed mainly in endometrial epithelial cells, its ligands IGF-I and IGF-II are expressed in endometrial stromal cells and their expression is associated with endometrial differentiation.[173,174] Estrogen-dependent activation of ER-α can up-regulate the expression of IGF-R.[175] McCampbell et al found increased IGF-R expression in biopsies from complex atypical hyperplasia and activated downstream components like increased pAkt levels independent of PTEN expression.[176] Specific binding sites for IGF-I were increased in endometrial cancer and IGF-R overexpression was found in 67% of endometrial cancers, independent of histologic type.[177-179] The role of autocrine IGF-R mediated growth regulation in endometrial cancer is still under discussion. In EC cells in vitro autocrine growth regulation was shown to be mediated by TGF-α and IGF, but not by EGF.[180] About 95% of IGF-I and IGF-II is associated with membrane-bound IGF binding proteins (IGFBP). Kleinman et al could show in endometrial cancer cells that IGF-R dependent stimulation of cell growth depends on IGF levels as well as levels of IGFBP subtypes. In these cells IGFBP levels were decreased and IGF-R levels increased by estradiol or tamoxifen stimulation.[181,182] These findings were underlined by various serum levels in EC patients showing decreased levels of IGFBP subtypes and increased IGF-1 levels.[183-187] Of note, obesity and diabetes mellitus are accepted risk factors for EC. It has been discussed whether increased insulin levels are associated with development of EC. High affinity binding-sites for insulin were demonstrated in EC cells and insulin stimulated cell growth.[188] However, clinical evaluations of C-peptide levels showed modest support to the hypothesis that hyperinsulinaemia is a risk factor for endometrial cancer.[189]

Angiogenic Factors

Angiogenesis is a multistep process essential for tumor growth, invasion and metastatic spread.[190] Microvessel density has been widely used as a measure of tumor-associated angiogenesis. Various studies have shown that high intratumor microvessel density in EC is associated with advanced clinical stage, increased risk of recurrent disease and poor prognosis.[191] In stage I endometrial carcinoma, greater depth of invasion and higher tumor grade are directly correlated with angiogenic intensity.[192] Vascular endothelial growth factor (VEGF) is the major stimulus for endothelial cell proliferation in EC and is, therefore, associated with high angiogenesis.[193] VEGF is an independent predictor of poor prognosis, particularly within stage I endometrial disease.[194] However, VEGF expression did not correlate with histological grade or the number of microvessels in the tumor area. Since the stimulating effect of VEGF on endothelial cells is basically dependent on the presence of VEGF receptors, i.e., flk-1, the detection of a functionally intact angiogenic pathway VEGF/flk-1 is a more reliable and independent prognostic parameter.[195] The expression of another angiogenic factor, thymidine phosphorylase (TP), correlates with increased microvessel density in EC.[196] TP expression is related to the adverse histopathological variables of the type II EC, such as high tumor grade, deep myometrial invasion and advanced stage of disease.[195] Stefansson et al have recently examined the significance of vascular proliferation and the degree of pericyte coverage in a large and population-based series of EC with complete follow-up.[197] They found that vascular proliferation is the strongest angiogenic marker independent of other prognostic factors. Decreased pericyte coverage was significantly associated with vascular invasion by tumor cells and reduced patient survival.[197] Additionally, in the same study peritumoral lymphatic vessel density was shown to contribute to the clinical progress of EC.[197]

Hormone Receptors and Aromatase

Estrogen Receptor

The steroid receptors for estrogen (ER) are composed of six functional domains. The DNA-binding domain (DBD) is relatively conserved and targets the receptors to the estrogen responsive elements (EREs). The E region of the steroid receptors contains a multifunctional domain and is involved in ligand-binding, receptor dimerization, nuclear localization, nuclear coactivator/corepressor interaction and ligand-dependent activating function.[198] The two main isoforms of the ER, ER-α and ER-β, show structural differences resulting in distinct ligand affinities and physiologic properties. For example, tamoxifen exhibits partial agonist activities after binding to ER-α whereas it acts mainly as pure antagonist when bound to ER-β.[199] ER-α is the predominant ER isoform in endometrium.[200] Both isoforms are capable of forming ER-α/ER-β heterodimers and thus influence each other function.[201,202] In this context, ER-β has been shown to function as a dominant inhibitor of ER-α.[203] In addition, both ER-α and ER-β are represented by several isoforms resulting from alternative splicing and these splice variants can exhibit altered hormone-binding effects on EREs and/or transcriptional properties.[204-206] Beside the described classic genomic activation of ER-α and ER-β, both receptors have been shown to regulate transcription by nonclassic genomic activation of components of the activating protein-1 (AP-1) pathway.[207] The nongenomic mechanism of ER action is cross-talk with the signal-transduction of growth-factor receptor cascades, for example via activation of MAP-kinase (ERK-1/2) and/or the PI3K/pAkt pathway.[208,209] One possible critical step in estrogen-dependent tumorigenesis might be an imbalance in ER-α and ER-β expression. Expression of ER-α decreases from hyperplastic and grade 1 endometrioid EC to grade 3 tumors. ER-α is rarely expressed in type 2 EC.[200,210,211] Expression levels of ER-β are low in normal endometrium and do not alter during tumor differentiation, suggesting a shift to decreased ER-α/ER-β ratio.[212,213] Transcriptional splicing errors for ER-α and ER-β have been described for EC, potentially leading to uncontrolled proliferation. Although there is no homogenous pattern in the development of EC for the described splice variants, some of them are found at increased levels in EC.[214-218] Recent investigations evaluated expression of steroid receptor cofactors 1-3 (SRC) in EC. Balmer et al found increased expression of SCR3 member AIB1 (amplified in breast cancer-1) in hyperplastic endometrium and in EC. Expression of AIB1 correlated with higher grade of carcinomas, potentially augmenting ER action in these tumors.[219] Kershah et al found increased levels of mRNA of SRC-1-3 in EC samples, whereas Uchikawa showed decreased levels of SCR-1 in EC topographically correlated with decreased ER expression, indicating sex steroid independent growth in these tumors.[220,221] ER activation can also be mediated in a ligand-independent way. For example, PTEN loss in endometrium activates Akt and results in increased phosphorylation of ER-α. ER-α phosphorylation even in the absence of ligand results in activation of EREs and transcription.[222] Estrogen-dependent growth in EC might also be mediated through G-protein coupled GPR30, inducing MAP-kinase and Akt activation.[150,223] Overexpression of GPR30 was shown in EC with down-regulated expression of ER-α/ER-β and PR and overexpression correlated with higher grade and lower survival.[149] The mechanisms of estrogen-dependent growth and potential antiestrogenic therapeutic strategies in EC are complex and require more global understanding of cross-talk action patterns between ER and its SRCs, the alternative estrogen receptor GPR30 and the signal-transduction of growth factor receptors to define subgroups of estrogen-dependent EC.

Progesterone Receptor

The steroid receptors for progesterone (PR) exist in two isoforms, PRA and PRB. These two receptors are almost identical, except that PRB contains a third transcription-activating functional domain, AF-3.[224,225] PRA has been shown to act in a dominant negative fashion and antagonizes the transcriptional activity of PRB and the ERs.[226] On simple progestin-responsive elements (PREs) PRA and PRB display similar transactivational activity, but PRA's transcriptional activity is more complex and cell and response element specific.[227] Loss of the inhibitory effects of PRA and disruption of the PRA/PRB ratio is thought to be involved in estrogen-induced endometrial hyperplasia and EC.[228-231] One factor for the disruption of the PRA/PRB ratio might be receptor gene polymorphism.[232] Low PR expression was shown to be associated with increased risk for tumor relapse, but in patients showing PR expression and PR gene polymorphism the risk was even higher.[233] Regarding the prognostic value of both PRs, only decrease of PRB expression seems to reflect poor prognosis in patients with EC.[234,235] PRB expression is found to be distributed in the cytoplasm in EC tissues, whereas PRA expression is only found in the nuclei, suggesting nongenomic actions of PRB.[236] Transfection of PRB and treatment with progestins in human endometrial cancer cells resulted in growth inhibition, inhibition of cyclin D1 expression, down-regulation of metalloproteases and down-regulation of cellular adhesion molecules.[237,238] PRB-expression is inversely correlated with p53 gene mutation and tumor grading.[235] Serial biopsies of patients with advanced type 1 EC treated with medroxyprogesterone showed no increased apoptosis but down-regulation of Ki-67 expression. Decreased Ki-67 expression was only observed in grade 1 and 2 tumors with high PR expression.[239] In EC cells ligand-bound PRB can inhibit the transcriptional activity of members of the AP-1 family and in particular, *c-jun*. Thus, progesterone might antagonize stimulatory effects of estrogens on AP-1.[240] In addition, ligand-bound PRB can inhibit NFκB activity through transcriptional control in EC cells.[241] Progestins are currently leading standard in the treatment of advanced type 1 EC. The PR isoforms, PRA and PRB, play important roles in growth control of EC and offer targets for novel therapeutic strategies. However, to understand the mechanisms of action of PRA and PRB in EC, especially regarding differences between type 1 and 2 EC, further evaluations are required.

Aromatase

There is no consistent evidence of increased concentrations of circulating endogenous estrogen in women with EC, but local concentration of estradiol in EC tissues was reported to be higher than that in blood and in normal endometrium.[46,242-246] These data suggest that endometrial cancer itself synthesizes estradiol as part of positive autocrine growth-regulation. CYP19 (aromatase) gene polymorphism has been discussed as potential risk factor in patients with EC. CYP19 genotypes containing the longest alleles A6 and A7 (A6A7/A6A6) were found to be over-represented in patients with EC and intratumoral aromatase activity was increased especially in patients with type II EC.[247-249] Aromatase expression could be demonstrated in more than 65% of EC tissues by PCR and IHC and tumor aromatase expression did not correlate with ER/PR expression or prognosis.[250-252] Aromatase in stromal but not epithelial cells correlated positively with advanced surgical stage and poor survival.[253] In addition, aromatase expression was also demonstrated in low-grade endometrial stromal sarcomas.[254] Interestingly, very high intratumoral aromatase activity could be described preferably in poorly differentiated endometrioid carcinomas and in type II EC tissues, whereas negative aromatase activity could only be demonstrated in cases of low-risk type I EC.[255-257] Thus, although type II EC is considered as hormone-independent, increased ability of this tumor type to estrogen biosynthesis through cancer cell aromatase activity may lead to the reconsideration of such conclusion and warrants further investigation. Aromatase inhibitors showed moderate antiproliferative activity on endometrial cancer cells in vitro.[258,259] Safety data from the ATAC trial of postmenopausal women with breast cancer treated with aromatase inhibitor anastrozole indicated a preventive role of aromatase inhibitors by reducing the risk of EC.[260] A few case control studies and two phase II trials showed moderate activity of aromatase inhibitors in patients with advanced endometrial cancers.[256,261,262] Berstein et al treated 23 patients 2 weeks with aromatase inhibitors in the neoadjuvant setting and found in serial biopsies down-regulated PR expression, which was more pronounced in type II EC patients.[256] Burnett et al treated two obese premenopausal women with histologically confirmed grade 1 EC with a medroxyprogesterone/anastrozole combination up to six months leading to complete remission.[263] Although response rates in the phase II trials were low, aromatase inhibitors in the treatment of subgroups of patients, probably especially in patients with type II EC, might be useful. To define potential subgroups predictive factors for response, for example the role of intratumoral aromatase activity, are required.

GnRH Receptor

A series of papers from different laboratories has demonstrated the expression of gonadotropin-releasing hormone (GnRH, GnRH-I) in almost 100% of ECs and the expression of the GnRH receptor (GnRH-R, GnRH-I-R) in about 80% of ECs.[264, 265] Recently, the expression of a second human GnRH (GnRH-II) was reported.[266] The existence of a functional active type II GnRH receptor (GnRH-II-R) in the human being is under discussion, but there is an increasing evidence that a functionally active GnRH-II-R exists in human EC.[265, 267-270] In EC, GnRH-I, GnRH-II and their receptors are parts of a negative autocrine regulatory system of cell proliferation.[264, 267] Agonists of GnRH-I and GnRH-II inhibit the mitogenic signal transduction of growth factor receptors and related oncogene products associated with tyrosine kinase activity via activation of a phosphotyrosine phosphatase resulting in down-regulation of cancer cell proliferation.[264, 267] Induction of apoptosis is not involved. The situation is different with GnRH-II antagonists. Treatment of human EC cells with GnRH-II antagonists induces apoptotic cell death via dose-dependent activation of caspase-3.[271] The fact that treatment with GnRH-II antagonists resulted in an increase of caspase-3 activity and a loss of mitochondrial membrane potential in cultured endometrial cancer cells suggests that GnRH-II antagonists induce apoptosis in these cells at least in part through activation of the intrinsic apoptotic pathway. The antitumor effects of the GnRH-II antagonists could be confirmed in nude mice. GnRH-II antagonists inhibited the growth of xenotransplants of human EC in nude mice significantly, without any apparent side effects.[271] Thus, GnRH-II antagonists seem to be suitable drugs for an efficacious and less toxic endocrine therapy for EC.

Future Perspective

Despite the great effort made to unravel the molecular alterations associated with endometrial cancer, tumors lacking MSI phenotype or mutations in any of the studied genes suggest the existence of unrecognized pathways in the development of EC. Hopefully, ongoing and future research will help to understand better the mechanisms leading to the formation of these cancers. New technologies such as the cDNA microarray technology for identifying differences in gene expression patterns in individual ECs will make more clear a distinctions in the biology and clinical outcome of these neoplasms. The increased knowledge of the molecular pathology of the individual EC will assist to develop techniques to identify premalignant diseases, improve disease management and treatment and invent specific target therapies based on molecular pathways.

References

1. Parazzini F, La Vecchia C, Bocciolone L et al. The epidemiology of endometrial cancer. Gynecol Oncol 1991; 41(1):1-16.
2. Amant F, Moerman P, Neven P et al. Endometrial cancer. Lancet 6-12 2005; 366(9484):491-505.

3. Bokhman JV. Two pathogenetic types of endometrial carcinoma. Gynecol Oncol 1983; 15(1):10-17.
4. Sherman ME. Theories of endometrial carcinogenesis: a multidisciplinary approach. Mod Pathol 2000; 13(3):295-308.
5. Emons G, Fleckenstein G, Hinney B et al. Hormonal interactions in endometrial cancer. Endocr Relat Cancer 2000; 7(4):227-242.
6. ACOG practice bulletin, clinical management guidelines for obstetrician-gynecologists, number 65, August 2005: management of endometrial cancer. Obstet Gynecol 2005; 106(2):413-425.
7. Beral V, Bull D, Reeves G. Endometrial cancer and hormone-replacement therapy in the Million Women Study. Lancet 2005; 365(9470):1543-1551.
8. Deligdisch L, Cohen CJ. Histologic correlates and virulence implications of endometrial carcinoma associated with adenomatous hyperplasia. Cancer 1985; 56(6):1452-1455.
9. Deligdisch L, Holinka CF. Progesterone receptors in two groups of endometrial carcinoma. Cancer 1986; 57(7):1385-1388.
10. Nyholm HC, Nielsen AL, Norup P. Endometrial cancer in postmenopausal women with and without previous estrogen replacement treatment: comparison of clinical and histopathological characteristics. Gynecol Oncol 1993; 49(2):229-235.
11. Cohen CJ, Rahaman J. Endometrial cancer. Management of high risk and recurrence including the tamoxifen controversy. Cancer 1995; 76(10 Suppl):2044-2052.
12. Nyholm HC, Nielsen AL, Lyndrup J et al. Plasma oestrogens in postmenopausal women with endometrial cancer. Br J Obstet Gynaecol 1993; 100(12):1115-1119.
13. Sivridis E, Fox H, Buckley CH. Endometrial carcinoma: two or three entities? Int J Gynecol Cancer 1998; 8:183-188.
14. Pothuri B, Ramondetta L, Eifel P et al. Radiation-associated endometrial cancers are prognostically unfavorable tumors: a clinicopathologic comparison with 527 sporadic endometrial cancers. Gynecol Oncol 2006; 103(3):948-951.
15. Sherman ME, Bur ME, Kurman RJ. p53 in endometrial cancer and its putative precursors: evidence for diverse pathways of tumorigenesis. Hum Pathol 1995; 26(11):1268-1274.
16. Faquin WC, Fitzgerald JT, Boynton KA et al. Intratumoral genetic heterogeneity and progression of endometrioid type endometrial adenocarcinomas. Gynecol Oncol 2000; 78(2):152-157.
17. Esteller M, Levine R, Baylin SB et al. MLH1 promoter hypermethylation is associated with the microsatellite instability phenotype in sporadic endometrial carcinomas. Oncogene 1998; 17(18):2413-2417.
18. Mutter GL. Pten, a protean tumor suppressor. Am J Pathol 2001; 158(6):1895-1898.
19. Matias-Guiu X, Catasus L, Bussaglia E et al. Molecular pathology of endometrial hyperplasia and carcinoma. Hum Pathol 2001; 32(6):569-577.
20. Coller HA, Grandori C, Tamayo P et al. Expression analysis with oligonucleotide microarrays reveals that MYC regulates genes involved in growth, cell cycle, signaling and adhesion. Proc Natl Acad Sci USA 2000; 97(7):3260-3265.
21. Gusberg SB. Precursors of corpus carcinoma, estrogens and adenomatous hyperplasia. Am J Obstet Gynecol 1947; 52:3-9.
22. Ehrlich CE, Young PC, Cleary RE. Cytoplasmic progesterone and estradiol receptors in normal, hyperplastic and carcinomatous endometria: therapeutic implications. Am J Obstet Gynecol 1981; 141(5):539-546.
23. Kurman RJ, Kaminski PF, Norris HJ. The behavior of endometrial hyperplasia. A long-term study of "untreated" hyperplasia in 170 patients. Cancer 1985; 56(2):403-412.
24. Mutter GL, Boynton KA, Faquin WC et al. Allelotype mapping of unstable microsatellites establishes direct lineage continuity between endometrial precancers and cancer. Cancer Res 1996; 56(19):4483-4486.
25. Duggan BD, Felix JC, Muderspach LI et al. Microsatellite instability in sporadic endometrial carcinoma. J Natl Cancer Inst 1994; 86(16):1216-1221.
26. Catasus L, Bussaglia E, Rodrguez I et al. Molecular genetic alterations in endometrioid carcinomas of the ovary: similar frequency of beta-catenin abnormalities but lower rate of microsatellite instability and PTEN alterations than in uterine endometrioid carcinomas. Hum Pathol 2004; 35(11):1360-1368.
27. Risinger JI, Berchuck A, Kohler MF et al. Genetic instability of microsatellites in endometrial carcinoma. Cancer Res 1993; 53(21):5100-5103.
28. Mutter GL, Lin MC, Fitzgerald JT et al. Altered PTEN expression as a diagnostic marker for the earliest endometrial precancers. J Natl Cancer Inst 2000; 92(11):924-930.
29. Gurin CC, Federici MG, Kang L et al. Causes and consequences of microsatellite instability in endometrial carcinoma. Cancer Res 1999; 59(2):462-466.
30. Levine RL, Cargile CB, Blazes MS et al. PTEN mutations and microsatellite instability in complex atypical hyperplasia, a precursor lesion to uterine endometrioid carcinoma. Cancer Res 1998; 58(15):3254-3258.

31. Maxwell GL, Risinger JI, Gumbs C et al. Mutation of the PTEN tumor suppressor gene in endometrial hyperplasias. Cancer Res 1998; 58(12):2500-2503.
32. Risinger JI, Hayes AK, Berchuck A et al. PTEN/MMAC1 mutations in endometrial cancers. Cancer Res 1997; 57(21):4736-4738.
33. Tashiro H, Blazes MS, Wu R et al. Mutations in PTEN are frequent in endometrial carcinoma but rare in other common gynecological malignancies. Cancer Res 1997; 57(18):3935-3940.
34. Mutter GL, Wada H, Faquin WC et al. K-ras mutations appear in the premalignant phase of both microsatellite stable and unstable endometrial carcinogenesis. Mol Pathol 1999; 52(5):257-262.
35. Enomoto T, Inoue M, Perantoni AO et al. K-ras activation in premalignant and malignant epithelial lesions of the human uterus. Cancer Res 1991; 51(19):5308-5314.
36. Fujimoto I, Shimizu Y, Hirai Y et al. Studies on ras oncogene activation in endometrial carcinoma. Gynecol Oncol 1993; 48(2):196-202.
37. Sakamoto T, Murase T, Urushibata H et al. Microsatellite instability and somatic mutations in endometrial carcinomas. Gynecol Oncol 1998; 71(1):53-58.
38. Swisher EM, Peiffer-Schneider S, Mutch DG et al. Differences in patterns of TP53 and KRAS2 mutations in a large series of endometrial carcinomas with or without microsatellite instability. Cancer 1999; 85(1):119-126.
39. Schlosshauer PW, Pirog EC, Levine RL et al. Mutational analysis of the CTNNB1 and APC genes in uterine endometrioid carcinoma. Mod Pathol 2000; 13(10):1066-1071.
40. Mirabelli-Primdahl L, Gryfe R, Kim H et al. Beta-catenin mutations are specific for colorectal carcinomas with microsatellite instability but occur in endometrial carcinomas irrespective of mutator pathway. Cancer Res 1999; 59(14):3346-3351.
41. Fukuchi T, Sakamoto M, Tsuda H et al. Beta-catenin mutation in carcinoma of the uterine endometrium. Cancer Res 1998; 58(16):3526-3528.
42. Carcangiu ML, Chambers JT. Uterine papillary serous carcinoma: a study on 108 cases with emphasis on the prognostic significance of associated endometrioid carcinoma, absence of invasion and concomitant ovarian carcinoma. Gynecol Oncol 1992; 47(3):298-305.
43. Slomovitz BM, Burke TW, Eifel PJ et al. Uterine papillary serous carcinoma (UPSC): a single institution review of 129 cases. Gynecol Oncol 2003; 91(3):463-469.
44. Abeler VM, Kjorstad KE. Clear cell carcinoma of the endometrium: a histopathological and clinical study of 97 cases. Gynecol Oncol 1991; 40(3):207-217.
45. Ambros RA, Sherman ME, Zahn CM et al. Endometrial intraepithelial carcinoma: a distinctive lesion specifically associated with tumors displaying serous differentiation. Hum Pathol 1995; 26(11):1260-1267.
46. Sherman ME, Sturgeon S, Brinton LA et al. Risk factors and hormone levels in patients with serous and endometrioid uterine carcinomas. Mod Pathol 1997; 10(10):963-968.
47. Berchuck A, Boyd J. Molecular basis of endometrial cancer. Cancer 1995; 76(10 Suppl):2034-2040.
48. Tashiro H, Isacson C, Levine R et al. p53 gene mutations are common in uterine serous carcinoma and occur early in their pathogenesis. Am J Pathol 1997; 150(1):177-185.
49. Silverberg SG, Major FJ, Blessing JA et al. Carcinosarcoma (malignant mixed mesodermal tumor) of the uterus. A Gynecologic Oncology Group pathologic study of 203 cases. Int J Gynecol Pathol 1990; 9(1):1-19.
50. McCluggage WG. Malignant biphasic uterine tumours: carcinosarcomas or metaplastic carcinomas? J Clin Pathol 2002; 55(5):321-325.
51. Bitterman P, Chun B, Kurman RJ. The significance of epithelial differentiation in mixed mesodermal tumors of the uterus. A clinicopathologic and immunohistochemical study. Am J Surg Pathol 1990; 14(4):317-328.
52. Emoto M, Iwasaki H, Kikuchi M et al. Characteristics of cloned cells of mixed mullerian tumor of the human uterus. Carcinoma cells showing myogenic differentiation in vitro. Cancer 1993; 71(10):3065-3075.
53. Wada H, Enomoto T, Fujita M et al. Molecular evidence that most but not all carcinosarcomas of the uterus are combination tumors. Cancer Res 1997; 57(23):5379-5385.
54. Kounelis S, Jones MW, Papadaki H et al. Carcinosarcomas (malignant mixed mullerian tumors) of the female genital tract: comparative molecular analysis of epithelial and mesenchymal components. Hum Pathol 1998; 29(1):82-87.
55. Abeln EC, Smit VT, Wessels JW et al. Molecular genetic evidence for the conversion hypothesis of the origin of malignant mixed mullerian tumours. J Pathol 1997; 183(4):424-431.
56. Fujii H, Yoshida M, Gong ZX et al. Frequent genetic heterogeneity in the clonal evolution of gynecological carcinosarcoma and its influence on phenotypic diversity. Cancer Res 2000; 60(1):114-120.

57. Goodfellow PJ, Buttin BM, Herzog TJ et al. Prevalence of defective DNA mismatch repair and MSH6 mutation in an unselected series of endometrial cancers. Proc Natl Acad Sci USA 2003; 100(10):5908-5913.

58. Amant F, Dorfling CM, Dreyer L et al. Microsatellite instability in uterine sarcomas. Int J Gynecol Cancer 2001; 11(3):218-223.

59. Risinger JI, Umar A, Boyer JC et al. Microsatellite instability in gynecological sarcomas and in hMSH2 mutant uterine sarcoma cell lines defective in mismatch repair activity. Cancer Res 1995; 55(23):5664-5669.

60. Taylor NP, Gibb RK, Powell MA et al. Defective DNA mismatch repair and XRCC2 mutation in uterine carcinosarcomas. Gynecol Oncol 2006; 100(1):107-110.

61. Thapar R, Williams JG, Campbell SL. NMR characterization of full-length farnesylated and nonfarnesylated H-Ras and its implications for Raf activation. J Mol Biol 2004; 343(5):1391-1408.

62. Wang Y, Zhang Z, Lubet R et al. Tobacco smoke-induced lung tumorigenesis in mutant A/J mice with alterations in K-ras, p53, or Ink4a/Arf. Oncogene 2005; 24(18):3042-3049.

63. Murua Escobar H, Gunther K, Richter A et al. Absence of ras-gene hot-spot mutations in canine fibrosarcomas and melanomas. Anticancer Res 2004; 24(5A):3027-3028.

64. Tanoguchi K, Yaegashi N, Jiko K et al. K-ras point mutations in spontaneously occurring endometrial adenocarcinomas in the Donryu rat. Tohoku J Exp Med 1999; 189(2):87-93.

65. Semczuk A, Schneider-Stock R, Berbec H et al. K-ras exon 2 point mutations in human endometrial cancer. Cancer Lett 2001; 164(2):207-212.

66. Semczuk A, Skomra D, Cybulski M et al. Immunohistochemical analysis of MIB-1 proliferative activity in human endometrial cancer. Correlation with clinicopathological parameters, patient outcome, retinoblastoma immunoreactivity and K-ras codon 12 point mutations. Histochem J 2001; 33(4):193-200.

67. Lax SF, Kendall B, Tashiro H et al. The frequency of p53, K-ras mutations and microsatellite instability differs in uterine endometrioid and serous carcinoma: evidence of distinct molecular genetic pathways. Cancer 2000; 88(4):814-824.

68. Sasaki H, Nishii H, Takahashi H et al. Mutation of the Ki-ras protooncogene in human endometrial hyperplasia and carcinoma. Cancer Res 1993; 53(8):1906-1910.

69. Lagarda H, Catasus L, Arguelles R et al. K-ras mutations in endometrial carcinomas with microsatellite instability. J Pathol 2001; 193(2):193-199.

70. Tu Z, Gui L, Wang J et al. Tumorigenesis of K-ras mutation in human endometrial carcinoma via upregulation of estrogen receptor. Gynecol Oncol 2006; 101(2):274-279.

71. Niederacher D, An HX, Cho YJ et al. Mutations and amplification of oncogenes in endometrial cancer. Oncology 1999; 56(1):59-65.

72. Tashiro H, Lax SF, Gaudin PB et al. Microsatellite instability is uncommon in uterine serous carcinoma. Am J Pathol 1997; 150(1):75-79.

73. Duggan BD, Felix JC, Muderspach LI et al. Early mutational activation of the c-Ki-ras oncogene in endometrial carcinoma. Cancer Res 1994; 54(6):1604-1607.

74. Caduff RF, Johnston CM, Frank TS. Mutations of the Ki-ras oncogene in carcinoma of the endometrium. Am J Pathol 1995; 146(1):182-188.

75. Shiozawa T, Miyamoto T, Kashima H et al. Estrogen-induced proliferation of normal endometrial glandular cells is initiated by transcriptional activation of cyclin D1 via binding of c-Jun to an AP-1 sequence. Oncogene 2004; 23(53):8603-8610.

76. Yamashita S, Takayanagi A, Shimizu N. Temporal and cell-type specific expression of c-fos and c-jun protooncogenes in the mouse uterus after estrogen stimulation. Endocrinology 1996; 137(12):5468-5475.

77. Webb DK, Moulton BC, Khan SA. Estrogen induced expression of the C-jun proto-oncogene in the immature and mature rat uterus. Biochem Biophys Res Commun 1990; 168(2):721-726.

78. Morishita S, Niwa K, Ichigo S et al. Overexpressions of c-fos/jun mRNA and their oncoproteins (Fos/Jun) in the mouse uterus treated with three natural estrogens. Cancer Lett 1995; 97(2):225-231.

79. Fujimoto J, Hori M, Ichigo S et al. Clinical implication of fos and jun expressions and protein kinase activity in endometrial cancers. Eur J Gynaecol Oncol 1995; 16(2):138-146.

80. Bai MK, Costopoulos JS, Christoforidou BP et al. Immunohistochemical detection of the c-myc oncogene product in normal, hyperplastic and carcinomatous endometrium. Oncology 1994; 51(4):314-319.

81. Bircan S, Ensari A, Ozturk S et al. Immunohistochemical analysis of c-myc, c-jun and estrogen receptor in normal, hyperplastic and neoplastic endometrium. Pathol Oncol Res 2005; 11(1):32-39.

82. Geisler JP, Geisler HE, Manahan KJ et al. Nuclear and cytoplasmic c-myc staining in endometrial carcinoma and their relationship to survival. Int J Gynecol Cancer 2004; 14(1):133-137.

83. Williams JA Jr, Wang ZR, Parrish RS et al. Fluorescence in situ hybridization analysis of HER-2/neu, c-myc and p53 in endometrial cancer. Exp Mol Pathol 1999; 67(3):135-143.

84. Holt SE, Shay JW. Role of telomerase in cellular proliferation and cancer. J Cell Physiol 1999; 180(1):10-18.
85. Granger MP, Wright WE, Shay JW. Telomerase in cancer and aging. Crit Rev Oncol Hematol 2002; 41(1):29-40.
86. Cong YS, Wright WE, Shay JW. Human telomerase and its regulation. Microbiol Mol Biol Rev 2002; 66(3):407-425, table of contents.
87. Stewart SA, Weinberg RA. Telomerase and human tumorigenesis. Semin Cancer Biol 2000; 10(6):399-406.
88. Mutter GL, Lin MC, Fitzgerald JT et al. Changes in endometrial PTEN expression throughout the human menstrual cycle. J Clin Endocrinol Metab 2000; 85(6):2334-2338.
89. Horikawa I, Barrett JC. Transcriptional regulation of the telomerase hTERT gene as a target for cellular and viral oncogenic mechanisms. Carcinogenesis 2003; 24(7):1167-1176.
90. Kyo S, Takakura M, Kanaya T et al. Estrogen activates telomerase. Cancer Res 1999; 59(23):5917-5921.
91. Wang Z, Kyo S, Takakura M et al. Progesterone regulates human telomerase reverse transcriptase gene expression via activation of mitogen-activated protein kinase signaling pathway. Cancer Res 2000; 60(19):5376-5381.
92. Soda H, Raymond E, Sharma S et al. Effects of androgens on telomerase activity in normal and malignant prostate cells in vitro. Prostate 2000; 43(3):161-168.
93. Wang Z, Kyo S, Maida Y et al. Tamoxifen regulates human telomerase reverse transcriptase (hTERT) gene expression differently in breast and endometrial cancer cells. Oncogene 2002; 21(22):3517-3524.
94. Chen XJ, Zheng W, Chen LL et al. Telomerase antisense inhibition for the proliferation of endometrial cancer in vitro and in vivo. Int J Gynecol Cancer 2006; 16(6):1987-1993.
95. Zhou C, Boggess JF, Bae-Jump V et al. Induction of apoptosis and inhibition of telomerase activity by arsenic trioxide (As(2)O(3)) in endometrial carcinoma cells. Gynecol Oncol 2007; 105(1):218-222.
96. Potter E, Bergwitz C, Brabant G. The cadherin-catenin system: implications for growth and differentiation of endocrine tissues. Endocr Rev 1999; 20(2):207-239.
97. Gumbiner BM. Cell adhesion: the molecular basis of tissue architecture and morphogenesis. Cell 1996; 84(3):345-357.
98. Giles RH, van Es JH, Clevers H. Caught up in a Wnt storm: Wnt signaling in cancer. Biochim Biophys Acta 2003; 1653(1):1-24.
99. Bullions LC, Levine AJ. The role of beta-catenin in cell adhesion, signal transduction and cancer. Curr Opin Oncol 1998; 10(1):81-87.
100. Palacios J, Gamallo C. Mutations in the beta-catenin gene (CTNNB1) in endometrioid ovarian carcinomas. Cancer Res 1998; 58(7):1344-1347.
101. Wu R, Zhai Y, Fearon ER et al. Diverse mechanisms of beta-catenin deregulation in ovarian endometrioid adenocarcinomas. Cancer Res 2001; 61(22):8247-8255.
102. Morin PJ, Sparks AB, Korinek V et al. Activation of beta-catenin-Tcf signaling in colon cancer by mutations in beta-catenin or APC. Science 1997; 275(5307):1787-1790.
103. Arce L, Yokoyama NN, Waterman ML. Diversity of LEF/TCF action in development and disease. Oncogene 2006; 25(57):7492-7504.
104. Machin P, Catasus L, Pons C et al. CTNNB1 mutations and beta-catenin expression in endometrial carcinomas. Hum Pathol 2002; 33(2):206-212.
105. Saegusa M, Hashimura M, Yoshida T et al. beta- Catenin mutations and aberrant nuclear expression during endometrial tumorigenesis. Br J Cancer 2001; 84(2):209-217.
106. Risinger JI, Maxwell GL, Chandramouli GV et al. Gene expression profiling of microsatellite unstable and microsatellite stable endometrial cancers indicates distinct pathways of aberrant signaling. Cancer Res 2005; 65(12):5031-5037.
107. Steck PA, Pershouse MA, Jasser SA et al. Identification of a candidate tumour suppressor gene, MMAC1, at chromosome 10q23.3 that is mutated in multiple advanced cancers. Nat Genet 1997; 15(4):356-362.
108. Li J, Yen C, Liaw D et al. PTEN, a putative protein tyrosine phosphatase gene mutated in human brain, breast and prostate cancer. Science 1997; 275(5308):1943-1947.
109. Cantley LC, Neel BG. New insights into tumor suppression: PTEN suppresses tumor formation by restraining the phosphoinositide 3-kinase/AKT pathway. Proc Natl Acad Sci USA 1999; 96(8):4240-4245.
110. Yuan XJ, Whang YE. PTEN sensitizes prostate cancer cells to death receptor-mediated and drug-induced apoptosis through a FADD-dependent pathway. Oncogene 2002; 21(2):319-327.
111. Wu X, Senechal K, Neshat MS et al. The PTEN/MMAC1 tumor suppressor phosphatase functions as a negative regulator of the phosphoinositide 3-kinase/Akt pathway. Proc Natl Acad Sci USA 1998; 95(26):15587-15591.

112. Latta E, Chapman WB. PTEN mutations and evolving concepts in endometrial neoplasia. Curr Opin Obstet Gynecol 2002; 14(1):59-65.
113. Oda K, Stokoe D, Taketani Y et al. High frequency of coexistent mutations of PIK3CA and PTEN genes in endometrial carcinoma. Cancer Res 2005; 65(23):10669-10673.
114. Velasco A, Bussaglia E, Pallares J et al. PIK3CA gene mutations in endometrial carcinoma: correlation with PTEN and K-RAS alterations. Hum Pathol 2006; 37(11):1465-1472.
115. Zhou C, Bae-Jump VL, Whang YE et al. The PTEN tumor suppressor inhibits telomerase activity in endometrial cancer cells by decreasing hTERT mRNA levels. Gynecol Oncol 2006; 101(2):305-310.
116. Veloso M, Wrba F, Kaserer K et al. p53 gene status and expression of p,53 mdm,2 and p21Wafl/Cip1 proteins in colorectal cancer. Virchows Arch 2000; 437(3):241-247.
117. Vousden KH, Prives C. P53 and prognosis: new insights and further complexity. Cell 2005; 120(1):7-10.
118. Soussi T, Kato S, Levy PP et al. Reassessment of the TP53 mutation database in human disease by data mining with a library of TP53 missense mutations. Hum Mutat 2005; 25(1):6-17.
119. Reich NC, Oren M, Levine AJ. Two distinct mechanisms regulate the levels of a cellular tumor antigen, p53. Mol Cell Biol 1983; 3(12):2143-2150.
120. Stewart RL, Royds JA, Burton JL et al. Direct sequencing of the p53 gene shows absence of mutations in endometrioid endometrial adenocarcinomas expressing p53 protein. Histopathology 1998; 33(5):440-445.
121. Alkushi A, Lim P, Coldman A et al. Interpretation of p53 immunoreactivity in endometrial carcinoma: establishing a clinically relevant cut-off level. Int J Gynecol Pathol 2004; 23(2):129-137.
122. Pijnenborg JM, van de Broek L, Dam de Veen GC et al. TP53 overexpression in recurrent endometrial carcinoma. Gynecol Oncol 2006; 100(2):397-404.
123. Kounelis S, Kapranos N, Kouri E et al. Immunohistochemical profile of endometrial adenocarcinoma: a study of 61 cases and review of the literature. Mod Pathol 2000; 13(4):379-388.
124. Moll UM, Chalas E, Auguste M et al. Uterine papillary serous carcinoma evolves via a p53-driven pathway. Hum Pathol 1996; 27(12):1295-1300.
125. Zheng W, Cao P, Zheng M et al. p53 overexpression and bcl-2 persistence in endometrial carcinoma: comparison of papillary serous and endometrioid subtypes. Gynecol Oncol 1996; 61(2):167-174.
126. Scully R, Livingston DM. In search of the tumour-suppressor functions of BRCA1 and BRCA2. Nature 2000; 408(6811):429-432.
127. Welcsh PL, King MC. BRCA1 and BRCA2 and the genetics of breast and ovarian cancer. Hum Mol Genet 2001; 10(7):705-713.
128. Thompson D, Easton DF. Cancer Incidence in BRCA1 mutation carriers. J Natl Cancer Inst 2002; 94(18):1358-1365.
129. Lavie O, Ben-Arie A, Pilip A et al. BRCA2 germline mutation in a woman with uterine serous papillary carcinoma—case report. Gynecol Oncol 2005; 99(2):486-488.
130. Lavie O, Hornreich G, Ben-Arie A et al. BRCA germline mutations in Jewish women with uterine serous papillary carcinoma. Gynecol Oncol 2004; 92(2):521-524.
131. Levine DA, Lin O, Barakat RR et al. Risk of endometrial carcinoma associated with BRCA mutation. Gynecol Oncol 2001; 80(3):395-398.
132. Goshen R, Chu W, Elit L et al. Is uterine papillary serous adenocarcinoma a manifestation of the hereditary breast-ovarian cancer syndrome? Gynecol Oncol 2000; 79(3):477-481.
133. Beiner ME, Finch A, Rosen B et al. The risk of endometrial cancer in women with BRCA1 and BRCA2 mutations. A prospective study. Gynecol Oncol 2007; 104(1):7-10.
134. Hornreich G, Beller U, Lavie O et al. Is uterine serous papillary carcinoma a BRCA1-related disease? Case report and review of the literature. Gynecol Oncol 1999; 75(2):300-304.
135. Salvesen HB, MacDonald N, Ryan A et al. Methylation of hMLH1 in a population-based series of endometrial carcinomas. Clin Cancer Res 2000; 6(9):3607-3613.
136. Risinger JI, Maxwell GL, Berchuck A et al. Promoter hypermethylation as an epigenetic component in Type I and Type II endometrial cancers. Ann NY Acad Sci 2003; 983:208-212.
137. Harris RC, Chung E, Coffey RJ. EGF receptor ligands. Exp Cell Res 2003; 284(1):2-13.
138. van der Geer P, Hunter T, Lindberg RA. Receptor protein-tyrosine kinases and their signal transduction pathways. Annu Rev Cell Biol 1994; 10:251-337.
139. Schlessinger J. Cell signaling by receptor tyrosine kinases. Cell 2000; 103(2):211-225.
140. Niikura H, Sasano H, Kaga K et al. Expression of epidermal growth factor family proteins and epidermal growth factor receptor in human endometrium. Hum Pathol 1996; 27(3):282-289.
141. Yokoyama Y, Takahashi Y, Hashimoto M et al. Immunohistochemical study of estradiol, epidermal growth factor, transforming growth factor alpha and epidermal growth factor receptor in endometrial neoplasia. Jpn J Clin Oncol 1996; 26(6):411-416.
142. Pfeiffer D, Spranger J, Al-Deiri M et al. mRNA expression of ligands of the epidermal-growth-factor-receptor in the uterus. Int J Cancer 7 1997; 72(4):581-586.

143. Jasonni VM, Amadori A, Santini D et al. Epidermal growth factor receptor (EGF-R) and transforming growth factor alpha (TGFA) expression in different endometrial cancers. Anticancer Res 1995; 15(4):1327-1332.

144. Jasonni VM, Santini D, Amadori A et al. Epidermal growth factor receptor expression and endometrial cancer histotypes. Ann NY Acad Sci 1994; 734:298-305.

145. Khalifa MA, Mannel RS, Haraway SD et al. Expression of EGFR, HER-2/neu, P53 and PCNA in endometrioid, serous papillary and clear cell endometrial adenocarcinomas. Gynecol Oncol 1994; 53(1):84-92.

146. Khalifa MA, Abdoh AA, Mannel RS et al. Prognostic utility of epidermal growth factor receptor overexpression in endometrial adenocarcinoma. Cancer 1994; 73(2):370-376.

147. Ejskjaer K, Sorensen BS, Poulsen SS et al. Expression of the epidermal growth factor system in endometrioid endometrial cancer. Gynecol Oncol 2007; 104(1):158-167.

148. Livasy CA, Reading FC, Moore DT et al. EGFR expression and HER2/neu overexpression/amplification in endometrial carcinosarcoma. Gynecol Oncol 2006; 100(1):101-106.

149. Smith HO, Leslie KK, Singh M et al. GPR30: a novel indicator of poor survival for endometrial carcinoma. Am J Obstet Gynecol 2007; 196(4):386 e381-389; discussion 386 e389-311.

150. Filardo EJ, Quinn JA, Bland KI et al. Estrogen-induced activation of Erk-1 and Erk-2 requires the G protein-coupled receptor homolog, GPR30 and occurs via trans-activation of the epidermal growth factor receptor through release of HB-EGF. Mol Endocrinol 2000; 14(10):1649-1660.

151. Albitar L, Laidler LL, Abdallah R et al. Regulation of signaling phosphoproteins by epidermal growth factor and Iressa (ZD1839) in human endometrial cancer cells that model type I and II tumors. Mol Cancer Ther 2005; 4(12):1891-1899.

152. Tang LL, Yokoyama Y, Wan X et al. PTEN sensitizes epidermal growth factor-mediated proliferation in endometrial carcinoma cells. Oncol Rep 2006; 15(4):855-859.

153. Dougall WC, Qian X, Peterson NC et al. The neu-oncogene: signal transduction pathways, transformation mechanisms and evolving therapies. Oncogene 1994; 9(8):2109-2123.

154. Ioffe OB, Papadimitriou JC, Drachenberg CB. Correlation of proliferation indices, apoptosis and related oncogene expression (bcl-2 and c-erbB-2) and p53 in proliferative, hyperplastic and malignant endometrium. Hum Pathol 1998; 29(10):1150-1159.

155. Halperin R, Zehavi S, Habler L et al. Comparative immunohistochemical study of endometrioid and serous papillary carcinoma of endometrium. Eur J Gynaecol Oncol 2001; 22(2):122-126.

156. Riben MW, Malfetano JH, Nazeer T et al. Identification of HER-2/neu oncogene amplification by fluorescence in situ hybridization in stage I endometrial carcinoma. Mod Pathol 1997; 10(8):823-831.

157. Rolitsky CD, Theil KS, McGaughy VR et al. HER-2/neu amplification and overexpression in endometrial carcinoma. Int J Gynecol Pathol 1999; 18(2):138-143.

158. Slomovitz BM, Broaddus RR, Burke TW et al. Her-2/neu overexpression and amplification in uterine papillary serous carcinoma. J Clin Oncol 2004; 22(15):3126-3132.

159. Morrison C, Zanagnolo V, Ramirez N et al. HER-2 is an independent prognostic factor in endometrial cancer: association with outcome in a large cohort of surgically staged patients. J Clin Oncol 2006; 24(15):2376-2385.

160. Wang D, Konishi I, Koshiyama M et al. Expression of c-erbB-2 protein and epidermal growth receptor in endometrial carcinomas. Correlation with clinicopathologic and sex steroid receptor status. Cancer 1993; 72(9):2628-2637.

161. Hetzel DJ, Wilson TO, Keeney GL et al. HER-2/neu expression: a major prognostic factor in endometrial cancer. Gynecol Oncol 1992; 47(2):179-185.

162. Saffari B, Jones LA, el-Naggar A et al. Amplification and overexpression of HER-2/neu (c-erbB2) in endometrial cancers: correlation with overall survival. Cancer Res 1995; 55(23):5693-5698.

163. Mariani A, Sebo TJ, Katzmann JA et al. HER-2/neu overexpression and hormone dependency in endometrial cancer: analysis of cohort and review of literature. Anticancer Res 2005; 25(4):2921-2927.

164. Bigsby RM, Li AX, Bomalaski J et al. Immunohistochemical study of HER-2/neu, epidermal growth factor receptor and steroid receptor expression in normal and malignant endometrium. Obstet Gynecol 1992; 79(1):95-100.

165. Santin AD, Bellone S, Gokden M et al. Overexpression of HER-2/neu in uterine serous papillary cancer. Clin Cancer Res 2002; 8(5):1271-1279.

166. Osipo C, Meeke K, Liu H et al. Trastuzumab therapy for tamoxifen-stimulated endometrial cancer. Cancer Res 2005; 65(18):8504-8513.

167. Treeck O, Diedrich K, Ortmann O. The activation of an extracellular signal-regulated kinase by oestradiol interferes with the effects of trastuzumab on HER2 signalling in endometrial adenocarcinoma cell lines. Eur J Cancer 2003; 39(9):1302-1309.

168. Villella JA, Cohen S, Smith DH et al. HER-2/neu overexpression in uterine papillary serous cancers and its possible therapeutic implications. Int J Gynecol Cancer 2006; 16(5):1897-1902.

169. Jewell E, Secord AA, Brotherton T et al. Use of trastuzumab in the treatment of metastatic endometrial cancer. Int J Gynecol Cancer 2006; 16(3):1370-1373.
170. Sepp-Lorenzino L. Structure and function of the insulin-like growth factor I receptor. Breast Cancer Res Treat 1998; 47(3):235-253.
171. Rutanen EM. Insulin-like growth factors in endometrial function. Gynecol Endocrinol 1998; 12(6):399-406.
172. LeRoith D, Roberts CT, Jr. The insulin-like growth factor system and cancer. Cancer Lett 2003; 195(2):127-137.
173. Rutanen EM. Insulin-like growth factors and insulin-like growth factor binding proteins in the endometrium. Effect of intrauterine levonorgestrel delivery. Hum Reprod 2000; 15 Suppl 3:173-181.
174. Zhou J, Dsupin BA, Giudice LC et al. Insulin-like growth factor system gene expression in human endometrium during the menstrual cycle. J Clin Endocrinol Metab 1994; 79(6):1723-1734.
175. Surmacz E, Bartucci M. Role of estrogen receptor alpha in modulating IGF-I receptor signaling and function in breast cancer. J Exp Clin Cancer Res 2004; 23(3):385-394.
176. McCampbell AS, Broaddus RR, Loose DS et al. Overexpression of the insulin-like growth factor I receptor and activation of the AKT pathway in hyperplastic endometrium. Clin Cancer Res 2006; 12(21):6373-6378.
177. Talavera F, Reynolds RK, Roberts JA et al. Insulin-like growth factor I receptors in normal and neoplastic human endometrium. Cancer Res 1990; 50(10):3019-3024.
178. Peiro G, Lohse P, Mayr D et al. Insulin-like growth factor-I receptor and PTEN protein expression in endometrial carcinoma. Correlation with bax and bcl-2 expression, microsatellite instability status and outcome. Am J Clin Pathol 2003; 120(1):78-85.
179. Nagamani M, Stuart CA, Dunhardt PA et al. Specific binding sites for insulin and insulin-like growth factor I in human endometrial cancer. Am J Obstet Gynecol 1991; 165(6 Pt 1):1865-1871.
180. Reynolds RK, Hu C, Baker VV. Transforming growth factor-alpha and insulin-like growth factor-I, but not epidermal growth factor, elicit autocrine stimulation of mitogenesis in endometrial cancer cell lines. Gynecol Oncol 1998; 70(2):202-209.
181. Kleinman D, Karas M, Roberts CT Jr et al. Modulation of insulin-like growth factor I (IGF-I) receptors and membrane-associated IGF-binding proteins in endometrial cancer cells by estradiol. Endocrinology 1995; 136(6):2531-2537.
182. Kleinman D, Karas M, Danilenko M et al. Stimulation of endometrial cancer cell growth by tamoxifen is associated with increased insulin-like growth factor (IGF)-I induced tyrosine phosphorylation and reduction in IGF binding proteins. Endocrinology 1996; 137(3):1089-1095.
183. Ayabe T, Tsutsumi O, Sakai H et al. Increased circulating levels of insulin-like growth factor-I and decreased circulating levels of insulin-like growth factor binding protein-1 in postmenopausal women with endometrial cancer. Endocr J 1997; 44(3):419-424.
184. Oh JC, Wu W, Tortolero-Luna G et al. Increased plasma levels of insulin-like growth factor 2 and insulin-like growth factor binding protein 3 are associated with endometrial cancer risk. Cancer Epidemiol Biomarkers Prev 2004; 13(5):748-752.
185. Weiderpass E, Brismar K, Bellocco R et al. Serum levels of insulin-like growth factor-I, IGF-binding protein 1 and 3 and insulin and endometrial cancer risk. Br J Cancer 2003; 89(9):1697-1704.
186. Lacey JV Jr, Potischman N, Madigan MP et al. Insulin-like growth factors, insulin-like growth factor-binding proteins and endometrial cancer in postmenopausal women: results from a U.S. case-control study. Cancer Epidemiol Biomarkers Prev 2004; 13(4):607-612.
187. Augustin LS, Dal Maso L, Franceschi S et al. Association between components of the insulin-like growth factor system and endometrial cancer risk. Oncology 2004; 67(1):54-59.
188. Nagamani M, Stuart CA. Specific binding and growth-promoting activity of insulin in endometrial cancer cells in culture. Am J Obstet Gynecol 1998; 179(1):6-12.
189. Cust AE, Allen NE, Rinaldi S et al. Serum levels of C-peptide, IGFBP-1 and IGFBP-2 and endometrial cancer risk; Results from the European prospective investigation into cancer and nutrition. Int J Cancer 2007; 120(12):2656-2664.
190. Hanahan D, Folkman J. Patterns and emerging mechanisms of the angiogenic switch during tumorigenesis. Cell 1996; 86(3):353-364.
191. Kirschner CV, Alanis-Amezcua JM, Martin VG et al. Angiogenesis factor in endometrial carcinoma: a new prognostic indicator? Am J Obstet Gynecol 1996; 174(6):1879-1882; discussion 1882-1874.
192. Abulafia O, Triest WE, Sherer DM et al. Angiogenesis in endometrial hyperplasia and stage I endometrial carcinoma. Obstet Gynecol 1995; 86(4 Pt 1):479-485.
193. Ferrara N. Role of vascular endothelial growth factor in the regulation of angiogenesis. Kidney Int 1999; 56(3):794-814.
194. Sivridis E, Giatromanolaki A, Anastasiadis P et al. Angiogenic co-operation of VEGF and stromal cell TP in endometrial carcinomas. J Pathol 2002; 196(4):416-422.

195. Sivridis E. Angiogenesis and endometrial cancer. Anticancer Res 2001; 21(6B):4383-4388.
196. Mazurek A, Kuc P, Terlikowski S et al. Evaluation of tumor angiogenesis and thymidine phosphorylase tissue expression in patients with endometrial cancer. Neoplasma 2006; 53(3):242-246.
197. Stefansson IM, Salvesen HB, Akslen LA. Vascular proliferation is important for clinical progress of endometrial cancer. Cancer Res 2006; 66(6):3303-3309.
198. Kumar V, Green S, Stack G et al. Functional domains of the human estrogen receptor. Cell 1987; 51(6):941-951.
199. Barkhem T, Carlsson B, Nilsson Y et al. Differential response of estrogen receptor alpha and estrogen receptor beta to partial estrogen agonists/antagonists. Mol Pharmacol 1998; 54(1):105-112.
200. Geisinger KR, Homesley HD, Morgan TM et al. Endometrial adenocarcinoma. A multiparameter clinicopathologic analysis including the DNA profile and the sex steroid hormone receptors. Cancer 1986; 58(7):1518-1525.
201. Taylor AH, Al-Azzawi F. Immunolocalisation of oestrogen receptor beta in human tissues. J Mol Endocrinol 2000; 24(1):145-155.
202. Pace P, Taylor J, Suntharalingam S et al. Human estrogen receptor beta binds DNA in a manner similar to and dimerizes with estrogen receptor alpha. J Biol Chem 1997; 272(41):25832-25838.
203. Hall JM, McDonnell DP. The estrogen receptor beta-isoform (ERbeta) of the human estrogen receptor modulates ERalpha transcriptional activity and is a key regulator of the cellular response to estrogens and antiestrogens. Endocrinology 1999; 140(12):5566-5578.
204. Rice LW, Jazaeri AA, Shupnik MA. Estrogen receptor mRNA splice variants in pre- and postmenopausal human endometrium and endometrial carcinoma. Gynecol Oncol 1997; 65(1):149-157.
205. Ogawa S, Inoue S, Watanabe T et al. Molecular cloning and characterization of human estrogen receptor betacx: a potential inhibitor ofestrogen action in human. Nucleic Acids Res 1998; 26(15):3505-3512.
206. Zhang QX, Hilsenbeck SG, Fuqua SA et al. Multiple splicing variants of the estrogen receptor are present in individual human breast tumors. J Steroid Biochem Mol Biol 1996; 59(3-4):251-260.
207. Paech K, Webb P, Kuiper GG et al. Differential ligand activation of estrogen receptors ERalpha and ERbeta at AP1 sites. Science 1997; 277(5331):1508-1510.
208. Bunone G, Briand PA, Miksicek RJ et al. Activation of the unliganded estrogen receptor by EGF involves the MAP kinase pathway and direct phosphorylation. EMBO J 1996; 15(9):2174-2183.
209. Migliaccio A, Castoria G, Di Domenico M et al. Sex steroid hormones act as growth factors. J Steroid Biochem Mol Biol 2002; 83(1-5):31-35.
210. Wu W, Slomovitz BM, Celestino J et al. Coordinate expression of Cdc25B and ER-alpha is frequent in low-grade endometrioid endometrial carcinoma but uncommon in high-grade endometrioid and nonendometrioid carcinomas. Cancer Res 2003; 63(19):6195-6199.
211. Jazaeri AA, Nunes KJ, Dalton MS et al. Well-differentiated endometrial adenocarcinomas and poorly differentiated mixed mullerian tumors have altered ER and PR isoform expression. Oncogene 2001; 20(47):6965-6969.
212. Saegusa M, Okayasu I. Changes in expression of estrogen receptors alpha and beta in relation to progesterone receptor and pS2 status in normal and malignant endometrium. Jpn J Cancer Res 2000; 91(5):510-518.
213. Mylonas I, Jeschke U, Shabani N et al. Normal and malignant human endometrium express immunohistochemically estrogen receptor alpha (ER-alpha), estrogen receptor beta (ER-beta) and progesterone receptor (PR). Anticancer Res 2005; 25(3A):1679-1686.
214. Horvath G, Leser G, Hahlin M et al. Exon deletions and variants of human estrogen receptor mRNA in endometrial hyperplasia and adenocarcinoma. Int J Gynecol Cancer 2000; 10(2):128-136.
215. Critchley HO, Henderson TA, Kelly RW et al. Wild-type estrogen receptor (ERbeta1) and the splice variant (ERbetacx/beta2) are both expressed within the human endometrium throughout the normal menstrual cycle. J Clin Endocrinol Metab 2002; 87(11):5265-5273.
216. Skrzypczak M, Bieche I, Szymczak S et al. Evaluation of mRNA expression of estrogen receptor beta and its isoforms in human normal and neoplastic endometrium. Int J Cancer 2004; 110(6):783-787.
217. Bryant W, Snowhite AE, Rice LW et al. The estrogen receptor (ER)alpha variant Delta5 exhibits dominant positive activity on ER-regulated promoters in endometrial carcinoma cells. Endocrinology 2005; 146(2):751-759.
218. Chakravarty D, Srinivasan R, Ghosh S et al. Estrogen receptor beta1 and the beta2/betacx isoforms in nonneoplastic endometrium and in endometrioid carcinoma. Int J Gynecol Cancer. 2007.
219. Balmer NN, Richer JK, Spoelstra NS et al. Steroid receptor coactivator AIB1 in endometrial carcinoma, hyperplasia and normal endometrium: Correlation with clinicopathologic parameters and biomarkers. Mod Pathol 2006; 19(12):1593-1605.
220. Kershah SM, Desouki MM, Koterba KL et al. Expression of estrogen receptor coregulators in normal and malignant human endometrium. Gynecol Oncol 2004; 92(1):304-313.

221. Uchikawa J, Shiozawa T, Shih HC et al. Expression of steroid receptor coactivators and corepressors in human endometrial hyperplasia and carcinoma with relevance to steroid receptors and Ki-67 expression. Cancer 2003; 98(10):2207-2213.

222. Vilgelm A, Lian Z, Wang H et al. Akt-mediated phosphorylation and activation of estrogen receptor alpha is required for endometrial neoplastic transformation in Pten+/- mice. Cancer Res 2006; 66(7):3375-3380.

223. Vivacqua A, Bonofiglio D, Recchia AG et al. The G protein-coupled receptor GPR30 mediates the proliferative effects induced by 17beta-estradiol and hydroxytamoxifen in endometrial cancer cells. Mol Endocrinol 2006; 20(3):631-646.

224. Kastner P, Krust A, Turcotte B et al. Two distinct estrogen-regulated promoters generate transcripts encoding the two functionally different human progesterone receptor forms A and B. EMBO J 1990; 9(5):1603-1614.

225. Sartorius CA, Melville MY, Hovland AR et al. A third transactivation function (AF3) of human progesterone receptors located in the unique N-terminal segment of the B-isoform. Mol Endocrinol 1994; 8(10):1347-1360.

226. Huse B, Verca SB, Matthey P et al. Definition of a negative modulation domain in the human progesterone receptor. Mol Endocrinol 1998; 12(9):1334-1342.

227. Graham JD, Clarke CL. Expression and transcriptional activity of progesterone receptor A and progesterone receptor B in mammalian cells. Breast Cancer Res 2002; 4(5):187-190.

228. Arnett-Mansfield RL, deFazio A, Wain GV et al. Relative expression of progesterone receptors A and B in endometrioid cancers of the endometrium. Cancer Res 2001; 61(11):4576-4582.

229. De Vivo I, Huggins GS, Hankinson SE et al. A functional polymorphism in the promoter of the progesterone receptor gene associated with endometrial cancer risk. Proc Natl Acad Sci USA 2002; 99(19):12263-12268.

230. Saito S, Ito K, Nagase S et al. Progesterone receptor isoforms as a prognostic marker in human endometrial carcinoma. Cancer Sci 2006; 97(12):1308-1314.

231. Hanekamp EE, Kuhne LM, Grootegoed JA et al. Progesterone receptor A and B expression and progestagen treatment in growth and spread of endometrial cancer cells in nude mice. Endocr Relat Cancer 2004; 11(4):831-841.

232. Junqueira MG, da Silva ID, Nogueira-de-Souza NC et al. Progesterone receptor (PROGINS) polymorphism and the risk of endometrial cancer development. Int J Gynecol Cancer 2007; 17(1):229-232.

233. Pijnenborg JM, Romano A, Dam-de Veen GC et al. Aberrations in the progesterone receptor gene and the risk of recurrent endometrial carcinoma. J Pathol 2005; 205(5):597-605.

234. Sakaguchi H, Fujimoto J, Hong BL et al. Drastic decrease of progesterone receptor form B but not A mRNA reflects poor patient prognosis in endometrial cancers. Gynecol Oncol 2004; 93(2):394-399.

235. Miyamoto T, Watanabe J, Hata H et al. Significance of progesterone receptor-A and -B expressions in endometrial adenocarcinoma. J Steroid Biochem Mol Biol 2004; 92(3):111-118.

236. Leslie KK, Stein MP, Kumar NS et al. Progesterone receptor isoform identification and subcellular localization in endometrial cancer. Gynecol Oncol 2005; 96(1):32-41.

237. Saito T, Mizumoto H, Tanaka R et al. Overexpressed progesterone receptor form B inhibit invasive activity suppressing matrix metalloproteinases in endometrial carcinoma cells. Cancer Lett 2004; 209(2):237-243.

238. Dai D, Wolf DM, Litman ES et al. Progesterone inhibits human endometrial cancer cell growth and invasiveness: down-regulation of cellular adhesion molecules through progesterone B receptors. Cancer Res 2002; 62(3):881-886.

239. Dahmoun M, Boman K, Cajander S et al. Intratumoral effects of medroxy-progesterone on proliferation, apoptosis and sex steroid receptors in endometrioid endometrial adenocarcinoma. Gynecol Oncol 2004; 92(1):116-126.

240. Dai D, Litman ES, Schonteich E et al. Progesterone regulation of activating protein-1 transcriptional activity: a possible mechanism of progesterone inhibition of endometrial cancer cell growth. J Steroid Biochem Mol Biol 2003; 87(2-3):123-131.

241. Davies S, Dai D, Feldman I et al. Identification of a novel mechanism of NF-kappaB inactivation by progesterone through progesterone receptors in Hec50co poorly differentiated endometrial cancer cells: induction of A20 and ABIN-2. Gynecol Oncol 2004; 94(2):463-470.

242. Naitoh K, Honjo H, Yamamoto T et al. Estrone sulfate and sulfatase activity in human breast cancer and endometrial cancer. J Steroid Biochem 1989; 33(6):1049-1054.

243. Vermeulen-Meiners C, Jaszmann LJ, Haspels AA et al. The endogenous concentration of estradiol and estrone in normal human postmenopausal endometrium. J Steroid Biochem 1984; 21(5):607-612.

244. Vermeulen-Meiners C, Poortman J, Haspels AA et al. The endogenous concentration of estradiol and estrone in pathological human postmenopausal endometrium. J Steroid Biochem 1986; 24(5):1073-1078.

245. Potischman N, Hoover RN, Brinton LA et al. Case-control study of endogenous steroid hormones and endometrial cancer. J Natl Cancer Inst 1996; 88(16):1127-1135.
246. Berstein LM, Tchernobrovkina AE, Gamajunova VB et al. Tumor estrogen content and clini-comorphological and endocrine features of endometrial cancer. J Cancer Res Clin Oncol 2003; 129(4):245-249.
247. Berstein LM, Imyanitov EN, Suspitsin EN et al. CYP19 gene polymorphism in endometrial cancer patients. J Cancer Res Clin Oncol 2001; 127(2):135-138.
248. Berstein LM, Imyanitov EN, Kovalevskij AJ et al. CYP17 and CYP19 genetic polymorphisms in endometrial cancer: association with intratumoral aromatase activity. Cancer Lett 2004; 207(2):191-196.
249. Berstein L, Zimarina T, Imyanitov E et al. Hormonal imbalance in two types of endometrial cancer and genetic polymorphism of steroidogenic enzymes. Maturitas 2006; 54(4):352-355.
250. Pathirage N, Di Nezza LA, Salmonsen LA et al. Expression of aromatase, estrogen receptors and their coactivators in patients with endometrial cancer. Fertil Steril 2006; 86(2):469-472.
251. Bulun SE, Economos K, Miller D et al. CYP19 (aromatase cytochrome P450) gene expression in human malignant endometrial tumors. J Clin Endocrinol Metab 1994; 79(6):1831-1834.
252. Fowler JM, Ramirez N, Cohn DE et al. Correlation of cyclooxygenase-2 (COX-2) and aromatase expression in human endometrial cancer: tissue microarray analysis. Am J Obstet Gynecol 2005; 192(4):1262-1271; discussion 1271-1263.
253. Segawa T, Shozu M, Murakami K et al. Aromatase expression in stromal cells of endometrioid endo-metrial cancer correlates with poor survival. Clin Cancer Res 2005; 11(6):2188-2194.
254. Reich O, Regauer S. Aromatase expression in low-grade endometrial stromal sarcomas: an immunohis-tochemical study. Mod Pathol 2004; 17(1):104-108.
255. Jongen VH, Thijssen JH, Hollema H et al. Is aromatase cytochrome P450 involved in the pathogenesis of endometrioid endometrial cancer? Int J Gynecol Cancer 2005; 15(3):529-536.
256. Berstein L, Zimarina T, Kovalevskij A et al. CYP19 gene expression and aromatase activity in endometrial cancer tissue: importance of the type of the disease. Neoplasma 2005; 52(2):115-118.
257. Berstein L, Kovalevskij A, Zimarina T et al. Aromatase and comparative response to its inhibitors in two types of endometrial cancer. J Steroid Biochem Mol Biol 2005; 95(1-5):71-74.
258. Sasano H, Sato S, Ito K et al. Effects of aromatase inhibitors on the pathobiology of the human breast, endometrial and ovarian carcinoma. Endocr Relat Cancer 1999; 6(2):197-204.
259. Yamamoto T, Kitawaki J, Urabe M et al. Estrogen productivity of endometrium and endometrial cancer tissue; influence of aromatase on proliferation of endometrial cancer cells. J Steroid Biochem Mol Biol 1993; 44(4-6):463-468.
260. Duffy S, Jackson TL, Lansdown M et al. The ATAC adjuvant breast cancer trial in postmenopausal women: baseline endometrial subprotocol data. BJOG 2003; 110(12):1099-1106.
261. Rose PG, Brunetto VL, VanLe L et al. A phase II trial of anastrozole in advanced recurrent or persistent endometrial carcinoma: a Gynecologic Oncology Group study. Gynecol Oncol 2000; 78(2):212-216.
262. Ma BB, Oza A, Eisenhauer E et al. The activity of letrozole in patients with advanced or recurrent endometrial cancer and correlation with biological markers—a study of the National Cancer Institute of Canada Clinical Trials Group. Int J Gynecol Cancer 2004; 14(4):650-658.
263. Burnett AF, Bahador A, Amezcua C. Anastrozole, an aromatase inhibitor and medroxyprogesterone acetate therapy in premenopausal obese women with endometrial cancer: a report of two cases success-fully treated without hysterectomy. Gynecol Oncol 2004; 94(3):832-834.
264. Gründker C, Günthert AR, Westphalen S et al. Biology of the gonadotropin-releasing hormone system in gynecological cancers. Eur J Endocrinol 2002; 146(1):1-14.
265. Cheng CK, Leung PC. Molecular biology of gonadotropin-releasing hormone (GnRH)-I, GnRH-II and their receptors in humans. Endocr Rev 2005; 26(2):283-306.
266. White RB, Eisen JA, Kasten TL et al. Second gene for gonadotropin-releasing hormone in humans. Proc Natl Acad Sci USA 1998; 95(1):305-309.
267. Eicke N, Günthert AR, Emons G et al. GnRH-II agonist [D-Lys6]GnRH-II inhibits the EGF-induced mitogenic signal transduction in human endometrial and ovarian cancer cells. Int J Oncol 2006; 29(5):1223-1229.
268. Eicke N, Günthert AR, Viereck V et al. GnRH-II receptor-like antigenicity in human placenta and in cancers of the human reproductive organs. Eur J Endocrinol 2005; 153(4):605-612.
269. Gründker C, Günthert AR, Millar RP et al. Expression of gonadotropin-releasing hormone II (GnRH-II) receptor in human endometrial and ovarian cancer cells and effects of GnRH-II on tumor cell prolifera-tion. J Clin Endocrinol Metab 2002; 87(3):1427-1430.
270. Gründker C, Schlotawa L, Viereck V et al. Antiproliferative effects of the GnRH antagonist cetrorelix and of GnRH-II on human endometrial and ovarian cancer cells are not mediated through the GnRH type I receptor. Eur J Endocrinol 2004; 151(1):141-149.
271. Fister S, Günthert AR, Emons G et al. Gonadotropin-releasing hormone type II antagonists induce apoptotic cell death in human endometrial and ovarian cancer cells in vitro and in vivo. Cancer Res 2007; 67(4):1750-1756.

CHAPTER 12

Cell Cycle Machinery:
Links with Genesis and Treatment of Breast Cancer

Alison J. Butt, C. Elizabeth Caldon, Catriona M. McNeil, Alexander
Swarbrick, Elizabeth A. Musgrove and Robert L. Sutherland*

Abstract

Loss of normal growth control is a hallmark of cancer. Thus, understanding the mechanisms of tissue-specific, normal growth regulation and the changes that occur during tumorigenesis may provide insights of both diagnostic and therapeutic importance. Control of cell proliferation in the normal mammary gland is steroid hormone (estrogen and progestin)-dependent, involves complex interactions with other hormones, growth factors and cytokines and ultimately converges on activation of three proto-oncogenes (c-Myc, cyclin D1 and cyclin E1) that are rate limiting for the G1 to S phase transition during normal cell cycle progression. Mammary epithelial cell-specific overexpression of these genes induces mammary carcinoma in mice, while cyclin D1 null mice have arrested mammary gland development and are resistant to carcinoma induced by the *neu/erbB2* and *ras* oncogenes. Furthermore, c-Myc, cyclins D1, E1 and E2 are commonly overexpressed in primary breast cancer where elevated expression is often associated with a more aggressive disease phenotype and an adverse patient outcome. This may be due in part to overexpression of these genes conferring resistance to endocrine therapies since in vitro studies provide compelling evidence that overexpression of c-Myc and to a lesser extent cyclin D1 and cyclin E1, attenuate the growth inhibitory effects of SERMS, antiestrogens and progestins in breast cancer cells. Thus, abnormal regulation of the expression of cell cycle molecules, involved in the steroidal control of cell proliferation in the mammary gland, are likely to be directly involved in the development, progression and therapeutic responsiveness of breast cancer. Furthermore, a more detailed understanding of these pathways may identify new targets for therapeutic intervention particularly in endocrine-unresponsive and endocrine-resistant disease.

Introduction

Loss of normal growth control, including aberrations in the homeostatic mechanisms that ensure integrity of cell cycle progression, is a hallmark of cancer.[1] A pivotal regulatory pathway determining rates of cell cycle transition from G_1 to S phase is the cyclin/cyclin-dependent kinase (CDK)/p16^{INK4A}/retinoblastoma protein (Rb) pathway.[2] Alterations to different components of this pathway through overexpression, mutation and epigenetic gene silencing are almost universal in human cancer.[3] Interestingly, there appears to be a degree of tissue specificity in the particular genetic abnormalities within the Rb pathway in different cancers with aberrations in the expression of cyclins D1, E1 and the CDK inhibitor p27^{Kip1} common in breast cancer.

In the mammary gland the sex steroid hormones, estrogen and progesterone and their cognate receptors, ER and PR, are essential for normal development and physiological function. There is now an expansive literature documenting the molecular mechanisms through which these

*Corresponding Author: RL Sutherland—Cancer Research Program, Garvan Institute of Medical Research, 384 Victoria St, Darlinghurst, NSW 2010, Australia. Email: r.sutherland@garvan.org.au

Innovative Endocrinology of Cancer, edited by Lev M. Berstein and Richard J. Santen.
©2008 Landes Bioscience and Springer Science+Business Media.

hormones exert their mitogenic effects both in the normal mammary gland and in breast cancer. These data show that estrogen/progestin action converges on a number of molecules with pivotal roles in the regulation of the Rb pathway and thus, in the G_1 to S phase transition of the cell cycle. These include the proto-oncogenes c-Myc, cyclins D1, D3, E1 and E2 and the CDK inhibitors, p21[WAF1/Cip1] and p27[Kip1]. Furthermore, the expression of several of these molecules changes significantly during breast tumorigenesis and is associated with distinct breast cancer phenotypes and patient outcome. Thus, aberrant expression and/or function of cell cycle regulatory molecules involved in the normal physiological response to sex steroid hormones is a common feature of breast cancer and may be intimately involved mechanistically in the disease process.

This review briefly summarizes contemporary literature addressing the functions of selected cell cycle regulatory genes in mammary epithelial cells and their potential roles in the development and progression of human breast cancer.

Cell Cycle Control Mechanisms and Their Regulation in Breast Cancer Cells

Mechanisms of Cell Cycle Control

Cyclins are the regulatory subunits of holoenzymes whose catalytic subunit is a CDK. Cyclins share a sequence motif termed the 'cyclin box' that mediates binding to a similarly well-conserved region on the CDK.[4] Members of this family of serine/threonine kinases were originally characterized by virtue of their roles in cell cycle control, although more recently identified cyclin-CDK complexes have roles in transcriptional control.[5] In addition, cyclin D1 can act as a transcriptional cofactor, a function which is CDK-independent.[6] As the name suggests, CDKs lack kinase activity in the absence of cyclin association and thus, regulation of cyclin abundance is an important, but not the only, control mechanism for CDK activation.[4]

Progress through the cell cycle is accompanied by sequential accumulation of different cyclins that is correlated with the activation of specific cyclin-CDK complexes: cyclin E-CDK2 at the G_1/S phase boundary, cyclin A-CDK2 during S phase, cyclin A-CDK1 (CDC2) during G_2 and cyclin B-CDK1 during mitosis (Fig. 1). The D-type cyclins (cyclins D1-3) are less profoundly regulated during the cell cycle but are strongly mitogen-dependent. Consequently, the CDKs formed by association of D type cyclins and CDK4 or CDK6 can be viewed as 'mitogen sensors', that act during G_1 phase to link signals from the extracellular environment to other CDKs that comprise the 'core cell cycle machinery'.[7]

Several substrates for the different CDKs have been identified. A prevailing concept has been that each cyclin-CDK complex has a distinct substrate preference and that this specificity is a determinant in ordering cell cycle events. This is supported by several lines of evidence, for example the different spectra of cellular proteins phosphorylated by various recombinant cyclin-CDK complexes[8] and the distinct consensus sequences for phosphorylation by cyclin D1-CDK4 and cyclin E-CDK2 or cyclin A-CDK2.[9] However, the ability of cyclin E and cyclin D2 'knocked-in' to the cyclin D1 locus to complement defects in mice lacking cyclin D1 and the ability of fibroblasts lacking all three D-type cyclins or both E-type cyclins to proliferate, argue for significant functional redundancy between the cyclins.[10] Thus, an alternative view is that the spatial and temporal control of cyclin expression is a major determinant of specificity.[11]

The best-understood CDK substrate is Rb, the product of the retinoblastoma susceptibility gene. The importance of Rb as a CDK substrate is illustrated by the observation that cyclin D1 is not required for G_1 phase progression in cells lacking Rb.[12] However, cyclin D1-associated CDKs are not the only Rb kinases; there are 16 possible consensus sites for CDK phosphorylation within Rb and the protein is progressively phosphorylated by different CDKs during cell cycle progression.[2] Phosphorylation of Rb by cyclin D-CDK4 and/or cyclin D-CDK6 early in G_1 phase displaces histone deacetylases from Rb and allows subsequent phosphorylation of Rb by cyclin E-CDK2 and cyclin A-CDK2.[13] Phosphorylation by both sets of CDKs is necessary to

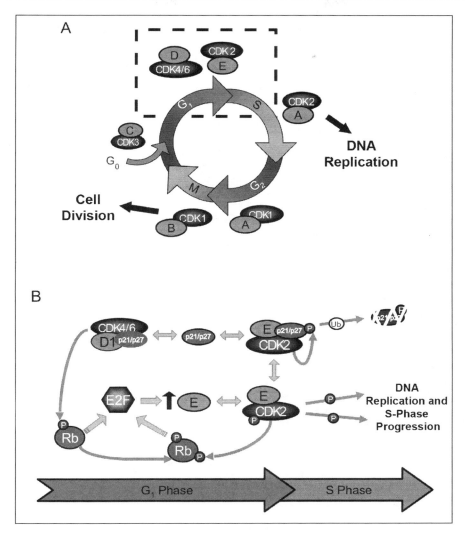

Figure 1. The eukaryotic cell cycle and phase-specific activation of cyclin-CDK complexes. A) the eukaryotic cell cycle involves the sequential action of cyclin-CDK complexes to move between the distinct phases of the cell cycle. The letters A, B, C, D and E denote each respective cyclin. B) The main features of G_1 to S phase progression. Briefly, sequential phosphorylation of Rb by cyclin D1-CDK4/6 and cyclin E-CDK2 allows E2F-mediated transcription of target genes including cyclin E and consequent progression into S phase. The distribution of the CDK inhibitors p21[WAF1/Cip1] and p27[Kip1] between these complexes provides an additional level of control over their activity. The levels of these CDK inhibitors are in part

completely overcome the growth inhibitory effects of Rb, release E2F transcription factors and allow initiation of DNA synthesis (Fig. 1).[13,14] Recent data also implicate another CDK, cyclin C-CDK3, in the phosphorylation of Rb during the transition from quiescence (G_0) to G_1.[15]

In addition to regulation of cyclin abundance there exist several other levels of regulation for CDK activity including a network of regulatory kinases and phosphatases,[4] and two families of endogenous small molecular weight CDK inhibitory proteins.[7] The INK4 family of CDK inhibitors (p15[INK4B], p16[INK4A], p18[INK4C], p19[INK4D]) specifically target CDK4 and CDK6.[7] The Cip/Kip family inhibitors (p21[WAF1/Cip1], p27[Kip1], p57[Kip2]) target a wider spectrum of CDKs. They profoundly inhibit the activity of cyclin E-CDK2 and cyclin A-CDK2, but also function as assembly factors for cyclin D-CDK complexes.[16] Like the cyclins, these inhibitors are mitogen-responsive. For example, p27[Kip1] expression provides a 'threshhold' that must be exceeded to allow CDK activation during mitogenic stimulation. One function of cyclin D1 appears to be sequestration of p27[Kip1]: alterations in cyclin D1 abundance not only directly affect the activity of CDK4 and CDK6 but can indirectly influence the activation of cyclin E-CDK2 by altering the availability of p27[Kip1].[7]

Steroid Regulation of Cell Cycle Progression

In the mammary gland the majority of development occurs postnatally under the influence of the ovarian sex steroid hormones, estrogen and progesterone. Although several other hormones, growth factors and cytokines regulate normal mammary gland physiology, the sex steroid hormones are required for mammary gland development, playing a pivotal role in side-branching and lobulo-alveolar development. These roles of the sex steroids carry over to breast cancer where estrogen action is essential for the development and maintenance of the majority of breast cancers[17] and the synthetic analogs of progesterone, progestins, exert both growth stimulatory and inhibitory effects depending on the stage of the disease process and the cellular phenotype.[18] Furthermore, progestins increase breast cancer risk when administered in HRT regimens and a PR allele that leads to the preferential expression of PR-B is associated with increased breast cancer risk.[19] Detailed analyses of the effects of sex steroids on breast cancer cell proliferation identify that both estrogens and progestins control this process by regulating the G_1 to S phase transition in the cell cycle.[20,21]

The effects of estrogen and progestins are mediated through ligand-activated transcription factors belonging to the nuclear receptor superfamily. Two ERs have been characterized, ERα and ERβ. Studies using ER knockout models have shown that ERα is the predominant mediator of the mitogenic effects of estrogen in the mammary gland,[22] while ERα appears to mediate the drive to proliferation in breast cancer cells but ERβ is growth inhibitory.[23] Although only one PR gene has been identified, there are two distinct isoforms of the receptors, PR-B and PR-A, that are generated from different transcriptional start sites. These isoforms have differential effects on mammary gland development and the regulation of breast cancer cell proliferation and differentiated function in vitro.[18]

Since both estrogens and progestins control G_1 to S phase progression much work has focused on the links between steroid hormone receptor signaling and the cell cycle machinery. This is most developed in the case of estrogen stimulation of breast cancer cell proliferation. One of the earliest transcriptional responses in the mitogenic response to estrogen is increased *MYC* expression, which occurs within 15 min of estrogen stimulation.[24] Similarly, acute downregulation of *MYC* expression is an early event in antiestrogen inhibition of breast cancer cells while downregulation of c-Myc with antisense oligonucleotides mimics the effect of antiestrogens on breast cancer cell cycle progression.[25] The DNA binding region of ERα is required for *MYC* induction and the P2 promoter region of the *MYC* gene contains an atypical ERE region.[26] Recently a strongly estrogen-inducible ER binding site 67 kb upstream of *MYC* has been identified which may also contribute to estrogen regulation of *MYC*, although its functional significance is yet to be characterized.[27]

The c-Myc protein is a nuclear transcription factor that has profound mitogenic effects on breast cancer cells through its ability to modulate regulators of cell cycle progression.[28] Inhibition of c-Myc expression abrogates estrogen-stimulated breast cancer cell proliferation and blocks cell cycle progression leading to a G_1 arrest.[29] Furthermore, induction of c-Myc can mimic the effects of estrogen and induce antiestrogen-arrested cells to reinitiate cell cycle progression,[30] implicating c-Myc as a prominent mediator of estrogen action in breast cancer cells. Numerous genetic targets of c-Myc activation and repression have been identified, including many cell cycle regulators (reviewed in ref. 31). Thus, a major mechanism governing c-Myc's effects on cell cycle progression in breast cancer cells is the activation of cyclin E-CDK2 via repression of the CDK inhibitor, p21$^{WAF1/Cip1}$.[30,32] In this respect, c-Myc's actions closely mimic those of estrogen,[33] again emphasizing its potential role as a major mediator of estrogen action in breast cancer cells.

The effects of estrogen on cell cycle progression are also tightly linked to increased expression of cyclin D1. Cyclin D1 induction in breast cancer cells shortens G_1 and can rescue growth factor-deprived and antiestrogen-arrested cells enabling them to complete the cell cycle.[34] While estrogen rapidly induces cyclin D1 expresssion, antiestrogens have a converse acute inhibitory effect.[33,35,36] Furthermore, abrogation of cyclin D1 activity by cyclin D1 antibodies or the Cdk4 inhibitor p16^{INK4A} blocks estrogen-induced G_1-S phase progression,[37] indicating that estrogen acts, at least in part, through upregulation of cyclin D1 expression. Like c-Myc, inducible cyclin D1 expression can mimic the effects of estrogen allowing cell cycle re-entry in antiestrogen-arrested breast cancer cells.[30,36]

Estrogen also elicits rapid activation of cyclin E-CDK2 in breast cancer cells.[33,38,39] The mechanism governing this action is not fully elucidated, although it is known to involve estrogen-mediated inhibition of the CDK inhibitor, p21$^{WAF1/Cip1}$.[33,38] Overall, estrogen activation of cyclin D1 expression increases cyclin D1-CDK4 complex formation and sequestration of p21$^{WAF1/Cip1}$ and p27^{Kip1} at the expense of cyclin E-CDK2 complexes, thus activating the latter enzyme. The cyclin E-CDK2 complex binds hyperphosphorylated p130 in the absence of p21$^{WAF1/Cip1}$ and p27^{Kip1} binding, which may prevent reassociation with CDK inhibitors.[33] The activity of the cyclin E-CDK2 complex is further enhanced through upregulation of Cdc25A, which removes inhibitory phosphatases from the cyclin E-CDK2 complexes. Finally, p27^{Kip1} is relocalized from the nucleus to the cytoplasm by estrogen-induced ERK activation and simultaneously the degradation of p27^{Kip1} is increased through estrogen-mediated induction of Skp2.[40] Cyclin D1 expression also elicits effects on the activation of cyclin E-CDK2 similar to those of c-Myc.[30] However, in our MCF-7 model system overexpression of cyclin D1 did not induce c-Myc expression or vice versa, consistent with evidence that both *MYC* and *CCND1* are direct targets of the ER,[27,41] and further, suggesting that estrogen-stimulated cell cycle progression is mediated initially by distinct c-Myc and cyclin D1 pathways that converge on the activation of cyclin E-CDK2.[30] A summary of estrogen regulation of breast cancer cell cycle progression is presented in Figure 2.

In contrast to the stimulatory actions of estrogen in breast cancer cells in vitro, progesterone has a biphasic effect on cell proliferation, where it initially accelerates cells from G_1 to S phase but subsequently arrests cells in early G_1 following mitosis.[42] Progestins induce a similar effect to estrogen in the stimulatory phase of their action in that c-Myc and cyclin D1 are induced transiently within 2-3 hours of progestin treatment.[20] After the transient induction of S phase, cell proliferation is inhibited following a reduction in cyclin E-CDK2 and cyclin D-CDK4 activity.[20] This is mediated, in part, by a reduction in levels of cyclin D1 and cyclin E1, as well as increased expression of p18^{INK4c}, which disrupts cyclin D-CDK4/6 binding and hence, contributes to inactivation of CDK4/6.[43,44] The proportion of inactive cyclin E-CDK2 complexes bound by the CDK inhibitors p21$^{WAF1/Cip1}$ and p27^{Kip1} increases, due to both the upregulation of the CDK inhibitors and their redistribution from cyclin D-CDK4/6 complexes.[20,44] Inducible overexpression of cyclin D1 in progestin-pretreated cells restores the activity of cyclin E-CDK2 complexes,[44] emphasising the role of cyclin D1 abundance in regulating the availability of CDK inhibitors. A summary of these effects of progestins on the cell cycle machinery is presented in Figure 3.

Progestins regulate both proliferation and differentiation in breast cancer cells and there has been much interest in identifying progestin targets that may contribute to the co-ordination of these processes. One candidate is the HLH protein Id1, which is progestin-regulated and has roles in both the proliferation and differentiation of mammary epithelial cells. More recently, we have demonstrated a role for Wilms Tumor Protein 1 (Wt1) in mediating the growth inhibitory/differentiation-inducing effects of progestin action in breast cancer cells.[45] Progestin treatment of breast cancer cells leads to a rapid downregulation of Wt1 mRNA and protein. Conversely, overexpression of Wt1 attenuates progestin-mediated growth inhibition and activation of lipogenesis, a marker of differentiation in these cells. This is accompanied by the sustained expression of cyclin

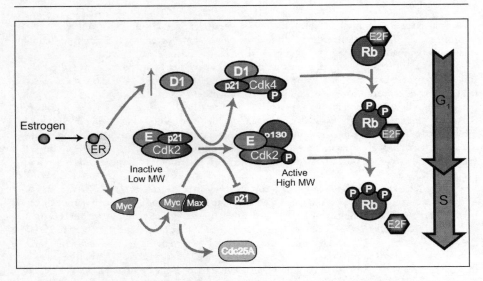

Figure 2. Estrogen action on the cell cycle machinery. Estrogen binding to the estrogen receptor activates parallel pathways through c-Myc and cyclin D1, resulting in the inhibition of p21$^{WAF1/Cip1}$. This leads to the activation of cyclin D1-CDK4 and cyclin E-CDK2 complexes and the subsequent phosphorylation of Rb, releasing E2F and allowing progression from G_1 to S phase. ER: estrogen receptor; D1: cyclin D1; E: cyclin E; P: phosphorylation.

D1 despite progestin treatment and increased levels of Rb phosphorylation at sites targeted by cyclin D1-CDK4 (Ser249/Thr252). Furthermore, Wt1 overexpression only modulates the effects of progestins and not either antiestrogens or androgens. These results indicate that Wt1 is an important early target of progestins that may co-ordinate proliferation and differentiation in breast cancer cells.

Cell Cycle Control Genes as Putative Breast Cancer Oncogenes/Tumor Suppressor Genes

Evidence that c-Myc and the cyclins are potential oncogenes and that the CDK inhibitors are potential tumor suppressor genes in breast cancer comes from both experimental model systems and studies of human breast cancer tissue.

Animal Models

c-Myc was one of the earliest characterised proto-oncogenes and the first oncogene demonstrated to induce mammary carcinoma in transgenic mouse models.[46] However, subsequent studies of various *MYC* transgenic mammary tumor models have demonstrated extended latencies and insufficiency of aberrant *MYC* expression alone to induce mammary tumorigenesis and have given support to the hypothesis that the acquisition of additional genetic lesions is a critical step in c-Myc-induced carcinogenesis. This may result from c-Myc-induced genomic destabilization through a dominant mutator phenotype and center upon suppression of the intrinsic apoptotic function of c-Myc. Indeed, transgene-mediated suppression of c-Myc-induced apoptosis (via expression of *ras*, *neu/erbB2*, *bcl-2* or *tgf-α*) in bitransgenic mouse models, leads to a potent accentuation of mammary tumorigenesis (reviewed in ref. 47).

Overexpression of cyclin D1 in the mammary gland leads to hyperplasia and eventually to carcinoma.[48] Similarly, cyclin E1 overexpression in mammary epithelium promotes tumor formation, but with low penetrance and long latency.[49] Thus, cyclin D1 and cyclin E1 are oncogenic in mice, although weakly so and it is likely that they co-operate with other oncogenes to mediate this effect.

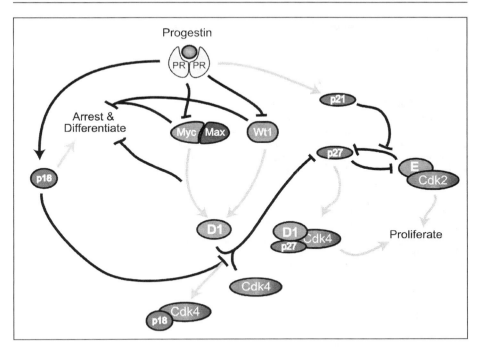

Figure 3. Progestin action on the cell cycle machinery. Progestin-mediated cell cycle arrest requires repression of c-Myc and upregulation of the CDK inhibitors p21[WAF1/Cip1] and p18[INK4C]. Downregulation of c-Myc then regulates the expression of numerous targets, including cyclin D1. Reduced cyclin D1 and increased p18[INK4C] expression then cooperate to inhibit the formation of cyclin D-CDK complexes. The loss of these complexes liberates sequestered p27[Kip1] which then cooperates with the induced p21[WAF1/Cip1] to inhibit cyclin E-CDK2 complexes. Grey lines indicate positive regulation, black lines represent repression. Dotted lines signify proposed pathways. PR: progesterone receptor; D1: cyclin D1; E: cyclin E.

Given its role as a target of mitogenic signaling, it is not surprising that cyclin D1 is implicated in the oncogenic actions of *ras* and *neu/erbB2*. In the mouse mammary gland, tumors induced by either oncogene display increased expression of cyclin D1.[50,51] Conversely, decreased cyclin D1 expression blocks the growth of tumors formed by mammary cells expressing activated *neu/erbB2*[50] and cyclin D1-null mice are resistant to tumor formation resulting from mammary-specific expression of *ras* or *neu/erbB2*.[51] Interestingly, although cyclin D1 has also been implicated as a target of Wnt signaling, *wnt*-stimulated oncogenesis was not impaired in cyclin D1-null mice.[51] In support of conclusions drawn from in vitro studies c-*myc* also induces mammary carcinoma independent of cyclin D1.

The observations that overexpression of p15[INK4b] and p16[INK4A], which target the cyclin D1-associated CDKs, can suppress *ras*-mediated transformation in vitro,[52] and that p16[INK4A] expression blocks *neu/erbB2*-induced mammary tumor formation in mice,[53] all indicate that the dependence on cyclin D1 is likely to be mediated by the ability of cyclin D1 to increase CDK activity, either by direct activation of CDK4 or by indirect activation of CDK2 through sequestration of CDK inhibitors. Although the formation of mammary tumors after expression of activated *neu/erbB2* is impaired in cyclin D1-null mice, some tumors do develop and these are characterized by increased cyclin E expression.[54] Similarly, mice that have cyclin E1 'knocked-in' to the cyclin D1 locus develop *neu/erbB2*-induced mammary tumors at a rate similar to wild-type, indicating that cyclin E1 expression can compensate for the absence of cyclin D1 during oncogenesis.[55] This is consistent with the idea that the requirement for cyclin D1 in mammary carcinoma reflects a need for CDK activity, or at least cell proliferation.

More recent experiments have addressed this issue directly. Development of *neu/erbB2*-induced mammary cancers is significantly impaired both in CDK4-null mice[56] and in knock-in mice where endogenous cyclin D1 is replaced with a 'kinase-dead' cyclin D1 point mutant that binds CDK4 and sequesters CDK inhibitors but is unable to activate the CDK4 kinase.[56,57] This does not simply result from failed mammary epithelial cell proliferation, since virgin CDK4-null mice display retarded mammary development but normal alveolar proliferation and differentiation occur during pregnancy and the 'kinase dead' cyclin D1 mutant is able to rescue the defects in pregnancy-associated mammary gland development in mice lacking cyclin D1. It is therefore clear that *neu/erbB2*-induced mammary oncogenesis requires active cyclin D1-CDK4, in contrast with mammary development, which is 'CDK-independent'. The ability of cyclin E1 to substitute for the function of cyclin D1 in mammary development as well as oncogenesis[55] suggests, however, that there is no absolute requirement for cyclin D1 and that the CDK independent function required for mammary development is likely to be sequestration of p27[Kip1] rather than the ability of cyclin D1 to regulate transcription.

The necessity for cyclin E1 in transformation has not been tested in vivo. However, in in vitro assays, fibroblasts lacking both cyclin E1 and E2 do not form foci in response to c-Myc or to Ras in combination with either c-Myc or dominant-negative p53. Although these fibroblasts display defects in cell cycle re-entry from quiescence, once proliferation is initiated it is only modestly impaired compared to controls with wild-type cyclin E, suggesting a specific requirement for cyclin E in oncogenic proliferation.[58] Thus, there is an emerging body of evidence, which is perhaps the most compelling for cyclin D1, that c-Myc and cyclins D1 and E1 are important for mammary tumorigenesis.

Deregulation in Breast Cancer

Studies of gene expression in human breast cancer tissue have provided substantial evidence for aberrant expression of c-Myc, several cyclins and p27[Kip1] in human breast cancer (Table 1). In clinical cohorts, *MYC* gene amplification is associated with the transition from in situ to invasive carcinoma, markers of an aggressive disease phenotype and poor prognosis in general.[59-61] *MYC* gene amplification occurs in approximately 15-20% of patients with breast cancer[60] but overexpression of *MYC* mRNA and c-Myc protein occurs more frequently, generally 30-50%, particularly in high-grade tumors.[60,62,63] Immunohistochemical studies have generally failed to demonstrate an association between c-Myc protein expression and outcome[64] but this may be due, in part, to difficulties in assessing c-Myc expression by immunohistochemistry with currently available antibodies. While some studies show an association between c-Myc overexpression and negative prognostic factors such as poor differentiation and high proliferation index,[62] at present it is difficult to draw definite conclusions regarding the prognostic significance of c-Myc protein overexpression in breast cancer.

Cyclin D1 protein is overexpressed in ~45% of breast cancers, predominantly in the ER-positive phenotypes.[65] The expression of cyclin D1 protein mirrors stages in the progression model of breast cancer, being expressed at low levels in normal breast, then at increasing levels in hyperplasia and ductal carcinoma in situ.[65] Amplification of the *CCND1* gene, as part of the 11q13 locus, partially accounts for the observed overexpression being present in ~13% of breast cancers. The overexpression of cyclin D1 protein in the remaining ~30% of breast cancer cases is probably due to alterations in transcriptional regulation and/or protein stabilisation that may in turn be due to deregulation of upstream mitogenic signaling pathways.

In contrast to cyclin D1 and cyclin D3 that are highly expressed,[66] cyclin D2 is not expressed in most cultured breast cancer cell lines or in breast cancer due to the cyclin D2 promoter being highly methylated.[67] The relationship of cyclin D3 expression to clinicopathological parameters has only been examined in a small series of studies. These indicate that cyclin D3 is overexpressed

Table 1. Aberrations of cell cycle regulators in breast cancer

	Frequency Range (%)	Mean (%)
MYC amplification	4-52	19
c-Myc overexpression	11-70	38
11q13 amplification	9-17	13
Cyclin D1 overexpression	28-81	45
Cyclin E overexpression	28-35	32
Decreased p27[Kip1] expression	50-63	57

in ~10% of breast cancers,[68] is not associated with gene amplification or ER status but often correlates with cyclin D1 overexpression.

Cyclin E1 is overexpressed in ~30% of breast cancers,[69] predominantly the ER-negative phenotype and is correlated with disease stage and markers of proliferation, i.e., Ki-67, PCNA and mitotic index.[70,71] Low molecular weight forms of cyclin E1 have been detected in breast cancer and were proposed as indicators of poor patient outcome.[72] Functionally, these isoforms may act through increased binding to CDK2 and decreased affinity for p21[WAF1/Cip1] and p27[Kip1],[73] as well as differential regulation by full-length cyclin E1. However, recently the relevance of these low molecular weight forms has been questioned since these isoforms were also identified in normal mammary epithelial cells in a similar ratio to that found in breast cancer tissue.[74]

Data concerning the role of the more recently described cyclin E2 in breast cancer, is less evolved. Some of the earliest publications on cyclin E2 documented its overexpression in breast cancers, but these were restricted to small numbers of samples with limited clinicopathological data. Transcript profiles of larger series of breast cancers have identified cyclin E2 as a component of several gene expression signatures associated with reduced survival.[75-77] Cyclin E2 is the only gene present in all three prognostic signatures and was among 60 genes associated with poor outcome in ER-positive patients.[76] These data prompted two recent qRT-PCR studies of the potential role of cyclin E2 as an individual prognostic marker compared with cyclin E1.[78,79] Although cyclin E2 levels were similar in ER-positive and -negative cancers, cyclin E1 was more highly expressed in ER-negative cancers while cyclin E2 was significantly associated with both grade and ER-positivity.

Of the Cip/Kip family of CDK inhibitors, p27[Kip1] has the strongest association with the disease process while there is conflicting evidence on the importance of p21[WAF1/Cip1] expression in breast tumorigenesis. p27[Kip1] is normally expressed at high levels in epithelial cells, but undergoes profound downregulation in breast cancer where it is strongly correlated with ER-negativity, high tumor grade and poor outcome. The downregulation of p27[Kip1] does not appear to occur through genetic mutation or loss of heterozygosity. Instead p27[Kip1] is downregulated through a combination of mechanisms including decreased stability of nuclear p27[Kip1] through the amplification of processes responsible for its degradation.[80] Both Skp2 and Cks1, which form part of the SCF[Skp2] complex that targets nuclear p27[Kip1] for degradation, are amplified or overexpressed in breast cancer,[81] and Skp2 overexpression correlates with low p27[Kip1] expression.[82]

Dysregulated signaling through growth factor pathways also decreases nuclear p27[Kip1] levels via cytoplasmic relocalisation and degradation. p27[Kip1] is targeted for phosphorylation and subsequent degradation by the ErbB2 and EGFR MEK/MAPK and Ras signaling pathways, leading to degradation.[83] Since these pathways are frequently altered in breast cancer, they are also likely to affect p27[Kip1] activity through upregulation of c-Myc and cyclin D1[83] leading in turn to decreased p27[Kip1] expression and increased levels of cyclin D-CDK4 complexes that sequester p27[Kip1] with resultant increased cyclin E-CDK2 activity. Finally, the PI3K/PKB pathway, which is also activated via ErbB2 and Ras, targets p27[Kip1] for cytoplasmic relocalization from the nucleus through phosphorylation of T157.[83] The activation of PI3K is opposed by PTEN, which also downregulates Skp2. PTEN is downregulated in breast cancer and is associated with low p27[Kip1] levels.[84]

While cytoplasmic p27[Kip1] is often degraded, it has been suggested that the presence of low levels of undegraded cytoplasmic p27[Kip1] may also provide an oncogenic feedback loop. Wu et al have identified that cytoplasmic p27[Kip1] enhances the assembly of cyclin D1-CDK4 complexes, as well as increasing AKT kinase levels.[85]

Of the INK4 family of inhibitors, only p16[INK4A] is altered in breast cancer predominantly through promoter hypermethylation in ~20-30% of cases.[86] p16[INK4A] inhibits cell cycle progression by disrupting cyclin D-CDK 4/6 complexes such that Rb phosphorylation is inhibited. Given that Rb is not usually directly mutated in breast cancer, the inactivation of p16[INK4A] may be important to overcome cell cycle arrest. Several recent reports have identified p16[INK4A] promoter methylation in normal breast and in early benign lesions, suggesting that p16[INK4A] downregulation may not associate with breast carcinogenesis.[86-88] However, there is compelling evidence that it is a subpopulation of normal breast cells that have p16[INK4A] methylation.[86] When cultured in vitro, this population escapes senescence and bear other characteristics of early carcinoma that are dependent on the p16[INK4A] methylation status, including upregulation of further methylation events and downregulation of p53.

Despite the importance of p16[INK4A] promoter methylation, it is actually the overexpression of p16[INK4A] that has been reported to be of prognostic significance in breast cancer. This has been examined in only a small series of studies, where overexpression of both p16[INK4A] mRNA and protein is associated with poor outcome.[89,90] In two studies, the high levels of p16[INK4A] protein have been observed to be primarily cytoplasmic, perhaps indicating functional inactivation through cytoplasmic sequestration, or oncogenic cytoplasmic functions of p16[INK4A].[87,91]

Thus, aberrant expression of several cell cycle regulatory genes is a common feature of breast cancer and often cosegregates with features of the pathophysiology of the disease e.g., disease phenotype and patient outcome. However, further work is required to determine if any of these will become biomarkers with clinical utility in the routine management of breast cancer.

Relationship of Cell Cycle Deregulation to Patient Outcome and Response to Endocrine Therapy

While there have been many studies in which archival tissue from breast cancer cohorts has been analyzed for expression of various cyclins, their relationship to response to endocrine therapy is not well defined. Thus, it is in cell culture systems that the evidence for the involvement of c-Myc and cyclins in the response to endocrine therapy, predominantly antiestrogens, is most compellingly demonstrated (Fig. 4).

The role of c-Myc in the proliferative response to estrogens is discussed above and importantly, provides evidence that c-Myc may play a role in the development of antiestrogen resistance. Inhibition of ER by estrogen withdrawal, aromatase inhibition, or treatment with tamoxifen or faslodex (ICI 182780), all downregulate *MYC* mRNA, which in turn induces cell cycle arrest.[25] Conversely, the acquisition of estrogen independence in MCF-7 cells maintained in estrogen-deprived medium is associated with the upregulation of selected estrogen-regulated genes including ER and *MYC*.[92] Furthermore, overexpression of c-Myc alone is capable of partially reversing the growth suppressive effects of antiestrogens in MCF-7 cells.[30,93]

The amplification of growth factor receptor signaling cascades can also converge on activation of c-Myc, thus potentially influencing endocrine responsiveness. High levels of ErbB2/ErbB3 signaling are frequently observed in breast cancer and lead to persistent Ras and Akt activity via amplification of the MAPK and PI-3 kinase signaling pathways. Ras phosphorylates c-Myc at serine-62 leading to protein stabilization and activation of the PI-3 kinase pathway stimulates translation of *MYC* mRNA and protein stabilization.[94,95] Furthermore, c-Myc protein levels are reduced by an ErbB2 inhibitor (PD153035) and this effect is reversed by ectopic expression of *MYC*.[96] This is consistent with the clinically observed antiestrogen resistance seen in breast cancers overexpressing ErbB2. A synergistic interaction between deregulated c-Myc and EGFR signaling has also been seen in mammary carcinomas in transgenic mice.[97] It is notable that co-amplification

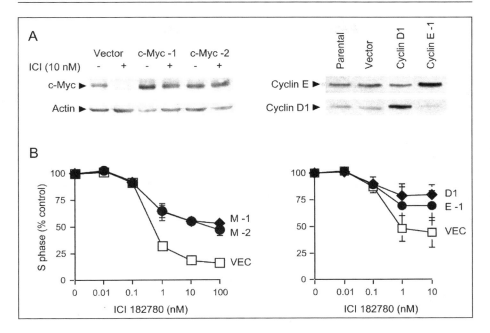

Figure 4. Overexpression of c-Myc, cyclin D1 or cyclin E1 modulates the response to antiestrogens. A), Western analysis of c-Myc, cyclin D1 and cyclin E1 expression in breast cancer cells stably transfected with empty vector, or human cDNAs for c-Myc, cyclin D1 or cyclin E1. B), Acute effects of c-Myc, cyclin D1 and cyclin E overexpression on the response to the pure antiestrogen, ICI 182780. After treatment of proliferating cells with ICI 182780 at the concentrations shown, cells were harvested and stained with ethidium bromide. The S phase fraction was determined by flow cytometry and represented relative to vehicle treated controls. Data points indicate mean of duplicate experiments ± S.D.

of *NEU/ERBB2* and *MYC* is associated with poorer survival in several clinical cohorts[98] although data are conflicting in this regard.[61]

At a clinical level, the impact of *MYC* amplification and expression on response to endocrine therapy is less clear than might be expected from in vitro studies and there are few data evaluating the relationship between *MYC* amplification and response to endocrine therapy. In a cohort of 181 patients with node-negative disease *MYC* amplification predicted recurrence but no differences were detected in the response to tamoxifen treatment among patients with and without gene amplification.[61] In another study, those patients with *MYC* amplification tended to have a slightly longer progression-free survival on endocrine therapy.[99] However, it is difficult to draw conclusions regarding the role of c-Myc from these small cohorts particularly because of the discrepancy between *MYC* amplification (~19%) and c-Myc protein overexpression (~38%). Further elucidation of the relationship between c-Myc overexpression and response to endocrine therapy must await more reliable immunohistochemical assessment in large cohorts of patients treated in the context of randomized treatment trials.

Similarly, in clinical cohorts the role of the c-Myc target gene and cell cycle regulator p21[WAF1/Cip1] in predicting overall outcome and response to antiestrogen therapy remains the subject of debate. Some investigators show that p21[WAF1/Cip1] expression predicts responsiveness to antiestrogens,[100] while others have shown no prognostic benefit in multivariate analyses.[101,102] In contrast, other investigators have shown a negative association between cytoplasmic p21[WAF1/Cip1] expression and outcome.[103,104] These conflicting data may reflect the fact that p21[WAF1/Cip1] function in breast cancer can also be influenced by p53 status, titration by cyclin-CDK complexes and intracellular localization which were not accounted for in these studies.

Like c-Myc, evidence demonstrating the role of cyclins in mediating the proliferative effects of estrogen, suggest they may also be involved in the development of endocrine resistance. Sustained expression of cyclin D1 is seen in breast cancer cells during their acquisition of tamoxifen-resistance.[105] In these cells ER expression and function remained intact and the pure antiestrogen, ICI 164,384 retained its anti-proliferative effects via suppression of cyclin D1. This is consistent with the clinical observation that patients with tamoxifen-resistant disease are able to derive benefit from second line therapy with ER downregulators.[106] Interestingly, overexpression of cyclin D1 confers complete resistance to the growth inhibitory effects of progestins.[107] Cyclin D1 can also potentiate the transcriptional activity of the ER independently of estradiol, with some evidence that this effect is not inhibited by antiestrogens.[108,109] This suggests a further mechanism by which the overexpression of cyclin D1 in breast cancers could lead to sustained ER signaling and endocrine resistance.

The situation is less clear when in vitro hypotheses derived from in vitro experiments are tested in a clinical setting. A large number of studies have examined the prognostic influence of changes in cyclin D1 expression and several show that a poor outcome is associated with amplification at the 11q13 locus.[110] Subsequent studies demonstrated a shortening of relapse-free survival in association with *CCND1* amplification.[111] However, many other studies have reported conflicting relationships between cyclin D1 overexpression and clinical outcome. Variation in methodologies, adjuvant treatment, ER assessment, size of the study cohort and the heterogeneity inherent in human populations may account for some of this variability. Certainly it is difficult to draw definitive conclusions about the relationship between cyclin D1 expression and prognosis from these studies.

When the more specific question of the potential role of cyclin D1 in endocrine responsiveness in the clinical setting is addressed, the data are again conflicting. There are reports of increased expression of cyclin D1 mRNA associated with a reduced response to tamoxifen treatment.[112,113] However, others have shown a trend towards superior response to tamoxifen in metastatic ER-positive tumors that overexpress cyclin D1.[114] Thus, the true impact of cyclin D1 on the response and resistance to antiestrogens in a clinical setting remains the subject of debate and is urgently in need of further study in large cohorts of known therapeutic responsiveness.

It is clear from the earlier discussion that cyclin E-CDK2 complexes are also crucial in mediating estrogen-induced progression through the G_1-S phase of the cell cycle and, as is the case for c-Myc and cyclin D1, there exist in vitro data supporting a role for cyclin E1 in the development of antiestrogen resistance. Studies in MCF-7 cells demonstrate that a three-fold overexpression of cyclin E1 can abrogate tamoxifen-mediated growth arrest.[115] Cyclin E1 overexpression also confers partial resistance to the acute, inhibitory effects of ICI 182,780, although to a lesser extent than that observed with cyclin D1 (Fig. 4).[116] Nonetheless, in clonogenic survival assays overexpression of both cyclin D1 and cyclin E1 confer significant resistance to the growth inhibitory effects of ICI 182,780.[116]

Cyclin E1 is overexpressed in ~30% of breast cancers (Table 1) and studies of protein expression in breast cancer tissue show that cyclin E1 levels correlate strongly with disease-specific and overall survival. In addition, the production of low-molecular weight isoforms of cyclin E1 confers resistance to the effects of the CDK inhibitors p21[WAF1/Cip1] and p27[Kip1] and to the effects of antiestrogens in MCF-7 cells.[117] It has also been noted that in experimental systems, overexpression of the low molecular weight isoforms of cyclin E1 is associated with a defect in progression through S phase with concomitant accumulation of chromosomal instability.[117] Importantly, the study on the role of full-length and low molecular weight isoforms of cyclin E1 demonstrated that cyclin E1 outperformed other independent clinical and pathological risk factors of recurrence and death and is consistent with the data from several other clinical studies showing adverse outcome in association with cyclin E1 overexpression.[72] However, on multivariate analysis a number of other clinical studies have failed to show any association between cyclin E1 expression and outcome.[70,118] There is some evidence that cyclin E1 expression is associated with poor relapse-free survival specifically in patients treated with endocrine therapy.[119] Other studies have shown that antiestrogen treatment has no influence on disease-specific survival among ER-positive cyclin E1 overexpressors, suggestive that cyclin E1 confers resistance to antiestrogens.[72] Again, more definitive conclusions on the role of cyclin E1 in endocrine resistance must await data from large, randomized treatment trials.

Conclusion

Female sex steroid hormones are essential for normal mammary gland development and physiological function through their regulation of cell proliferation, cell differentiation and cell death. These effects, which are retained in neoplastic breast tissue, are mediated, in part, by regulation of cell cycle regulatory molecules including cyclins, CDKs and CDK inhibition. There is compelling evidence that aberrant expression and regulation of these molecules accompanies the oncogenic process in breast tissue and may have a causative role in breast cancer development and progression. This, in turn, raises the possibility that cell cycle regulatory molecules may provide useful markers of disease progression and response to therapy and be targets for future therapeutic intervention. While there is strong preliminary data to support these concepts, more research is required to determine whether such goals are a likely clinical reality.

Acknowledgements

The authors thank Prof. Roger Daly (Garvan Institute) for useful discussions. Research in our laboratories is supported by grants from the following organizations: National Health and Medical Research Council of Australia (NH&MRC), Cancer Institute NSW, R.T. Hall Trust, Australian Cancer Research Foundation (ACRF) and Association for International Cancer Research (AICR). AJB and EAM are Cancer Institute NSW Fellows. AS is an NH&MRC CJ Martin Fellow. CEC and CMM are Cancer Institute NSW Scholars and CMM is also the recipient of an NH&MRC Postgraduate Scholarship. RLS is a Senior Principal Research Fellow of the NH&MRC.

References

1. Hanahan D, Weinberg RA. The hallmarks of cancer. Cell 2000; 100:57-70.
2. Harbour JW, Dean DC. Rb function in cell-cycle regulation and apoptosis. Nat Cell Biol 2000; 2:E65-7.
3. Malumbres M, Barbacid M. To cycle or not to cycle: a critical decision in cancer. Nat Rev Cancer 2001; 1:222-31.
4. Morgan DO. Cyclin-dependent kinases: engines, clocks and microprocessors. Annu Rev Cell Dev Biol 1997; 13:261-91.
5. Garriga J, Grana X. Cellular control of gene expression by T-type cyclin/CDK9 complexes. Gene 2004; 337:15-23.
6. Coqueret O. Linking cyclins to transcriptional control. Gene 2002; 299:35-55.
7. Sherr CJ, Roberts JM. CDK inhibitors: positive and negative regulators of G1-phase progression. Genes Dev 1999; 13:1501-12.
8. Sarcevic B, Lilischkis R, Sutherland RL. Differential phosphorylation of T-47D human breast cancer cell substrates by D1-, D3-, E- and A-type cyclin-CDK complexes. J Biol Chem 1997; 272:33327-37.
9. Kitagawa M, Higashi H, Jung HK et al. The consensus motif for phosphorylation by cyclin D1-Cdk4 is different from that for phosphorylation by cyclin A/E-Cdk2. EMBO J 1996; 15:7060-9.
10. Sherr CJ, Roberts JM. Living with or without cyclins and cyclin-dependent kinases. Genes Dev 2004; 18:2699-711.
11. Murray AW. Recycling the cell cycle: cyclins revisited. Cell 2004; 116:221-34.
12. Lukas J, Bartkova J, Rohde M et al. Cyclin D1 is dispensable for G1 control in retinoblastoma gene-deficient cells independently of cdk4 activity. Mol Cell Biol 1995; 15:2600-11.
13. Harbour JW, Luo RX, Dei Santi A et al. Cdk phosphorylation triggers sequential intramolecular interactions that progressively block Rb functions as cells move through G1. Cell 1999; 98:859-69.
14. Lundberg AS, Weinberg RA. Functional inactivation of the retinoblastoma protein requires sequential modification by at least two distinct cyclin-cdk complexes. Mol Cell Biol 1998; 18:753-61.
15. Ren S, Rollins BJ. Cyclin C/cdk3 promotes Rb-dependent G0 exit. Cell 2004; 117:239-51.
16. LaBaer J, Garrett MD, Stevenson LF et al. New functional activities for the p21 family of CDK inhibitors. Genes Dev 1997; 11:847-62.

17. Colditz GA. Relationship between estrogen levels, use of hormone replacement therapy and breast cancer. J Natl Cancer Inst 1998; 90:814-23.
18. Clarke CL, Sutherland RL. Progestin regulation of cellular proliferation. Endocr Rev 1990; 11:266-301.
19. De Vivo I, Hankinson SE, Colditz GA et al. A functional polymorphism in the progesterone receptor gene is associated with an increase in breast cancer risk. Cancer Res 2003; 63:5236-8.
20. Sutherland RL, Prall OW, Watts CK et al. Estrogen and progestin regulation of cell cycle progression. Journal of Mammary Gland Biology and Neoplasia 1998; 3:63-72.
21. Sutherland RL, Musgrove EA. Cyclins and breast cancer. J Mammary Gland Biol Neoplasia 2004; 9:95-104.
22. Hewitt SC, Harrell JC, Korach KS. Lessons in estrogen biology from knockout and transgenic animals. Annu Rev Physiol 2005; 67:285-308.
23. Ström A, Hartman J, Foster JS et al. Estrogen receptor beta inhibits 17beta-estradiol-stimulated proliferation of the breast cancer cell line T47D. Proc Natl Acad Sci USA 2004; 101:1566-71.
24. Dubik D, Shiu RP. Transcriptional regulation of c-myc oncogene expression by estrogen in hormone-responsive human breast cancer cells. J Biol Chem 1988; 263:12705-8.
25. Carroll JS, Swarbrick A, Musgrove EA et al. Mechanisms of growth arrest by c-myc antisense oligonucleotides in MCF-7 breast cancer cells: implications for the antiproliferative effects of antiestrogens. Cancer Res 2002; 62:3126-31.
26. Dubik D, Shiu RP. Mechanism of estrogen activation of c-myc oncogene expression. Oncogene 1992; 7:1587-94.
27. Carroll JS, CA M, J S et al. Genome-wide analysis of estrogen receptor binding sites. Nat Genet 2006; 38:1289-97.
28. Nass SJ, Dickson RB. Defining a role for c-Myc in breast tumorigenesis. Breast Cancer Research and Treatment 1997; 44:1-22.
29. Heikkila R, Schwab G, Wickstrom E et al. A c-myc antisense oligodeoxynucleotide inhibits entry into S phase but not progress from G0 to G1. Nature 1987; 328:445-9.
30. Prall OWJ, Rogan EM, Musgrove EA et al. c-Myc or cyclin D1 mimics estrogen effects on cyclin E-cdk2 activation and cell cycle reentry. Mol Cell Biol 1998; 18:4499-508.
31. Dang CV. c-Myc target genes involved in cell growth, apoptosis and metabolism. Molecular and Cellular Biology 1999; 19:1-11.
32. Mukherjee S, Conrad SE. C-Myc suppresses p21WAF1/CIP1 expression during estrogen signaling and antiestrogen resistance in human breast cancer cells. J Biol Chem 2005; 280:17617-25.
33. Prall OWJ, Sarcevic B, Musgrove EA et al. Estrogen-induced activation of cdk4 and cdk2 during G1-S phase progression is accompanied by increased cyclin D1 expression and decreased cyclin-dependent kinase inhibitor association with cyclin E-cdk2. J Biol Chem 1997; 272:10882-94.
34. Musgrove EA, Lee CS, Buckley MF et al. Cyclin D1 induction in breast cancer cells shortens G1 and is sufficient for cells arrested in G1 to complete the cell cycle. Proc Natl Acad Sci USA 1994; 91:8022-6.
35. Musgrove EA, Hamilton JA, Lee CS et al. Growth factor, steroid and steroid antagonist regulation of cyclin gene expression associated with changes in T-47D human breast cancer cell cycle progression. Mol Cell Biol 1993; 13:3577-87.
36. Wilcken NR, Prall OW, Musgrove EA et al. Inducible overexpression of cyclin D1 in breast cancer cells reverses the growth-inhibitory effects of antiestrogens. Clin Cancer Res 1997; 3:849-54.
37. Lukas J, Bartkova J, Bartek J. Convergence of mitogenic signalling cascades from diverse classes of receptors at the cyclin D-cyclin-dependent kinase-pRb-controlled G1 checkpoint. Molecular and Cellular Biology 1996; 16:6917-25.
38. Planas-Silva MD, Weinberg RA. Estrogen-dependent cyclin E-cdk2 activation through p21 redistribution. Molecular and Cellular Biology 1997; 17:4059-69.
39. Prall OW, Carroll JS, Sutherland RL. A low abundance pool of nascent p21WAF1/Cip1 is targeted by estrogen to activate cyclin E*Cdk2. J Biol Chem 2001; 276:45433-42.
40. Foster JS, Fernando RI, Ishida N et al. Estrogens down-regulate p27Kip1 in breast cancer cells through Skp2 and through nuclear export mediated by the ERK pathway. J Biol Chem 2003; 278:41355-66.
41. Eeckhoute J, Carroll JS, Geistlinger TR et al. A cell-type-specific transcriptional network required for estrogen regulation of cyclin D1 and cell cycle progression in breast cancer. Genes Dev 2006; 20:2513-26.
42. Musgrove EA, Lee CS, Sutherland RL. Progestins both stimulate and inhibit breast cancer cell cycle progression while increasing expression of transforming growth factor alpha, epidermal growth factor receptor, c-fos and c-myc genes. Mol Cell Biol 1991; 11:5032-43.
43. Swarbrick A, Lee CSL, Sutherland RL et al. Cooperation of p27[Kip1] and p18[INK4c] in progestin-mediated cell cycle arrest in T-47D breast cancer cells. Mol Cell Biol 2000; 20:2581-91.

44. Musgrove EA, Swarbrick A, Lee CS et al. Mechanisms of cyclin-dependent kinase inactivation by progestins. Mol Cell Biol 1998; 18:1812-25.
45. Caldon CE, Lee CS, Sutherland RL et al. Wilms' tumor protein 1: an early target of progestin regulation in T-47D breast cancer cells that modulates proliferation and differentiation. Oncogene 2007; doi: 10.1038/sj.onc.1210622.
46. Stewart TA, Pattengale PK, Leder P. Spontaneous mammary adenocarcinomas in transgenic mice that carry and express MTV/myc fusion genes. Cell 1984; 38:627-37.
47. Jamerson MH, Johnson MD, Dickson RB. Of mice and myc: c-Myc and mammary tumorigenesis. J Mammary Gland Biol Neoplasia 2004; 9:27-37.
48. Wang TC, Cardiff RD, Zukerberg L et al. Mammary hyperplasia and carcinoma in MMTV-cyclin D1 transgenic mice. Nature 1994; 369:669-71.
49. Bortner DM, Rosenberg MP. Induction of mammary gland hyperplasia and carcinomas in transgenic mice expressing human cyclin E. Mol Cell Biol 1997; 17:453-9.
50. Lee RJ, Albanese C, Fu M et al. Cyclin D1 is required for transformation by activated Neu and is induced through an E2F-dependent signaling pathway. Mol Cell Biol 2000; 20:672-83.
51. Yu Q, Geng Y, Sicinski P. Specific protection against breast cancers by cyclin D1 ablation. Nature 2001; 411:1017-21.
52. Serrano M, Gomez-Lahoz E, DePinho RA et al. Inhibition of ras-induced proliferation and cellular transformation by p16INK4. Science 1995; 267:249-52.
53. Yang C, Ionescu-Tiba V, Burns K et al. The role of the cyclin D1-dependent kinases in ErbB2-mediated breast cancer. Am J Pathol 2004; 164:1031-8.
54. Bowe DB, Kenney NJ, Adereth Y et al. Suppression of Neu-induced mammary tumor growth in cyclin D1 deficient mice is compensated for by cyclin E. Oncogene 2002; 21:291-8.
55. Geng Y, Whoriskey W, Park MY et al. Rescue of cyclin D1 deficiency by knockin cyclin E. Cell 1999; 97:767-77.
56. Yu Q, Sicinska E, Geng Y et al. Requirement for CDK4 kinase function in breast cancer. Cancer Cell 2006; 9:23-32.
57. Landis MW, Pawlyk BS, Li T et al. Cyclin D1-dependent kinase activity in murine development and mammary tumorigenesis. Cancer Cell 9:13-22.
58. Geng Y, Yu Q, Sicinska E et al. Cyclin E ablation in the mouse. Cell 2003; 114:431-43.
59. Robanus-Maandag EC, Bosch CA, Kristel PM et al. Association of C-MYC amplification with progression from the in situ to the invasive stage in C-MYC-amplified breast carcinomas. J Pathol 2003; 201:75-82.
60. Deming SL, Nass SJ, Dickson RB et al. C-myc amplification in breast cancer: a meta-analysis of its occurrence and prognostic relevance. Br J Cancer 2000; 83:1688-95.
61. Schlotter CM, Vogt U, Bosse U et al. C-myc, not HER-2/neu, can predict recurrence and mortality of patients with node-negative breast cancer. Breast Cancer Res 2003; 5:R30-6.
62. Naidu R, Wahab NA, Yadav M et al. Protein expression and molecular analysis of c-myc gene in primary breast carcinomas using immunohistochemistry and differential polymerase chain reaction. Int J Mol Med 2002; 9:189-96.
63. Blancato J, Singh B, Liu A et al. Correlation of amplification and overexpression of the c-myc oncogene in high-grade breast cancer: FISH, in situ hybridisation and immunohistochemical analyses. Br J Cancer 2004; 90:1612-9.
64. Callagy GM, Pharoah PD, Pinder SE et al. Bcl-2 is a prognostic marker in breast cancer independently of the Nottingham Prognostic Index. Clin Cancer Res 2006; 12:2468-75.
65. Alle KM, Henshall SM, Field AS et al. Cyclin D1 protein is overexpressed in hyperplasia and intraductal carcinoma of the breast. Clinical Cancer Research 1998; 4:847-54.
66. Buckley MF, Sweeney KJ, Hamilton JA et al. Expression and amplification of cyclin genes in human breast cancer. Oncogene 1993; 8:2127-33.
67. Evron E, Umbricht CB, Korz D et al. Loss of cyclin D2 expression in the majority of breast cancers is associated with promoter hypermethylation. Cancer Research 2001; 61:2782-7.
68. Bartkova J, Zemanova M, Bartek J. Abundance and subcellular localisation of cyclin D3 in human tumours. International Journal of Cancer 1996; 65:323-7.
69. Wang L, Shao ZM. Cyclin E expression and prognosis in breast cancer patients: a meta-analysis of published studies. Cancer Invest 2006; 24:581-7.
70. Rudolph P, Kühling H, Alm P et al. Differential prognostic impact of the cyclins E and B in premenopausal and postmenopausal women with lymph node-negative breast cancer. International Journal of Cancer 2003; 105:674-80.
71. Keyomarsi K, O'Leary N, Molnar G et al. Cyclin E, a potential prognostic marker for breast cancer. Cancer Research 1994; 54:380-5.

72. Keyomarsi K, Tucker SL, Buchholz TA et al. Cyclin E and survival in patients with breast cancer. N Engl J Med 2002; 347:1566-75.
73. Wingate H, Zhang N, McGarhen MJ et al. The tumor-specific hyperactive forms of cyclin E are resistant to inhibition by p21 and p27. J Biol Chem 2005; 280:15148-57.
74. Spruck C, Sun D, Fiegl H et al. Detection of low molecular weight derivatives of cyclin E1 Is a function of cyclin E1 protein levels in breast cancer. Cancer Res 2006; 66:7355-60.
75. van 't Veer LJ, Dai H, van de Vijver MJ et al. Gene expression profiling predicts clinical outcome of breast cancer. Nature 2002; 415:530-6.
76. Wang Y, Klijn JG, Zhang Y et al. Gene-expression profiles to predict distant metastasis of lymph-node-negative primary breast cancer. Lancet 2005; 365:671-9.
77. Sotiriou C, Wirapati P, Loi S et al. Gene expression profiling in breast cancer: understanding the molecular basis of histologic grade to improve prognosis. J Natl Cancer Inst 2006; 98:262-72.
78. Sieuwerts AM, Look MP, Meijer-van Gelder ME et al. Which cyclin E prevails as prognostic marker for breast cancer? Results from a retrospective study involving 635 lymph node-negative breast cancer patients. Clin Cancer Res 2006; 12:3319-28.
79. Desmedt C, Ouriaghli FE, Durbecq V et al. Impact of cyclins E, neutrophil elastase and proteinase 3 expression levels on clinical outcome in primary breast cancer patients. Int J Cancer 2006; 119:2539-45.
80. Alkarain A, Slingerland J. Deregulation of p27 by oncogenic signaling and its prognostic significance in breast cancer. Breast Cancer Research 2004; 6:13-21.
81. Chen C, Seth AK, Aplin AE. Genetic and expression aberrations of E3 ubiquitin ligases in human breast cancer. Molecular Cancer Research 2006; 4:695-707.
82. Zheng W-Q, Zheng J-M, Ma R et al. Relationship between levels of Skp2 and p27 in breast carcinomas and possible role of Skp2 as targeted therapy. Steroids 2005; 70:770-4.
83. Alkarain A, Jordan R, Slingerland J. p27 deregulation in breast cancer: prognostic significance and implications for therapy. Journal of Mammary Gland Biology & Neoplasia 2004; 9:67-80.
84. Tsutsui S, Inoue H, Yasuda K et al. Inactivation of PTEN is associated with a low p27^{Kip1} protein expression in breast carcinoma. Cancer 2005; 104:2048-53.
85. Wu FY, Wang SE, Sanders ME et al. Reduction of cytosolic p27^{Kip1} inhibits cancer cell motility, survival and tumorigenicity. Cancer Res 2006; 66:2162-72.
86. Tlsty TD, Crawford YG, Holst CR et al. Genetic and epigenetic changes in mammary epithelial cells may mimic early events in carcinogenesis. J Mammary Gland Biol Neoplasia 2004; 9:263-74.
87. Di Vinci A, Perdelli L, Banelli B et al. p16^{INK4a} promoter methylation and protein expression in breast fibroadenoma and carcinoma. International Journal of Cancer 2005; 114:414-21.
88. Huschtscha LI, Noble JR, Neumann AA et al. Loss of p16INK4 expression by methylation is associated with lifespan extension of human mammary epithelial cells. Cancer Res 1998; 58:3508-12.
89. Dublin EA, Patel NK, Gillett CE et al. Retinoblastoma and p16 proteins in mammary carcinoma: Their relationship to cyclin D1 and histopathological parameters. International Journal of Cancer 1998; 79:71-5.
90. Hui R, Macmillan RD, Kenny FS et al. INK4a gene expression and methylation in primary breast cancer: overexpression of p16^{INK4a} messenger RNA is a marker of poor prognosis. Clin Cancer Res 2000; 6:2777-87.
91. Emig R, Magener A, Ehemann V et al. Aberrant cytoplasmic expression of the p16 protein in breast cancer is associated with accelerated tumour proliferation. British Journal of Cancer 1998; 78:1661-8.
92. Jeng M-H, Shupnik MA, Bender TP et al. Estrogen receptor expression and function in long-term estrogen-deprived human breast cancer cells. Endocrinology 1998; 139:4164-74.
93. Venditti M, Iwasiow B, Orr FW et al. C-myc gene expression alone is sufficient to confer resistance to antiestrogen in human breast cancer cells. Int J Cancer 2002; 99:35-42.
94. Sears R, Lone G, DeGregori J et al. Ras enhances Myc protein stability. Molecular Cell 1999; 3:169-79.
95. Sears R, Nuckolls F, Haura E et al. Multiple Ras-dependent phosphorylation pathways regulate Myc protein stability. Genes and Development 2000; 14:2501-14.
96. Neve RM, Sutterluty H, Pullen N et al. Effects of oncogenic ErbB2 on G1 cell cycle regulators in breast tumour cells. Oncogene 2000; 19:1647-56.
97. Nass SJ, Dickson RB. Epidermal growth factor-dependent cell cycle progression is altered in mammary epithelial cells that overexpress c-myc. Clinical Cancer Research 1998; 4:1813-22.
98. Al-Kuraya K, Schraml P, Torhorst J et al. Prognostic relevance of gene amplifications and coamplifications in breast cancer. Cancer Res 2004; 64:8534-40.
99. Berns EM, Foekens JA, van Staveren IL et al. Oncogene amplification and prognosis in breast cancer: relationship with systemic treatment. Gene 1995; 159:11-8.

100. Pellikainen MJ, Pekola TT, Ropponen KM et al. p21WAF1 expression in invasive breast cancer and its association with p53, AP-2, cell proliferation and prognosis. J Clin Pathol 2003; 56:214-20.
101. Gohring UJ, Bersch A, Becker M et al. p21(waf) correlates with DNA replication but not with prognosis in invasive breast cancer. J Clin Pathol 2001; 54:866-70.
102. O'Hanlon DM, Kiely M, MacConmara M et al. An immunohistochemical study of p21 and p53 expression in primary node-positive breast carcinoma. Eur J Surg Oncol 2002; 28:103-7.
103. Caffo O, Doglioni C, Veronese S et al. Prognostic value of p21(WAF1) and p53 expression in breast carcinoma: an immunohistochemical study in 261 patients with long-term follow-up. Clin Cancer Res 1996; 2:1591-9.
104. Winters ZE, Leek RD, Bradburn MJ et al. Cytoplasmic p21WAF1/CIP1 expression is correlated with HER-2/ neu in breast cancer and is an independent predictor of prognosis. Breast Cancer Res 2003; 5:R242-9.
105. Kilker RL, Hartl MW, Rutherford TM et al. Cyclin D1 expression is dependent on estrogen receptor function in tamoxifen-resistant breast cancer cells. J Steroid Biochem Mol Biol 2004; 92:63-71.
106. Howell A, DeFriend D, Robertson J et al. Response to a specific antioestrogen (ICI 182780) in tamoxifen-resistant breast cancer. Lancet 1995; 345:29-30.
107. Musgrove EA, Hunter L-JK, Lee CSL et al. Cyclin D1 overexpression induces progestin resistance in T47D breast cancer cells despite p27KIP1 association with cyclin E-cdk2. Journal of Biological Chemistry 2001; 275:47675-83.
108. Neuman E, Ladha MH, Lin N et al. Cyclin D1 stimulation of estrogen receptor transcriptional activity independent of cdk4. Mol Cell Biol 1997; 17:5338-47.
109. Zwijsen RML, Wientjens E, Klompmaker R et al. CDK-independent activation of estrogen receptor by cyclin D1. Cell 1997; 88:405-15.
110. Dickson C, Fantl V, Gillett C et al. Amplification of chromosome band 11q13 and a role for cyclin D1 in human breast cancer. Cancer Lett 1995; 90:43-50.
111. Bieche I, Olivi M, Nogues C et al. Prognostic value of CCND1 gene status in sporadic breast tumours, as determined by real-time quantitative PCR assays. British Journal of Cancer 2002; 86:580-6.
112. Kenny FS, Hui R, Musgrove EA et al. Overexpression of cyclin D1 messenger RNA predicts for poor prognosis in estrogen receptor-positive breast cancer. Clin Cancer Res 1999; 5:2069-76.
113. Stendahl M, Kronblad A, Ryden L et al. Cyclin D1 overexpression is a negative predictive factor for tamoxifen response in postmenopausal breast cancer patients. Br J Cancer 2004; 90:1942-8.
114. Han S, Park K, Bae BN et al. Cyclin D1 expression and patient outcome after tamoxifen therapy in estrogen receptor positive metastatic breast cancer. Oncol Rep 2003; 10:141-4.
115. Dhillon NK, Mudryj M. Ectopic expression of cyclin E in estrogen responsive cells abrogates antiestrogen mediated growth arrest. Oncogene 2002; 21:4626-34.
116. Hui R, Finney GL, Carroll JS et al. Constitutive overexpression of cyclin D1 but not cyclin E confers acute resistance to antiestrogens in T-47D breast cancer cells. Cancer Res 2002; 62:6916-23.
117. Akli S, Zheng PJ, Multani AS et al. Tumor-specific low molecular weight forms of cyclin E induce genomic instability and resistance to p21, p27 and antiestrogens in breast cancer. Cancer Res 2004; 64:3198-208.
118. Bukholm IR, Bukholm G, Nesland JM. Over-expression of cyclin A is highly associated with early relapse and reduced survival in patients with primary breast carcinomas. Int J Cancer 2001; 93:283-7.
119. Span PN, Tjan-Heijnen VC, Manders P et al. Cyclin-E is a strong predictor of endocrine therapy failure in human breast cancer. Oncogene 2003; 22:4898-904.

CHAPTER 13

Selective Estrogen Modulators as an Anticancer Tool:
Mechanisms of Efficiency and Resistance

Surojeet Sengupta and V. Craig Jordan*

Abstract

The majority of breast cancers are estrogen receptor (ER) positive and depend on estrogen for growth. Therefore, blocking estrogen mediated actions remains the strategy of choice for the treatment and prevention of breast cancer. The selective estrogen receptor modulators (SERMs) are molecules that block estrogen action in breast cancer but can still potentially maintain the beneficial effects of estrogen in other tissues, such as bone and cardiovascular system. Tamoxifen, the prototypical drug of this class has been used extensively for the past 30 years to treat and prevent breast cancer. The target of drug action, ERs alpha and beta, are the two receptors which are responsible for the first step in estrogen and SERM action. The SERM binds to the ERs and confers a unique conformation to the complex. In a target site which expresses antiestrogenic actions, the conformation of the ER is distinctly different from estrogen bound ER. The complex recruits protein partners called corepressors to prevent the transcription of estrogen responsive genes. In contrast, at a predominantly estrogenic site coactivators for estrogen action are recruited. Unfortunately at an antiestrogenic site such as breast cancer, long term SERM therapy causes the development of acquired resistance. The breast and endometrial tumor cells selectively become SERM stimulated. Overexpression of receptor tyrosine kinases, HER-2, EGFR and IGFR and the signaling cascades following their activation are frequently involved in SERM resistant breast cancers. The aberrantly activated PI3K/AKT and MAPK pathways and their cross talk with the genomic components of the ER action are implicated in SERM resistance. Other down stream factors of HER-2 and EGFR signaling, such as PI3K/AKT, MAPK or mTOR pathways has also been found to be involved in resistance mechanisms. Blocking the actions of HER-2 and EGFR represent a rational strategy for treating SERM resistant phenotypes and may in fact restore the sensitivity to the SERMs. Another approach exploits the discovery that low dose estrogen will induce apoptosis in the SERM resistant breast cancers. Numerous clinical studies are addressing these issues.

Introduction

Selective estrogen receptor modulators (SERMs) are molecules which bind to estrogen receptors (ERs) and confer either estrogen-agonistic (estrogen-like) or estrogen-antagonistic (antiestrogen-like) actions in various estrogen target tissues and cells. In other words, the same SERM molecule can be estrogen agonistic in some tissues, as well as estrogen antagonistic in others, in the same organism at the same time. This pharmacology is unique and has allowed the SERMs

*Corresponding Author: V. Craig Jordan—Alfred G. Knudson Chair of Cancer Research, Fox Chase Cancer Center, 333 Cottman Avenue, Philadelphia, PA 19111-2497, USA. Email: v.craig.jordan@fccc.edu

Innovative Endocrinology of Cancer, edited by Lev M. Berstein and Richard J. Santen. ©2008 Landes Bioscience and Springer Science+Business Media.

to be not only valuable tools to dissect the subcellular action of estrogen but also has opened the door to important therapeutic applications. However, SERMs did not appear suddenly as a new drug group but were originally referred to as nonsteroidal antiestrogens[1] that have continuously evolved and been evaluated for different clinical application during the past 50 years.

Nonsteroidal antiestrogens were originally investigated as agents to modulate reproductive functions.[2] They were effective as post coital contraceptives in rats[3] but actually induced ovulation in subfertile women.[4] The failure of antiestrogen to become antifertility agents throughout the 1960's resulted in a decline in interest by the pharmaceutical industry in developing the drug group. Nevertheless, the molecules were of pharmacological interest and became important tools in endocrine research to decipher the actions of estradiol (Fig. 1). As a drug group, the nonsteroidal antiestrogens were noted to block estrogen binding to its target tissues e.g., uterus, vagina and some breast cancers[5-7] because they were competitive inhibitors of estradiol binding to ER.[8,9]

One compound ICI 46,474 was studied extensively because fashions in research changed significantly during the 1970s. There was a new focus on cancer research which, in this case, built on the prior experience with reproductive endocrinology.[10] ICI 46,474, the failed contraceptive was reinvented to become tamoxifen (Fig. 1), the first antiestrogen for the treatment of breast cancer.[11] This in turn caused an evaluation of the molecular mechanisms of its antitumor action. During 1970s a treatment strategy was developed in the laboratory so that tamoxifen was subsequently targeted to the patients with ER positive tumors, administered as a long term adjuvant therapy in early stage disease which resulted in a significant advance in cancer therapy with survival advantages for hundreds of thousands of patients.[12]

In the laboratory, the discovery that tamoxifen needed to be hydroxylated to 4-hydroxytamoxifen to achieve high binding affinity for the ER[13,14] created an important laboratory tool to examine antitumor actions in vitro, to study structure function relationships[1,15] and ultimately to discover the actual molecular mechanisms of antiestrogen action at the ER level.[16] Overall the SERMs have played a pioneering role in cancer treatment both as laboratory tools and targeted agents in cancer

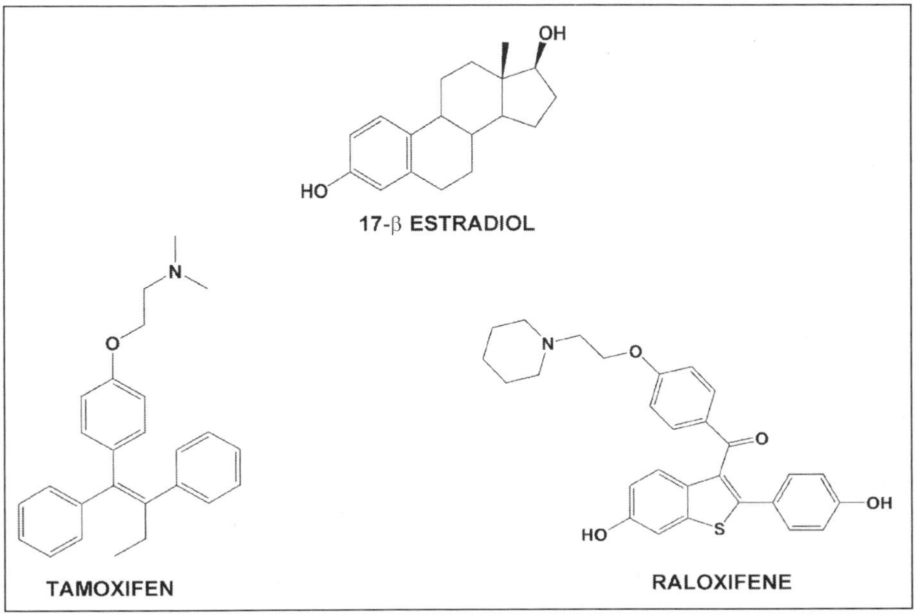

Figure 1. Chemical structures of 17-β estradiol, tamoxifen and raloxifene.

therapeutics. This chapter will trace their continuing development and current role in deciphering the complex signaling pathways that occur with the evolution of antihormonal drug resistance.

Estrogen, Tamoxifen and Cancer

As early as 1896, Dr. George Thomas Beatson noted that ablation of the ovarian stimulus (estrogen) restricted the growth of breast cancers.[17] Unfortunately only limited numbers of the breast cancer responded to the ablative surgery. More than 50 years later, the studies by Elwood Jensen,[18] that initially defined the target site specificity of estrogen action, helped further in understanding the requirement of the ER for the estrogen dependent growth of breast cancers.[19] The potential of tamoxifen (known as an anti-estrogen, at that time) to be used as an anti-breast cancer agent was recognized when it was reinvented from a failed contraceptive to become the first targeted drug for the treatment of breast cancer (see above).[11] Numerous studies using laboratory animals demonstrated the anti-tumor effects of tamoxifen. Early studies using a carcinogen-induced rat mammary tumor model revealed that tamoxifen was able to inhibit the growth as well as the tumor initiation.[20-24] However, long term therapy was stated to be the correct clinical strategy for the adjuvant treatment of breast cancer.[25,26] Similar findings were subsequently noted in xeno-transplanted ER positive breast cancer cells in the athymic (immuno-deficient) mice model. Tamoxifen was able to inhibit the estrogen-induced growth of the ER expressing breast tumors (MCF7 and ZR75) but not of ER negative (MDA-MB 231) tumors.[27,28] Overall these studies clearly indicated the anti-tumor effects of tamoxifen in ER positive breast cancers. The knowledge from the laboratory experiments, that tamoxifen could be used as a therapeutic agent to treat ER positive breast cancers, were successfully translated to clinical trials.[29,30] An early overview study combining 40 adjuvant tamoxifen trials noted highly significant benefits in both disease-free and overall survival.[31] A subsequent overview of randomized trials relevant to tamoxifen indicated that longer (5 years) duration treatments with tamoxifen are beneficial than shorter (1-2 years) treatments. Significant reduction in mortality was also observed with 5 years of treatment than shorter treatments.[12] Unfortunately treatment duration more than five years do not produce further benefits,[32] however, effective continuing reduction in breast cancer recurrence is noted for more than a decade after the termination of tamoxifen therapy.[12,33] The clinical trials for tamoxifen as an adjuvant therapy for breast cancer also revealed that 5 years of tamoxifen therapy reduces the recurrence of breast cancer and also the incidences of contralateral second primary breast tumors by fifty percent.[12,34] This led to the possibility that tamoxifen has potential as a chemo-preventive agent. However, the chemosuppresive actions of tamoxifen was already established earlier in experiments done in laboratory animals.[20,35] Several studies have now established that tamoxifen can significantly reduce the number of ER positive breast cancers in high risk group of both pre and post-menopausal women,[33,36-39] and is currently in use for therapeutic prevention of ER positive breast cancers in high risk population.

The idea that SERMs could be multifunctional medicines was based on the laboratory observations that a failed breast cancer drug keoxifene[40] (LY156758) actually maintained bone density in ovariectomized rats[41] and the same doses prevented mammary cancer in rats.[42] Most importantly, keoxifene was less estrogenic than tamoxifen in the rodent uterus[43] and was shown less active at stimulating human endometrial cancer growth in laboratory animals.[44] The publication of the idea[35,45] that nonsteroidal compounds of the same class as tamoxifen could be used to prevent osteoporosis in postmenopausal women but prevent breast cancer at the same time directly led to the subsequent re-examination of the pharmacology of keoxifene and the renaming of the compound into raloxifene (Fig. 1). The clinical investigation that a SERM could be used to prevent osteoporotic fractures but at the same time reduce the incidence of breast cancer[46] created a new dimension in chemoprevention.[47] Raloxifene was advanced for testing against the veteran tamoxifen to reduce breast cancer incidence in high risk postmenopausal women in the study of tamoxifen and raloxifene or STAR trial. Recent reports[48] demonstrate that raloxifene is equally effective as tamoxifen in preventing breast cancers in post-menopausal women. The study also showed lower incidence of endometrial cancer associated with raloxifene treatment than in case of tamoxifen.

Therefore, the clinical foundation to discover the ideal SERM has now been established. The SERM should prevent breast and endometrial cancer but increase bone density and reduce fractures. The challenge of molecular medicine for the future is to decipher the endocrine mediated control mechanisms for reversing or slowing the development of atherosclerosis, reducing hot flashes and defining the importance of estrogen regulated CNS function. To achieve these goals there is now a focused effort to understand the molecular modulation of estrogen action using SERMs as laboratory tools in estrogen target tissues and to understand SERM-stimulated drug resistance to optimize cancer control.

Molecular Mechanism of SERM Action

Mechanism of SERM action depends upon several factors. Essentially, SERMs bind to ERs α and/or β subtypes and confer a unique conformation to the ER. The complex further recruits coregulators and other accessory proteins at the estrogen-responsive elements of the promoters of specific genes to activate or repress transcription.[49] To completely understand the individual roles of these factors, we will discuss them separately.

Estrogen Receptors

Two sub-types of ERs α and β are responsible for the estrogen or SERM mediated effects. Different binding affinities of SERMs to these receptors and differential expression of these two sub-types in various target cells may account for selective modulation in some tissues.[50] In addition, hetero-dimerized ERs α and β may induce unique effects on estrogen- and tamoxifen-dependent gene expression.[51] A recent report also indicates that ER β mediates the effects on ER α induced transcription in ER positive breast cancer cells.[52]

Structurally, ER protein can be subdivided into six domains based on the function controlled by that region. The A/B domain contains one of the two transcriptional activation functions (AFs), known as AF1 which is largely involved in estrogen-independent activation of transcription. Another activation function domain, AF2, is located in the E domain which also harbors the ligand binding domain (LBD) and is involved in estrogen/ligand-dependent activation.[53] The structural studies of LBD of ERs α and β complexed with a SERM reveal that reorientation of the AF2 helix (helix 12) after the binding of the SERM to the hydrophobic pocket of the LBD and the interaction of amino acid asp351 of ERα with the alkylaminoethoxyphenyl side chain of tamoxifen are crucial for the corepressor recruitment to the surface of SERM-receptor complex.[16,54,55] Due to the usage of different mutants of ERα for the amino acid asp351 it is known that shielding and neutralization of asp351 by the side chain of raloxifene is critical in defining the antiestrogenicity of this SERM.[56] The involvement of the asp351 is further exemplified by changing the aspartate to glycine which abolishes the estrogen-agonist activity of tamoxifen, while retaining its antagonistic property.[57] AF2 region of the agonist-bound receptor is particularly important for the interactions of steroid receptor coactivators (SRCs 1-3) via the interacting amino acid motif LxxLL. Recruitment of these co-activator(s) to the promoters of estrogen responsive genes is also responsible for facilitating the activation of transcriptional machinery by chromatin remodeling. Additionally, SERMs may also show differential AF1 activity mediated by corepressor binding.[58] Using ERE-reporter constructs, it has been shown that AF1 domain of ERα is actively involved in agonist-induced gene expression whereas AF1 domain of ER β is involved very weakly.[59]

The activated ER binds to the specific estrogen responsive elements (ERE), found within the promoter region of responsive genes. Significantly, the nature of these DNA sequences also influences the recruitment of the coregulator proteins to the ER at the promoters. Using various ERE containing DNA sequences, it has been found that liganded ER α and β regulate the interaction of the coregulators depending upon the type of ERE, to which the receptor is bound.[60]

Coregulators

Interaction of particular coregulators (co-activators and corepressors) with the liganded estrogen receptors modulates the transcription of the responsive genes. Around 200 coactivators are currently known, which are associated with 48 nuclear receptors.[61] The coactivators undoubtedly play defining roles in the activity of SERMs by cell or tissue specific expression pattern of genes. Studies have indicated that the relative abundance of a co-activator, SRC1 (steroid coactivator 1) in uterine cells is responsible for the agonistic activity of tamoxifen in those cells, whereas tamoxifen acts as an estrogen antagonist in breast cancer cells where the SRC1 levels are low.[62] However, raloxifene, another related SERM, does not recruit SRC-1 even in the uterine cells,[62] underscoring the fact that the SERM induced conformation of estrogen receptor is crucial for the interaction of coregulators. Consistent with these findings, earlier studies have reported tamoxifen-induced growth of endometrial cancer cells but not of breast cancer cells in athymic mice[63] and also that raloxifene (keoxifene) is less estrogenic to endometrial cancer cells.[44] These finding translate to clinical experience.[48] Furthermore, SERMs can also increase the stability of the co-activators (SRC1 and SRC3) and thereby enhance the transcriptional capability of other nuclear receptors.[64] In addition to transcriptional regulation, relative abundance and stability of co-activators, post-translational modifications particularly, different phosphorylation and sumoylation states of the co-activators can also drastically influence the capacity to interact with ER and other members of the transcriptional complex and regulate the gene activation.[65,66]

Corepressors proteins, on the other hand are functional counterparts of co-activators, which are associated with transcriptionally inactive promoters and thus help repress the expression of genes.[67] There are fewer corepressors known than the co-activators. In the case of ER, the corepressors are known to interact with the unoccupied and antagonist bound receptor. Nuclear receptor corepressor (NCoR) and silencing mediator of retinoic acid and thyroid hormone receptor (SMRT) are the two most extensively studied corepressors in connection with ER. The ER bound to raloxifene or 4-hydroxytamoxifen (a potent antagonist metabolite of tamoxifen) is known to recruit NCoR and SMRT to the promoters of estrogen responsive genes and repress transcription.[62,68,69] It has been shown that inhibition of NCoR or SMRT by using antibodies can enhance the agonistic property of 4-hydroxytamoxifen.[70] Moreover, using fibroblasts from NCoR null mice, 4-hydroxytamoxifen was shown to be relatively potent ERα agonist.[71] The critical role of NCoR and SMRT in 4-hydroxytamoxifen-induced arrest of cell proliferation of ERα positive breast cancer cells was illustrated when 4-hydroxytamoxifen-stimulated cell cycle progression was noted in the breast cancer cells deficient in NCoR and SMRT.[72] However this study also found that not all estrogen responsive genes were activated by 4-hydroxytamoxifen in NCoR and SMRT deficient cells, clearly indicating that other molecules may also be important in SERM-induced repression of estrogen responsive genes. Indeed, there are several other corepressor proteins known for ER. Metastasis associated protein 1 (MTA 1) is a corepressor found to mediate the ER transcriptional repression.[73] Another corepressor, known as repressor of estrogen action (REA) was able to potentiate the inhibitory effects of anti-estrogens including 4-hydroxytamoxifen. It was also found that REA interacted with ER and competed with the co-activator SRC1 for binding to the estrogen bound ER.[74,75] This again emphasizes the fact that the relative levels of coregulators may be important in deciding the outcome of the SERM action. The proteasomal regulation of NCoR is another factor which may influence the SERM action. Degradation of NCoR by 26S proteasome is known and is mediated by seven in absentia homologue 2 (Siah2).[76] Interestingly, estrogen mediated up-regulation of Siah2 in ER positive breast cancer cells has been implicated in proteasomal degradation of NCoR and subsequent de-repression of NCoR regulated genes.[77]

In addition to acting as a "transcriptional adapter" between the receptors and the transcriptional machinery, the coregulator itself or its complex possess various enzymatic activities such as acetylation, phosphorylation, methylation or deacetylation by which they are able to modify the local chromatin structure such as to make the environment conducive for gene expression or repression. Intrinsic histone acetyl transferase activity was found to be associated with co-activator SRC1 which helps in the activation of transcriptional expression.[78] In contrast, the 4-hydroxytamoxifen bound ER complex which recruits the corepressors NCoR and SMRT is associated with histone deacetylases and other chromatin modifying enzymes. The deacetylase activity promotes transcriptional repression.[62,79] Interestingly, another enzyme in the coactivator complex, CARM1 (coactivator associated arginine methyltransferase 1) has recently been implicated in modifying the coactivator itself and inducing the degradation of the complex.[80] This suggests the ability of the enzymes in the complex to modify other proteins of its own complex apart from modification of the chromatin.

Evolution of SERM Resistant Breast Cancers

The preventive and therapeutic efficacy of SERMs for breast cancers is limited by the development of resistance for the SERMs. Initially, the development of SERM resistance was considered as overgrowth of ER negative cell population, over the growth arrested ER positive cells, by the antiestrogen (SERM) treatment.[81] However, we now know that there are various forms of SERM resistant breast cancer and studies of these resistant forms have led to novel therapeutic approaches. In general terms, SERM resistant breast cancers can be divided into two categories (a) de novo resistance and (b) acquired resistance. De novo resistance is defined as ER positive breast cancers which are nonresponsive to SERM therapy from the very beginning. De novo resistance can be demonstrated in the laboratory when ER positive MCF-7 breast cancer cells are stably transfected with the HER-2/neu gene. Tumors form very rapidly even during tamoxifen treatment.[82] Acquired resistance, on the other hand show those ER positive breast cancers which initially respond to SERM therapy, but do not continue to respond during long term therapy[81] (Fig. 2). This concept is illustrated in the laboratory if wild type MCF-7 breast cancer cells are inoculated into ovariectomized athymic mice and treated with tamoxifen. Initially most tumors do not grow but some tumors start to grow in the presence of the antiestrogen after about a year. If the growing tumors are transplanted into other athymic mice they will grow in response to either estrogen or tamoxifen.[83] Functional ER expression is still maintained in these SERM resistant cells. SERM resistance is unique because when the SERM is complexed with ER there is SERM stimulated growth. Examination of this form of SERM resistance in the clinic demonstrates that SERM resistant tumors can still respond to fulvestrant, a pure ER antagonist or the aromatase inhibitors which block the peripheral synthesis of estrogen in postmenopausal women.[84] This form of drug resistance i.e., SERM stimulated growth is referred to as phase I drug resistance (Fig. 2). Models for tamoxifen and raloxifene resistance are well described in the literature.[83,85]

Mechanism of SERM Resistance

Although the precise molecular mechanism for the SERM resistance is not completely understood, several genomic and extra-genomic factors are being shown to be involved in imparting resistance to SERMs or play a role in SERM induced growth of breast cancer cells. However, it is highly unlikely that any one particular mechanism is responsible for the SERM resistance in all patients. It could be possible that a combination of several factors may be responsible for the SERM resistance but for the sake of clarity these factors are discussed here individually.

Role of Epidermal Growth Factor Receptors (EGFRs) in SERM Resistant Breast Cancers

Signaling cascades originating from the cell surface of the cancer cells may drastically influence the genomic actions mediated by ER. One of the most prominent and well studied signaling pathway is the EGFR2, also known as HER-2/neu. HER-2, a receptor tyrosine kinase, is a member of the EGFR family and its amplification or overexpression is frequently associated with an aggressive phenotype of cancers.[86-88] Indeed, overexpressing HER-2 in ER positive MCF-7 breast cancer cells prevents the cells from responding to tamoxifen.[82,89] The mechanism by which HER-2 overexpression confers tamoxifen resistance and switches tamoxifen bound ER to an agonistic configuration has recently been described[90] (Fig. 3). An increased cross-talk between HER-2 and estrogen signaling pathways coupled with high SRC3 levels are responsible for subverting the ability of the tamoxifen bound ER to recruit corepressors. Instead the tamoxifen ER complex recruits coactivator SRC3.[90] Consistent with this conclusion, another study recently reported resensitization to tamoxifen by silencing the SRC3.[91] Additionally, in cells that overexpress HER-2, the agonistic activity of tamoxifen was reverted to an antagonist action by using inhibitors of HER-2

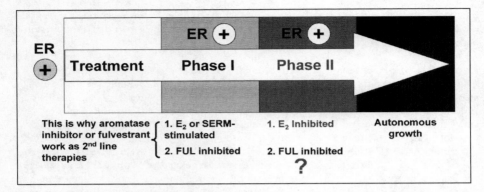

Figure 2. Diagram depicting different phases of SERM resistant breast cancers.

signaling.[82,90] This being the case, it is therefore important to understand the underlying mechanism of HER-2 initiated signaling cascades so that new therapeutic strategies can be formulated. Phosphatidylinositol-3-kinase (PI3K)/AKT and mitogen-activated protein kinases (MAPK) are the two critical signaling pathways which are activated aberrantly, in cells that overexpress HER-2.[92] Indeed, activation of AKT in ER positive breast cancer patients predicts decreased overall survival in tamoxifen treated patients.[93,94] Estrogen can rapidly activate AKT via the HER-2 pathway in cells expressing low levels of HER-2 and 4-hydroxytamoxifen can block this activation.[95] However, in breast cancer cells overexpressing HER-2, 4-hydroxytamoxifen can also activate AKT pathway in

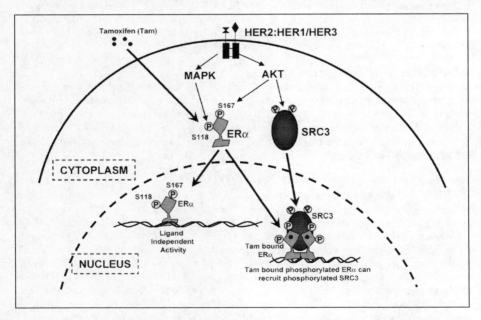

Figure 3. Schematic representation of cross talk between HER2 and estrogen signaling pathways. High HER2 expression activates AKT and MAPK pathways which can phosphorylate estrogen receptor (ER) and steroid coactivator 3 (SRC3). Phosphorylated ER can activate transcription independent of ligand. Tamoxifen bound phosphorylated ER can recruit phosphorylated SRC3 instead of corepressors and act as an estrogen agonist.

a HER-2 dependent manner,[90] exemplifying the conversion of 4-hydroxytamoxifen to an agonist. Both AKT and MAPK pathways can phosphorylate ER as well as the coactivator AIB1 (SRC3). Serine 167 residue of ER can be phosphorylated by AKT,[96] whereas serine 118 residue of ER can be phosphorylated by the MAPK pathway, both resulting in ligand-independent activation of estrogen receptor.[97,98] Not surprisingly, breast cancers with high levels of SRC3 along with HER-2 over-expression are associated with worse outcome following tamoxifen therapy, indicating resistance.[99] A recent study have also reported that specific phosphorylation of ER can modify the binding ability of ligands and also modulate its capacity to interact with co-activators.[100] In addition to HER-2, elevated level of EGFR/HER-1, another member of the EGFR family, is also correlated with poor prognosis and has been implicated in SERM resistant breast cancers.[101,102] Different members of EGFR family can dimerize, autophosphorylate and activate different signaling pathways. Long term treatment with tamoxifen, resulting in resistance, is also associated with increased translocation of ER α out of the nucleus and enhanced interaction with EGFR.[103] Similarly, high levels of HER-2 were found to increase the relocalization of ER α from nucleus to cytoplasm.[104] It is therefore evident from these findings that aberrant signaling cascades initiated by over-expressing EGFR and HER-2, particularly involving PI3K/AKT and MAPK pathways, are critically involved in cross talk with the genomic components of ER responses. All of these events may merge to create resistance to SERM treatment.

Other Factors Involved in SERM Resistant Breast Cancers

In addition to aberrant activation of AKT and MAPK pathways in SERM resistant breast cancers, several other factors have also been reported. The mammalian target of rapamycin (mTOR), which is a downstream target of PI3K/AKT and MAPK pathway,[105,106] is found to be involved in estrogen induced proliferation of ER positive breast cancer cells.[107,108] Furthermore, specific inhibitors of the mTOR pathway restore sensitivity to tamoxifen in a tamoxifen resistant cell line, both in vitro and in vivo.[109]

Another downstream target of EGFR and HER-2, is c-Src which phosphorylates p27 and impairs its inhibitory action on cyclin dependent kinase 2 (Cdk2) resulting in increased mitogenic activity. This mechanism is also implicated in tamoxifen resistance, as inhibition of c-Src was found to restore tamoxifen sensitivity.[110]

A rather novel approach to reversing tamoxifen resistance is to use disulfide benzamide (DIBA) that disrupts the zinc fingers of ER DNA binding domain and prevents the association of coactivators with 4-hydroxytamoxifen bound ER. DIBA was able to restore the tamoxifen sensitivity in several different tamoxifen resistant cells. However, this effect was achieved without altering the phosphorylation statuses of HER-2, MAPK, AKT and AIB1 in these cells.[111] It is possible that the use of DIBA with an inhibitor of phosphorylation would be a reasonable strategy for long term therapeutic use.

Therapeutic Options for SERM Resistant Breast Cancers

Since EGFR and HER-2 mediated signaling events play important roles in SERM resistant phenotype of breast cancers, blocking these pathways represent a logical approach in combating SERM resistance. Indeed, several laboratory studies have used selective inhibitors of HER-2 and/or EGFR in SERM resistant cells and reported beneficial outcomes, including reversal of SERM resistance.[90] A recent study[112] demonstrates that using a combination of three drugs, all targeting the HER2 by different mechanisms, along with tamoxifen or estrogen deprivation could effectively block the growth of HER2 overexpressing ER positive breast cancer in athymic mice. In another study using raloxifene resistant breast cancer cells, blocking of HER-2 activation by trastuzumab (humanized monoclonal antibody against HER-2) was found to decrease the growth of the resistant tumors in laboratory animals.[85] This approach was particularly effective in preventing the growth of tamoxifen stimulated endometrial cancers.[113] Clinical efforts are therefore directed towards using either small molecule inhibitors against EGFR and HER-2 or humanized monoclonal antibody against HER-2 as a monotherapy or in combination with other therapies including SERMs, in patients not responding to endocrine therapies.[114] As mentioned earlier aromatase inhibitors or fulvestrant are equally effective at treating breast cancer patients who are already resistant to tamoxifen. However, laboratory studies[115] now show that the initial inhibition of tumor growth, by either fulvestrant or estrogen deprivation is quickly followed by resistance and all the resistant tumors exhibit elevated levels of phosphorylated AKT and MAPK.[115] Tumor control by fulvestrant or estrogen deprivation is enhanced when this approach is combined with therapy that inhibits the EGFR/HER-2 signaling. These findings further underscore the idea that inhibiting the downstream targets of AKT and MAPK pathway, like mTOR, may be of significant importance in attenuation of SERM resistance.[109]

Resistance to Long Term Antihormone Therapy

The laboratory models and mechanisms discussed so far really represent the early stages of drug resistance to SERMs. The models replicate treatment of metastatic breast cancer with tamoxifen and do not replicate the strategy of long term adjuvant therapy with 5 years of tamoxifen. To address this deficiency tamoxifen-stimulated breast tumors have been repeatedly transplanted into tamoxifen-treated athymic mice to replicate micrometastases that grow in a tamoxifen environment for years. Remarkably, the signal transduction pathways in tumor cells become reconfigured so that estrogen is no longer a survival signal but triggers apoptosis in phase II resistant breast cancer cells[116-118] (Fig. 2).

Estrogen Induced Apoptosis

Phase II tamoxifen stimulated tumors are dependent upon tamoxifen for growth and are cross resistant with raloxifene.[119] Indeed the converse is also true. Raloxifene-resistant breast cancer cells can be grown into tumors in athymic mice by treatment with either raloxifene or tamoxifen.[118] However, it is the dramatic antitumor effect of estrogen as a major factor in breast tumor cell survival that is intriguing. High dose estrogen therapy was originally used as a palliative treatment for postmenopausal metastatic breast cancer before tamoxifen, an antiestrogen, was developed during the 1970's.[11] Alexander Haddow[120] reported that high doses of synthetic estrogens would produce a 30% response rate in unselected patients and the responses would last about one year. Despite the fact that treatment with high dose estrogen therapy has slipped into disuse with the ubiquitous use of tamoxifen and new aromatase inhibitors, recent laboratory studies indicate that low dose, rather than high dose, estrogen could again find a place in the treatment paradigm of metastatic breast cancer. The first indication that this was true occurred when the findings that physiologic level of circulating estradiol could cause tumor regression in long term tamoxifen resistant tumors (phase II).[116,117] The idea is now being advanced to the clinic as there is every reason to believe that the concept will translate as a treatment for antihormone resistant breast cancer. It is already known that high dose estrogen produces a 30% response rate in patients whose tumors are refractory following exhaustive antihormonal therapy.[121]

Additionally the paradoxical effect of estrogen to induce apoptosis is not limited to SERM resistant breast cancer cells, but has also been observed in estrogen deprived breast cancer cells.[122,123] Although the precise mechanism of estrogen induced apoptosis is under intense investigation, studies have indicated the involvement of mitochondrial pathway of apoptosis in estrogen deprived cells,[124] and a different mechanism in raloxifene resistant cells.[118] Most importantly, laboratory studies have shown that the breast cancer cells that become resistant to estrogen induced apoptosis regain the sensitivity for SERM therapy.[117] Therefore, it is possible that cyclical treatments with SERM and estrogen may help to control breast cancer growth for a prolonged period.[125]

Conclusion

Currently, tamoxifen, the prototypical SERM, can be used to treat all stages of ER positive breast cancers and for chemoprevention in high risk women. The effectiveness of this class of drugs is based on selectively blocking the estrogen mediated effects in the breast cancer. The fact that the ER is such an important target and that majority of breast tumors are ER positive has made ER blockade such a significant therapeutic success. This clinical success has led to the development of other SERMs in the group, like raloxifene, with fewer undesirable effects. However, despite significant advances the use of long term SERM treatment is ultimately associated with acquired breast cancer resistance. Nevertheless, studies during the past decade have identified specific signaling pathways that are involved in the cross talk with ER signaling, thereby creating resistance to SERMs. Although encouraging results and strategies are being developed to employ inhibitors of phosphorylation pathways it may be that the tumors develop too many signaling options to use a single approach to block resistance. In this regard the novel finding that estrogen will eventually induce apoptosis in SERM resistant breast cancer cells merits further detailed study for its wider therapeutic use. It may be that the skill of the ER to activate apoptosis can be used to identify an apoptotic trigger to kill cancer cells selectively.

References

1. Jordan VC. Biochemical pharmacology of antiestrogen action. Pharmacol Rev 1984; 36(4):245-276.
2. Harper MJ, Walpole AL. A new derivative of triphenylethylene: effect on implantation and mode of action in rats. J Reprod Fertil 1967; 13(1):101-119.
3. Harper MJ, Walpole AL. Mode of action of I.C.I. 46,474 in preventing implantation in rats. J Endocrinol 1967; 37(1):83-92.
4. Klopper A, Hall M. New synthetic agent for the induction of ovulation: preliminary trials in women. Br Med J 1971; 1(5741):152-154.
5. Jordan VC. Prolonged antioestrogenic activity of ICI 46,474 in the ovariectomized mouse. J Reprod Fertil 1975; 42(2):251-258.
6. Lippman M, Bolan G, Huff K. Interactions of antiestrogens with human breast cancer in long-term tissue culture. Cancer Treat Rep 1976; 60(10):1421-1429.
7. Jordan VC, Koerner S. Tamoxifen (ICI 46,474) and the human carcinoma 8S oestrogen receptor. Eur J Cancer 1975; 11(3):205-206.
8. Skidmore J, Walpole AL, Woodburn J. Effect of some triphenylethylenes on oestradiol binding in vitro to macromolecules from uterus and anterior pituitary. J Endocrinol 1972; 52(2):289-298.
9. Jordan VC. Antiestrogenic and antitumor properties of tamoxifen in laboratory animals. Cancer Treat Rep 1976; 60(10):1409-1419.
10. Jordan VC, Brodie AM. Development and evolution of therapies targeted to the estrogen receptor for the treatment and prevention of breast cancer. Steroids 2007; 72(1):7-25.
11. Jordan VC. Tamoxifen: a most unlikely pioneering medicine. Nat Rev Drug Discov 2003; 2(3):205-213.
12. Tamoxifen for early breast cancer: an overview of the randomised trials. Early Breast Cancer Trialists' Collaborative Group. Lancet 1998; 351(9114):1451-467.
13. Jordan VC, Collins MM, Rowsby L et al. A monohydroxylated metabolite of tamoxifen with potent antioestrogenic activity. J Endocrinol 1977; 75(2):305-316.
14. Allen KE, Clark ER, Jordan VC. Evidence for the metabolic activation of nonsteroidal antioestrogens: a study of structure-activity relationships. Br J Pharmacol 1980; 71(1):83-91.
15. Jordan VC, Murphy CS. Endocrine pharmacology of antiestrogens as antitumor agents. Endocr Rev 1990; 11(4):578-610.
16. Shiau AK, Barstad D, Loria PM et al. The structural basis of estrogen receptor/coactivator recognition and the antagonism of this interaction by tamoxifen. Cell 1998; 95(7):927-937.
17. Beatson GT. On the treatmnet of inoperable cases of carcinoma of the mamma: suggestions for a new method of treatment, with illustrative cases. Lancet 1896; 148:104-107, 162-167.
18. Jensen EV, Jacobson HI. Basic guide to the mechanism of estrogen action. Recent Progress in Hormone Research 1962; 18:387-414.
19. Jensen EV, Block GE, Smith S et al. Estrogen receptors and breast cancer response to adrenalectomy. Natl Cancer Inst Monogr 1971; 34:55-70.
20. Jordan VC. Effect of tamoxifen (ICI 46,474) on initiation and growth of DMBA-induced rat mammary carcinomata. Eur J Cancer 1976; 12(6):419-424.
21. Jordan VC, Koerner S. Tamoxifen as an anti-tumour agent: role of oestradiol and prolactin. J Endocrinol 1976; 68(02):305-311.
22. Jordan VC, Dowse LJ. Tamoxifen as an anti-tumour agent: effect on oestrogen binding. J Endocrinol 1976; 68(02):297-303.
23. Jordan VC, Jaspan T. Tamoxifen as an anti-tumour agent: oestrogen binding as a predictive test for tumour response. J Endocrinol 1976; 68(3):453-460.

24. Nicholson RI, Golder MP. The effect of synthetic anti-oestrogens on the growth and biochemistry of rat mammary tumours. Eur J Cancer 1975; 11(8):571-579.

25. Jordan VC, Dix CJ, Allen KE. The effectiveness of long term tamoxifen treatment in a laboratory model for adjuvant hormone therapy of breast cancer. In: Salmon SE, Jones SE, eds. Adjuvant Therapy of Cancer. Vol 2. New York: Grune & Stratton, Inc; 1979:19-26.

26. Jordan VC, Allen KE. Evaluation of the antitumour activity of the nonsteroidal antioestrogen monohydroxytamoxifen in the DMBA-induced rat mammary carcinoma model. Eur J Cancer 1980; 16(2):239-251.

27. Osborne CK, Hobbs K, Clark GM. Effect of estrogens and antiestrogens on growth of human breast cancer cells in athymic nude mice. Cancer Res 1985; 45(2):584-590.

28. Gottardis MM, Robinson SP, Jordan VC. Estradiol-stimulated growth of MCF-7 tumors implanted in athymic mice: a model to study the tumoristatic action of tamoxifen. J Steroid Biochem 1988; 30(1-6):311-314.

29. Kiang DT, Kennedy BJ. Tamoxifen (antiestrogen) therapy in advanced breast cancer. Ann Intern Med 1977; 87(6):687-690.

30. Baum M, Brinkley DM, Dossett JA et al. Improved survival among patients treated with adjuvant tamoxifen after mastectomy for early breast cancer. Lancet 1983; 2(8347):450.

31. Systemic treatment of early breast cancer by hormonal, cytotoxic, or immune therapy. 133 randomised trials involving 31,000 recurrences and 24,000 deaths among 75,000 women. Early Breast Cancer Trialists' Collaborative Group. Lancet 1992; 339(8785):71-85.

32. Fisher B, Dignam J, Bryant J et al. Five versus more than five years of tamoxifen for lymph node-negative breast cancer: updated findings from the National Surgical Adjuvant Breast and Bowel Project B-14 randomized trial. J Natl Cancer Inst 2001; 93(9):684-690.

33. Powles TJ, Ashley S, Tidy A et al. Twenty-year follow-up of the Royal Marsden randomized, double-blinded tamoxifen breast cancer prevention trial. J Natl Cancer Inst 2007; 99(4):283-290.

34. Adjuvant tamoxifen in the management of operable breast cancer: the Scottish Trial. Report from the Breast Cancer Trials Committee, Scottish Cancer Trials Office (MRC), Edinburgh. 1987; 2(8552):171-175.

35. Jordan VC. Chemosuppression of breast cancer with tamoxifen: laboratory evidence and future clinical investigations. Cancer Invest 1988; 6(5):589-595.

36. Fisher B, Costantino JP, Wickerham DL et al. Tamoxifen for the prevention of breast cancer: current status of the National Surgical Adjuvant Breast and Bowel Project P-1 study. J Natl Cancer Inst 2005; 97(22):1652-1662.

37. Cuzick J, Forbes J, Edwards R et al. First results from the International Breast Cancer Intervention Study (IBIS-I): a randomised prevention trial. Lancet 2002; 360(9336):817-824.

38. Fisher B, Costantino JP, Wickerham DL et al. Tamoxifen for prevention of breast cancer: report of the National Surgical Adjuvant Breast and Bowel Project P-1 Study. J Natl Cancer Inst 1998; 90(18):1371-1388.

39. Cuzick J, Forbes JF, Sestak I et al. Long-term results of tamoxifen prophylaxis for breast cancer—96-month follow-up of the randomized IBIS-I trial. J Natl Cancer Inst 2007; 99(4):272-282.

40. Buzdar AU, Marcus C, Holmes F et al. Phase II evaluation of Ly156758 in metastatic breast cancer. Oncology 1988; 45(5):344-345.

41. Jordan VC, Phelps E, Lindgren JU. Effects of anti-estrogens on bone in castrated and intact female rats. Breast Cancer Res Treat 1987; 10(1):31-35.

42. Gottardis MM, Jordan VC. Antitumor actions of keoxifene and tamoxifen in the N-nitrosomethylurea-induced rat mammary carcinoma model. Cancer Res 1987; 47(15):4020-4024.

43. Black LJ, Jones CD, Falcone JF. Antagonism of estrogen action with a new benzothiophene derived antiestrogen. Life Sci 1983; 32(9):1031-1036.

44. Gottardis MM, Ricchio ME, Satyaswaroop PG et al. Effect of steroidal and nonsteroidal antiestrogens on the growth of a tamoxifen-stimulated human endometrial carcinoma (EnCa101) in athymic mice. Cancer Res 1990; 50(11):3189-3192.

45. Lerner LJ, Jordan VC. The development of antiestrogens for the treatment of breast cancer. Cancer Res 1990; 50:4177-4189.

46. Cummings SR, Eckert S, Krueger KA et al. The effect of raloxifene on risk of breast cancer in postmenopausal women: results from the MORE randomized trial. Multiple Outcomes of Raloxifene Evaluation. JAMA 1999; 281(23):2189-2197.

47. Jordan VC. Optimising endocrine approaches for the chemoprevention of breast cancer beyond the Study of Tamoxifen and Raloxifene (STAR) trial. Eur J Cancer 2006; 42(17):2909-2913.

48. Vogel VG, Costantino JP, Wickerham DL et al. Effects of tamoxifen vs raloxifene on the risk of developing invasive breast cancer and other disease outcomes: the NSABP Study of Tamoxifen and Raloxifene (STAR) P-2 trial. JAMA 2006; 295(23):2727-2741.

49. Jordan VC. Chemoprevention of breast cancer with selective oestrogen-receptor modulators. Nat Rev Cancer 2007; 7(1):46-53.
50. Kuiper GG, Carlsson B, Grandien K et al. Comparison of the ligand binding specificity and transcript tissue distribution of estrogen receptors alpha and beta. Endocrinology 1997; 138(3):863-870.
51. Monroe DG, Secreto FJ, Subramaniam M et al. Estrogen receptor alpha and beta heterodimers exert unique effects on estrogen- and tamoxifen-dependent gene expression in human U2OS osteosarcoma cells. Mol Endocrinol 2005; 19(6):1555-1568.
52. Matthews J, Wihlen B, Tujague M et al. Estrogen receptor (ER) beta modulates ERalpha-mediated transcriptional activation by altering the recruitment of c-Fos and c-Jun to estrogen-responsive promoters. Mol Endocrinol 2006; 20(3):534-543.
53. Tsai MJ, O'Malley BW. Molecular mechanisms of action of steroid/thyroid receptor superfamily members. Annu Rev Biochem 1994; 63:451-486.
54. Brzozowski AM, Pike AC, Dauter Z et al. Molecular basis of agonism and antagonism in the oestrogen receptor. Nature 1997; 389(6652):753-758.
55. Pike AC, Brzozowski AM, Hubbard RE et al. Structure of the ligand-binding domain of oestrogen receptor beta in the presence of a partial agonist and a full antagonist. EMBO J 1999; 18(17):4608-4618.
56. Liu H, Park WC, Bentrem DJ et al. Structure function relationships of the raloxifene-estrogen receptor-alpha complex for regulating transforming growth factor-alpha expression in breast cancer cells. J Biol Chem 2002; 277(11):9189-9198.
57. MacGregor Schafer J, Liu H, Bentrem DJ et al. Allosteric silencing of activating function 1 in the 4-hydroxytamoxifen estrogen receptor complex is induced by substituting glycine for aspartate at amino acid 351. Cancer Res 2000; 60(18):5097-5105.
58. Webb P, Nguyen P, Kushner PJ. Differential SERM effects on corepressor binding dictate ERalpha activity in vivo. J Biol Chem 2003; 278(9):6912-6920.
59. Hall JM, McDonnell DP. The estrogen receptor beta-isoform (ERbeta) of the human estrogen receptor modulates ERalpha transcriptional activity and is a key regulator of the cellular response to estrogens and antiestrogens. Endocrinology 1999; 140(12):5566-5578.
60. Hall JM, McDonnell DP, Korach KS. Allosteric regulation of estrogen receptor structure, function and coactivator recruitment by different estrogen response elements. Mol Endocrinol 2002; 16(3):469-486.
61. Lonard DM, O'Malley BW. The expanding cosmos of nuclear receptor coactivators. Cell 2006; 125(3):411-414.
62. Shang Y, Brown M. Molecular determinants for the tissue specificity of SERMs. Science 2002; 295(5564):2465-2468.
63. Gottardis MM, Robinson SP, Satyaswaroop PG et al. Contrasting actions of tamoxifen on endometrial and breast tumor growth in the athymic mouse. Cancer Res 1988; 48(4):812-815.
64. Lonard DM, Tsai SY, O'Malley BW. Selective estrogen receptor modulators 4-hydroxytamoxifen and raloxifene impact the stability and function of SRC-1 and SRC-3 coactivator proteins. Mol Cell Biol 2004; 24(1):14-24.
65. Wu RC, Smith CL, O'Malley BW. Transcriptional regulation by steroid receptor coactivator phosphorylation. Endocr Rev 2005; 26(3):393-399.
66. Smith CL, O'Malley BW. Coregulator function: a key to understanding tissue specificity of selective receptor modulators. Endocr Rev 2004; 25(1):45-71.
67. McKenna NJ, Lanz RB, O'Malley BW. Nuclear receptor coregulators: cellular and molecular biology. Endocr Rev 1999; 20(3):321-344.
68. Shang Y, Hu X, DiRenzo J et al. Cofactor dynamics and sufficiency in estrogen receptor-regulated transcription. Cell 2000; 103(6):843-852.
69. Smith CL, Nawaz Z, O'Malley BW. Coactivator and corepressor regulation of the agonist/antagonist activity of the mixed antiestrogen, 4-hydroxytamoxifen. Mol Endocrinol 1997; 11(6):657-666.
70. Lavinsky RM, Jepsen K, Heinzel T et al. Diverse signaling pathways modulate nuclear receptor recruitment of N-CoR and SMRT complexes. Proc Natl Acad Sci USA 1998; 95(6):2920-2925.
71. Jepsen K, Hermanson O, Onami TM et al. Combinatorial roles of the nuclear receptor corepressor in transcription and development. Cell 2000; 102(6):753-763.
72. Keeton EK, Brown M. Cell cycle progression stimulated by tamoxifen-bound estrogen receptor-alpha and promoter-specific effects in breast cancer cells deficient in N-CoR and SMRT. Mol Endocrinol 2005; 19(6):1543-1554.
73. Mazumdar A, Wang RA, Mishra SK et al. Transcriptional repression of oestrogen receptor by metastasis-associated protein 1 corepressor. Nat Cell Biol 2001; 3(1):30-37.
74. Montano MM, Ekena K, Delage-Mourroux R et al. An estrogen receptor-selective coregulator that potentiates the effectiveness of antiestrogens and represses the activity of estrogens. Proc Natl Acad Sci USA 1999; 96(12):6947-6952.

75. Delage-Mourroux R, Martini PG, Choi I et al. Analysis of estrogen receptor interaction with a repressor of estrogen receptor activity (REA) and the regulation of estrogen receptor transcriptional activity by REA. J Biol Chem 2000; 275(46):35848-35856.

76. Zhang J, Guenther MG, Carthew RW et al. Proteasomal regulation of nuclear receptor corepressor-mediated repression. Genes Dev 1998; 12(12):1775-1780.

77. Frasor J, Danes JM, Funk CC et al. Estrogen down-regulation of the corepressor N-CoR: mechanism and implications for estrogen derepression of N-CoR-regulated genes. Proc Natl Acad Sci USA 2005; 102(37):13153-13157.

78. Spencer TE, Jenster G, Burcin MM et al. Steroid receptor coactivator-1 is a histone acetyltransferase. Nature 1997; 389(6647):194-198.

79. Liu XF, Bagchi MK. Recruitment of distinct chromatin-modifying complexes by tamoxifen-complexed estrogen receptor at natural target gene promoters in vivo. J Biol Chem 2004; 279(15):15050-15058.

80. Feng Q, Yi P, Wong J et al. Signaling within a coactivator complex: methylation of SRC-3/AIB1 is a molecular switch for complex disassembly. Mol Cell Biol 2006; 26(21):7846-7857.

81. Jordan VC. Selective estrogen receptor modulation: concept and consequences in cancer. Cancer Cell 2004; 5(3):207-213.

82. Benz CC, Scott GK, Sarup JC et al. Estrogen-dependent, tamoxifen-resistant tumorigenic growth of MCF-7 cells transfected with HER2/neu. Breast Cancer Res Treat 1992; 24(2):85-95.

83. Gottardis MM, Jordan VC. Development of tamoxifen-stimulated growth of MCF-7 tumors in athymic mice after long-term antiestrogen administration. Cancer Res 1988; 48(18):5183-5187.

84. Howell A, Robertson JF, Quaresma Albano J et al. Fulvestrant, formerly ICI 182,780, is as effective as anastrozole in postmenopausal women with advanced breast cancer progressing after prior endocrine treatment. J Clin Oncol 2002; 20(16):3396-3403.

85. O'Regan RM, Osipo C, Ariazi E et al. Development and therapeutic options for the treatment of raloxifene-stimulated breast cancer in athymic mice. Clin Cancer Res 2006; 12(7 Pt 1):2255-2263.

86. Konecny G, Pauletti G, Pegram M et al. Quantitative association between HER-2/neu and steroid hormone receptors in hormone receptor-positive primary breast cancer. J Natl Cancer Inst 2003; 95(2):142-153.

87. Slamon DJ, Clark GM, Wong SG et al. Human breast cancer: correlation of relapse and survival with amplification of the HER-2/neu oncogene. Science 1987; 235(4785):177-182.

88. Yu D, Hung MC. Overexpression of ErbB2 in cancer and ErbB2-targeting strategies. Oncogene 2000; 19(53):6115-6121.

89. Kurokawa H, Lenferink AE, Simpson JF et al. Inhibition of HER2/neu (erbB-2) and mitogen-activated protein kinases enhances tamoxifen action against HER2-overexpressing, tamoxifen-resistant breast cancer cells. Cancer Res 2000; 60(20):5887-5894.

90. Shou J, Massarweh S, Osborne CK et al. Mechanisms of tamoxifen resistance: increased estrogen receptor-HER2/neu cross-talk in ER/HER2-positive breast cancer. J Natl Cancer Inst 2004; 96(12):926-935.

91. Mc Ilroy M, Fleming FJ, Buggy Y et al. Tamoxifen-induced ER-alpha-SRC-3 interaction in HER2 positive human breast cancer; a possible mechanism for ER isoform specific recurrence. Endocr Relat Cancer 2006; 13(4):1135-1145.

92. Schiff R, Massarweh SA, Shou J et al. Cross-talk between estrogen receptor and growth factor pathways as a molecular target for overcoming endocrine resistance. Clin Cancer Res 2004; 10(1 Pt 2):331S-336S.

93. Tokunaga E, Kataoka A, Kimura Y et al. The association between Akt activation and resistance to hormone therapy in metastatic breast cancer. Eur J Cancer 2006; 42(5):629-635.

94. Kirkegaard T, Witton CJ, McGlynn LM et al. AKT activation predicts outcome in breast cancer patients treated with tamoxifen. J Pathol 2005; 207(2):139-146.

95. Stoica GE, Franke TF, Wellstein A et al. Estradiol rapidly activates Akt via the ErbB2 signaling pathway. Mol Endocrinol 2003; 17(5):818-830.

96. Campbell RA, Bhat-Nakshatri P, Patel NM et al. Phosphatidylinositol 3-kinase/AKT-mediated activation of estrogen receptor alpha: a new model for anti-estrogen resistance. J Biol Chem 2001; 276(13):9817-9824.

97. Bunone G, Briand PA, Miksicek RJ et al. Activation of the unliganded estrogen receptor by EGF involves the MAP kinase pathway and direct phosphorylation. EMBO J 1996; 15(9):2174-2183.

98. Kato S, Endoh H, Masuhiro Y et al. Activation of the estrogen receptor through phosphorylation by mitogen-activated protein kinase. Science 1995; 270(5241):1491-1494.

99. Osborne CK, Bardou V, Hopp TA et al. Role of the estrogen receptor coactivator AIB1 (SRC-3) and HER-2/neu in tamoxifen resistance in breast cancer. J Natl Cancer Inst 2003; 95(5):353-361.

100. Likhite VS, Stossi F, Kim K et al. Kinase-specific phosphorylation of the estrogen receptor changes receptor interactions with ligand, deoxyribonucleic acid and coregulators associated with alterations in estrogen and tamoxifen activity. Mol Endocrinol 2006; 20(12):3120-3132.
101. Knowlden JM, Hutcheson IR, Jones HE et al. Elevated levels of epidermal growth factor receptor/c-erbB2 heterodimers mediate an autocrine growth regulatory pathway in tamoxifen-resistant MCF-7 cells. Endocrinology 2003; 144(3):1032-1044.
102. Tsutsui S, Ohno S, Murakami S et al. Prognostic value of epidermal growth factor receptor (EGFR) and its relationship to the estrogen receptor status in 1029 patients with breast cancer. Breast Cancer Res Treat 2002; 71(1):67-75.
103. Fan P, Wang J, Santen RJ et al. Long-term treatment with tamoxifen facilitates translocation of estrogen receptor alpha out of the nucleus and enhances its interaction with EGFR in MCF-7 breast cancer cells. Cancer Res 2007; 67(3):1352-1360.
104. Yang Z, Barnes CJ, Kumar R. Human epidermal growth factor receptor 2 status modulates subcellular localization of and interaction with estrogen receptor alpha in breast cancer cells. Clin Cancer Res 2004; 10(11):3621-3628.
105. Altomare DA, Testa JR. Perturbations of the AKT signaling pathway in human cancer. Oncogene 2005; 24(50):7455-7464.
106. Ma L, Chen Z, Erdjument-Bromage H et al. Phosphorylation and functional inactivation of TSC2 by Erk implications for tuberous sclerosis and cancer pathogenesis. Cell 2005; 121(2):179-193.
107. Chang SB, Miron P, Miron A et al. Rapamycin inhibits proliferation of estrogen-receptor-positive breast cancer cells. J Surg Res 2007; 138(1):37-44.
108. Yue W, Wang J, Li Y et al. Farnesylthiosalicylic acid blocks mammalian target of rapamycin signaling in breast cancer cells. Int J Cancer 2005; 117(5):746-754.
109. deGraffenried LA, Friedrichs WE, Russell DH et al. Inhibition of mTOR activity restores tamoxifen response in breast cancer cells with aberrant Akt Activity. Clin Cancer Res 2004; 10(23):8059-8067.
110. Chu I, Sun J, Arnaout A et al. p27 phosphorylation by Src regulates inhibition of cyclin E-Cdk2. Cell 2007; 128(2):281-294.
111. Wang LH, Yang XY, Zhang X et al. Disruption of estrogen receptor DNA-binding domain and related intramolecular communication restores tamoxifen sensitivity in resistant breast cancer. Cancer Cell 2006; 10(6):487-499.
112. Arpino G, Gutierrez C, Weiss H et al. Treatment of human epidermal growth factor receptor 2-overexpressing breast cancer xenografts with multiagent HER-targeted therapy. J Natl Cancer Inst 2007; 99(9):694-705.
113. Osipo C, Meeke K, Liu H et al. Trastuzumab therapy for tamoxifen-stimulated endometrial cancer. Cancer Res 2005; 65(18):8504-8513.
114. Johnston SR. Clinical efforts to combine endocrine agents with targeted therapies against epidermal growth factor receptor/human epidermal growth factor receptor 2 and mammalian target of rapamycin in breast cancer. Clin Cancer Res 2006; 12(3 Pt 2):1061s-1068s.
115. Massarweh S, Osborne CK, Jiang S et al. Mechanisms of Tumor Regression and Resistance to Estrogen Deprivation and Fulvestrant in a Model of Estrogen Receptor-Positive, HER-2/neu-Positive Breast Cancer. Cancer Res 2006; 66(16):8266-8273.
116. Wolf DM, Jordan VC. A laboratory model to explain the survival advantage observed in patients taking adjuvant tamoxifen therapy. Recent Results Cancer Res 1993; 127:23-33.
117. Yao K, Lee ES, Bentrem DJ et al. Antitumor action of physiological estradiol on tamoxifen-stimulated breast tumors grown in athymic mice. Clin Cancer Res 2000; 6(5):2028-2036.
118. Liu H, Lee ES, Gajdos C et al. Apoptotic action of 17beta-estradiol in raloxifene-resistant MCF-7 cells in vitro and in vivo. J Natl Cancer Inst 2003; 95(21):1586-1597.
119. O'Regan RM, Gajdos C, Dardes RC et al. Effects of raloxifene after tamoxifen on breast and endometrial tumor growth in athymic mice. J Natl Cancer Inst 2002; 94(4):274-283.
120. Haddow A, Watkinson J, Paterson E. Influence of synthetic oestrogens upon advanced malignant disease. Br Med J 1944; 2:393-398.
121. Lonning PE, Taylor PD, Anker G et al. High-dose estrogen treatment in postmenopausal breast cancer patients heavily exposed to endocrine therapy. Breast Cancer Res Treat 2001; 67(2):111-116.
122. Song RX, Mor G, Naftolin F et al. Effect of long-term estrogen deprivation on apoptotic responses of breast cancer cells to 17beta-estradiol. J Natl Cancer Inst 2001; 93(22):1714-1723.
123. Lewis JS, Osipo C, Meeke K et al. Estrogen-induced apoptosis in a breast cancer model resistant to long-term estrogen withdrawal. J Steroid Biochem Mol Biol 2005; 94(1-3):131-141.
124. Lewis JS, Meeke K, Osipo C et al. Intrinsic mechanism of estradiol-induced apoptosis in breast cancer cells resistant to estrogen deprivation. J Natl Cancer Inst 2005; 97(23):1746-1759.
125. Jordan VC, Lewis JS, Osipo C et al. The apoptotic action of estrogen following exhaustive antihormonal therapy: a new clinical treatment strategy. Breast 2005; 14(6):624-630.

CHAPTER 14

Pharmacogenomics of Endocrine Therapy in Breast Cancer

Richard Weinshilboum*

Abstract

The treatment of breast cancer with selective estrogen receptor modulators such as tamoxifen and with aromatase inhibitors represents a major advance in cancer chemotherapy. However, there are large variations among patients in both the therapeutic efficacy and side effects of these drugs. Pharmacogenomics is the study of the role of inheritance in this variation and genetic variation in tamoxifen response represents one of the most striking examples of the potential clinical importance of pharmacogenomics. Tamoxifen requires "metabolic activation" catalyzed by cytochrome P450 2D6 (CYP2D6) to form hydroxylated metabolites—4-hydroxytamoxifen and endoxifen (N-desmethyl-4-hydroxytamoxifen)—both of which are much more potent than is the parent drug. However, *CYP2D6* is genetically polymorphic. Approximately 5-8% of Caucasian subjects are CYP2D6 "poor metabolizers" on a genetic basis and, as a result, are relatively unable to catalyze tamoxifen hydroxylation. These same subjects appear to have poorer outcomes when treated with tamoxifen than do CYP2D6 "extensive metabolizers". These data led the US Food and Drug Administration (FDA) to hold public hearings in 2006 on the inclusion of this pharmacogenomic information in tamoxifen labeling. However, a series of important questions still remains to be addressed with regard to tamoxifen pharmacogenomics. There have also been preliminary attempts to study the pharmacogenomics of aromatase inhibitors, including the application of a genotype-to-phenotype research strategy designed to explore the nature and extent of common DNA sequence variation in the *CYP19* gene that encodes aromatase. Those results—together with our current level of understanding of tamoxifen pharmacogenomics—will be reviewed in this chapter and both will be placed within the context of the overall development of pharmacogenomics.

Introduction

Pharmacogenomics is the study of the role of inheritance in individual differences in drug response.[1] The therapy of breast cancer with selective estrogen receptor modulators (SERMs) such as tamoxifen and with aromatase inhibitors represents a major advance in the drug therapy of cancer.[2] That advance is part of a "therapeutic revolution" which occurred during the latter half of the twentieth and continues into the twenty-first century.[3] The convergence of that revolution with the dramatic advances that occurred at the same time in human genomics[4,5] makes it possible to apply the techniques of modern genomic science in an attempt to understand the contribution of inheritance to variation in drug response phenotypes. That variation can range from adverse drug reactions at one end of the spectrum to lack of the desired therapeutic effect at the other. Pharmacogenomics is a major component of efforts to "individualize" medicine and one of the

*Richard Weinshilboum—Mayo Clinic College of Medicine-Mayo Clinic-Mayo Foundation Rochester, MN 55905, USA. Email: weinshilboum.richard@mayo.edu

Innovative Endocrinology of Cancer, edited by Lev M. Berstein and Richard J. Santen.
©2008 Landes Bioscience and Springer Science+Business Media.

most striking examples of the potential of pharmacogenomics to influence clinical practice involves the use of tamoxifen to treat breast cancer.

Pharmacogenomic effects are often classified as those that alter factors which influence the concentration of drug reaching its target, so-called "pharmacokinetic (PK)" factors and those that involve the drug target itself, "pharmacodynamic (PD)" factors.[1] When a drug such as tamoxifen is administered to a patient, it must be absorbed, distributed to its site of action, interact with its target(s), undergo metabolism and, finally, be excreted.[6] Absorption, distribution, metabolism and excretion can all influence "PK"—the concentration of drug or, in the case of tamoxifen, the concentrations of active metabolites of the drug, that finally reach the target. Genetic variation can also occur in the drug target itself or in signaling cascades downstream from the target, in this case involving "PD" factors. Historically, pharmacogenomic studies began with the observation of variation in phenotype, for example, the occurrence of an adverse drug reaction and then moved from clinical phenotype to biochemical cause, e.g., inherited lack of a drug-metabolizing enzyme and, ultimately, to the genome, in a "phenotype-to-genotype" progression. However, in today's post-genomic world, application of a genotype-to-phenotype research strategy is also possible. In the subsequent discussion of the endocrine therapy of breast cancer, both approaches will be illustrated.

The therapy of breast cancer patients with tamoxifen, as mentioned previously, represents a striking example of the potential clinical importance of pharmacogenomics—and the development of our knowledge of tamoxifen pharmacogenomics will be outlined subsequently. Studies have also been initiated of the pharmacogenomics of aromatase inhibitors, although they are not as well developed as is tamoxifen pharmacogenomics. Some of those latter studies began with an attempt to define common variation in the sequence of the aromatase gene (*CYP19*), the gene that encodes the target for aromatase inhibitors. In subsequent paragraphs, the observations and insights that resulted in our present understanding of tamoxifen pharmacogenomics will be described, followed by a brief overview of initial efforts to study the pharmacogenomics of aromatase inhibitors. Finally, both of these efforts involving the endocrine therapy of breast cancer will be considered within the context of the development of pharmacogenomics as a discipline, developments that promise to soon make it possible to query the entire human genome in order to better individualize drug therapy.

Tamoxifen Pharmacogenomics

Tamoxifen therapy of breast cancer patients represents one of the most striking and clinically relevant examples of the application of pharmacogenomics in an attempt to "personalize" pharmacologic therapy. It also illustrates the way in which knowledge of drug metabolism, a topic often regarded by students and practitioners alike as arcane or even "boring", provided important, clinically relevant insights. Although tamoxifen is itself a SERM, it is also a "pro-drug" that can be metabolized to form 4-hydroxy and N-desmethyl-4-hydroxy metabolites that are much more potent than is the parent compound (Fig. 1).[7] During the past decade, a series of events converged that resulted in the hypothesis that genetic variation in the CYP2D6-catalyzed hydroxylation of tamoxifen might represent a major factor responsible for individual variation in clinical response to that drug. Those events included a great deal of work which indicated that the selective serotonin reuptake inhibitors (SSRIs) used to treat depression were also effective in treating "hot flashes" induced by tamoxifen therapy;[8-10] the realization that many of those agents were—like tamoxifen—metabolized by CYP2D6; the characterization of a novel active metabolite of tamoxifen (endoxifen),[11-13] and clinical epidemiologic data in support of the hypothesis that CYP2D6 genotype was associated with tamoxifen efficacy.[14-16] In the text that follows, each of these topics will be addressed in turn—and presently unanswered questions with regard to tamoxifen pharmacogenomics will also be summarized.

Hot flashes are a common side effect of tamoxifen therapy, occurring in 50-70% of patients treated with this drug, but it is obviously not possible to treat this side effect in breast cancer patients with exogenous estrogens.[17] Therefore, when anecdotal reports appeared that hot flashes might

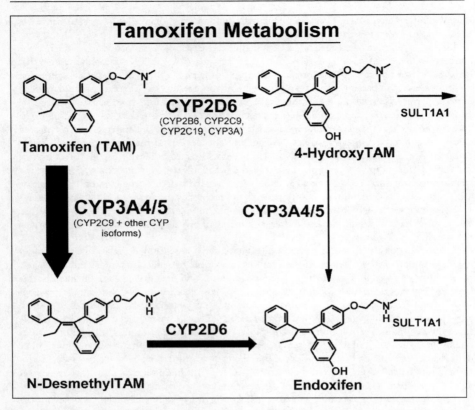

Figure 1. Tamoxifen (TAM) metabolism. Cytochrome P450 (CYP)3A4/5 catalyzes the formation of N-desmethyltamoxifen, while the generation of 4-hydroxytamoxifen and endoxifen are catalyzed predominantly by CYP2D6.[46] It has also been suggested that SULT1A1 may play a role in endoxifen clearance. The relative importance of each reaction is indicated by the size of the arrows (modified from Jin Y, Desta Z, Stearns V et al. J Natl Cancer Inst 2005; 97(1):30-39).[22]

respond to treatment with the SSRI drugs used to treat depression, those reports were followed by a series of clinical trials in which specific SSRIs were used to treat hot flashes. Included among the drugs studied in that fashion were venlafaxine, fluoxetine and paroxetine.[8-10] For example, 81 women were randomized to 20 mg of fluoxetine or placebo in one study and the "hot flash score" decreased by 50% in the fluoxetine arm versus 36% in the placebo arm.[9] In a similar study of 191 women treated with venlafaxine, hot flash scores were reduced 27% in the placebo arm and 61% in the 150 mg of venlafaxine arm.[8] It was a study of this type using paroxetine that led to the recognition of a potent active metabolite of tamoxifen and focused attention squarely on CYP2D6 and its pharmacogenomic variation as a potentially important factor in variation in response to tamoxifen therapy among patients with breast cancer.[7,10]

At that time, it was believed that the most therapeutically relevant tamoxifen metabolite was 4-hydroxytamoxifen—which was approximately 100 times as potent as the parent drug in its effect on the estrogen receptor.[18,19] Two studies published by Stearns and coworkers in 2003 were designed to test the hypothesis that paroxetine might be useful in the treatment of hot flashes in patients treated with tamoxifen.[7,10] The approach taken in those studies utilized a "drug metabolism perspective", with the use of HPLC assays of tamoxifen and its metabolites based, in part, on the hypothesis the SSRIs might compete for and inhibit CYP2D6-catalyzed tamoxifen hydroxylation. Those investigators observed a metabolite that resulted from both 4-hydroxylation and N-demethylation—a metabolite that they named "endoxifen".[7] As shown in Figure 1, the formation of 4-hydroxytamoxifen and endoxifen is catalyzed predominantly by CYP2D6, while the N-demethylation step is catalyzed by CYP3A4/5. These were important observations because CYP2D6 is one of the most genetically polymorphic and one of the most intensively studied drug-metabolizing enzymes in all of pharmacogenomics.[20]

The gene encoding CYP2D6 includes functionally significant single nucleotide polymorphisms (SNPs); but the gene can also be deleted and it can undergo amplification, with up to 13 active copies.[20] Prior to the cloning and characterization of the *CYP2D6* gene, its genetic variation was explored by the use of "pro-drugs" such as the antihypertensive agent debrisoquine. In those studies, debrisoquine would be administered to a group of subjects and its CYP2D6-catalyzed 4-hydroxylation was monitored by assaying urinary 4-hydroxydebrisiquine and expressing the results as a "metabolic ratio", in which the parent drug concentration was divided by the concentration of the metabolite. Figure 2 shows debrisoquine "metabolic ratios" for 1,011 subjects studied at the Karolinska Institute.[21] At the far-right of the frequency distribution histogram the metabolic ratios for "poor metabolizers" (PMs)—subjects who either have inactive enzyme or the deletion of the *CYP2D6* gene—are shown, with a group of "extensive" metabolizers (EMs) in the center and, at the far-left, are data for ultra-rapid metabolizers (UMs)—some of whom have multiple

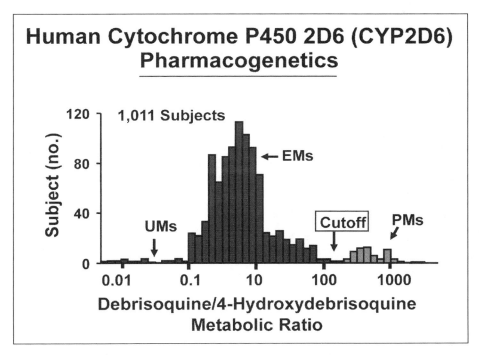

Figure 2. CYP2D6 pharmacogenetics. The figure shows the ratio of urinary debrisoquine to its metabolite, 4-hydroxydebrisoquine, in 1011 Swedish subjects. The formation of 4-hydroxydebrisoquine is catalyzed by CYP2D6. "PM" is "poor metabolizer"; "EM" is "extensive metabolizer"; and "UM" is "ultrarapid metabolizer". "Cutoff" is the demarcation between PMs and EMs (Reprinted by permission from Macmillan Publishers Ltd: Bertilsson L, Lou YQ, Du YL et al. Clin Pharmacol Ther 1992; 51:388-397.)

copies of the CYP2D6 gene. The next question addressed for tamoxifen was whether endoxifen was an active metabolite and whether its formation could be inhibited by other CYP2D6 substrates such as the SSRIs.

Stearns et al not only detected significant concentrations of endoxifen in the blood of patients treated with tamoxifen,[7] but this same group of investigators also showed that circulating endoxifen concentrations were reduced by paroxetine treatment.[7,22] Later studies demonstrated that plasma endoxifen concentrations were decreased by the administration of other SSRIs (Fig. 3)—in direct proportion to their metabolism by CYP2D6, i.e., these drugs could inhibit the formation of active metabolites of tamoxifen.[23] It was also demonstrated that endoxifen was an active metabolite that inhibited estradiol-stimulated MCF-7 cell proliferation.[7] Subsequent expression array studies showed that endoxifen had effects on global expression patterns in MCF-7 cells that were similar to those of 4-hydroxytamoxifen.[13] In addition, endoxifen concentrations in women treated with tamoxifen were approximately an order of magnitude higher than were 4-hydroxytamoxifen concentrations—indicating that endoxifen and not the 4-hydroxylated compound, might be the major active metabolite.[7,23] However, the formation of both 4-hydroxytamoxifen and endoxifen required CYP2D6. That fact raised a critical question with regard to the therapeutic efficacy of tamoxifen in the 5-8% of the Caucasian population who are relatively unable to catalyze the reaction required to form these active metabolites.[20] That question was addressed in a study of 94 patients on tamoxifen therapy who were genotyped for common variant CYP2D6 alleles. Those genotype-phenotype correlation data are depicted graphically in Figure 4 which shows the relationship between *CYP2D6* genotype and circulating endoxifen concentrations.[23] Patients without *CYP2D6* genes capable of encoding active enzyme has decreased endoxifen levels. The next

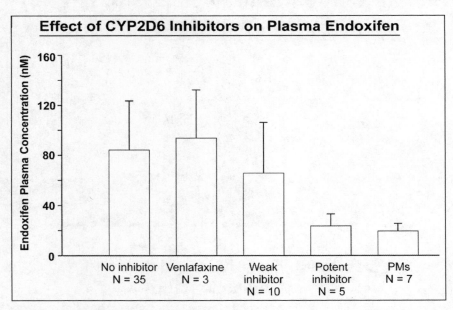

Figure 3. Effect of drugs that are CYP2D6 inhibitors on plasma endoxifen concentrations after 4 months of tamoxifen (20 mg/d). Bars represent mean ± SD. From left to right, the groups are composed of CYP2D6 EM/EMs who were taking neither CYP2D6 inhibitors nor venlafaxine, EM/EMs who were receiving venlafaxine, EM/EMs who were treated with drugs that are CYP2D6 inhibitors, EM/EMs who were receiving "potent" CYP2D6 inhibitors and PM/PMs who were not taking any CYP2D6 inhibitors (Reprinted by permission from Macmillan Publishers Ltd: Borges S, Desta Z, Li L et al. Clin Pharmacol Ther 2006; 80(1):61-74.)

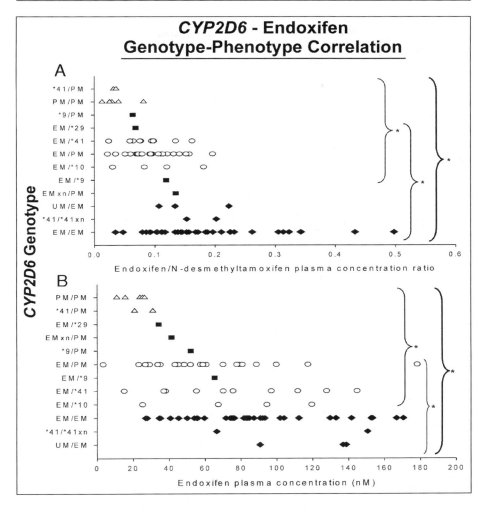

Figure 4. *CYP2D6*-endoxifen genotype-phenotype correlation. (A) Association of *CYP2D6* genotype with endoxifen/N-desmethyltamoxifen ratio in 94 breast cancer patients after 4 months of tamoxifen treatment (20 mg/d) without concomitant CYP2D6 inhibitors. Genotype groups are ranked on the basis of their mean values, from lowest (top) to highest (bottom). Genotypes represented by only one patient were excluded from group comparisons. Triangles indicate patients without any fully functional *CYP2D6* allele (mean, 0.04 ± 0.02), circles indicate patients carrying only one fully functional *CYP2D6* allele (mean, 0.09 ± 0.04), diamonds indicate patients with two or more copies of any functional or dysfunctional *CYP2D6* allele (mean, 0.18 ± 0.09) and squares indicate patients excluded from the group comparisons. * = $P < .001$. (B) Association of *CYP2D6* genotype with endoxifen concentration in the same breast cancer patients pictured in (A). Triangles indicate patients without any fully functional *CYP2D6* allele (mean, 21.9 ± 6.8 nmol/L), circles indicate patients with only one fully functional *CYP2D6* allele (mean, 64.2 ± 38.2 nmol/L), diamonds indicate patients with two or more copies of any functional or dysfunctional *CYP2D6* allele (mean, 88.6 ± 39.6 nmol/L) and squares indicate patients excluded from the group comparisons. * = $P < .05$ (Reprinted by permission from Macmillan Publishers Ltd: Borges S, Desta Z, Li L et al. Clin Pharmacol Ther 2006; 80(1):61-74.)

question to be addressed was whether there might be a relationship between CYP2D6 genotype and clinically relevant endpoints such as disease-free survival after the treatment of breast cancer with tamoxifen.

It would have taken years to complete prospective trials to test the hypothesis that tamoxifen response in patients with breast cancer might be influenced by *CYP2D6* genotype. Fortunately, paraffin block breast cancer tissue from which DNA could be extracted was available from previous tamoxifen clinical trials—many of which were initiated in the mid- or late-1980s. As a result, a series of retrospective studies was performed using that type of material. The results of the first of those studies, a study based on an NCI North Central Cancer Treatment Group (NCCTG) trial initiated in the 1980s, showed that patients with the most common "loss of function" *CYP2D6* allele, *CYP2D6*4*, had less favorable outcomes than did patients with the "wild type" genotype (Fig. 5).[14] Those results were confirmed by data for a small group of patients included in the Italian Tamoxifen Trial.[15] A recent follow-up study of these same NCCTG patients indicated that women who were treated with drugs that could compete for CYP2D6-catalyzed metabolism, drugs such as fluoxetine, also had a higher frequency of disease recurrence.[16] These reports stimulated a flurry of editorial comment,[24-27] review articles[28-30] and, in October 2006—US Food and Drug Administration (FDA) public hearings on the possible inclusion of CYP2D6 pharmacogenomic data in tamoxifen labeling.[25]

After those public hearings, the Clinical Pharmacology Subcommittee of the FDA Advisory Committee for Pharmaceutical Science recommended that tamoxifen labeling should inform prescribers that patients who are CYP2D6 "poor metabolizers" have an increased risk for disease recurrence.[25] They also recommended that the label should warn that certain antidepressants can inhibit a patient's ability to metabolize tamoxifen to form active metabolites.[25] It should be noted that these original positive studies were retrospective and that their results remain the subject of controversy. That is true because two retrospective studies published by a Swedish group reported not only that *CYP2D6*4* was not a risk factor for breast cancer recurrence, but that this genotype was actually protective—although the results were not statistically significant.[31,32] In addition, a retrospective study from the United States failed to observe a relationship between *CYP2D6* genotype and clinical outcome in breast cancer patients treated with tamoxifen.[33] However, a very recent study from Germany that genotyped additional *CYP2D6* alleles which are associated with decreased enzyme function confirmed and extended the original observations that genotypes with lower CYP2D6 enzyme activity are associated with poorer clinical outcomes in breast cancer patients treated with tamoxifen.[34]

In summary, tamoxifen illustrates the potential clinical importance of pharmacogenomics—as well as the challenges involved in "translating" this type of biomedical research into the clinic. It also raises a series of important questions. First, all of the present clinical data for tamoxifen pharmacogenomics were obtained (for obvious practical reasons) from retrospective studies, so this area of research cries out for a carefully designed prospective study. Second, all of the clinical data available thus far were obtained from Caucasian subjects and there are many examples of ethnic variation in pharmacogenomic response,[1] so studies in additional ethnic groups will be required. Not surprisingly, there have already been publications in which the ethical aspects of genomic testing for *CYP2D6* have been examined,[35] and this entire discussion needs to be placed within a context in which the development of aromatase inhibitors presents a practical alternative to tamoxifen therapy—at least in postmenopausal women. That is, have these pharmacogenomic results appeared too late in the "life span" of tamoxifen to be of any practical value or clinical relevance?[26] No matter what the answers to these questions might be, the tamoxifen "story" serves to demonstrate both the potential clinical importance of pharmacogenomics and the many challenges that we face if this aspect of personalized medicine is to move to the bedside—for even a single gene. It also brings us to the topic of aromatase inhibitors. What is known with regard to possible pharmacogenomic variation in clinical response to this class of drugs?

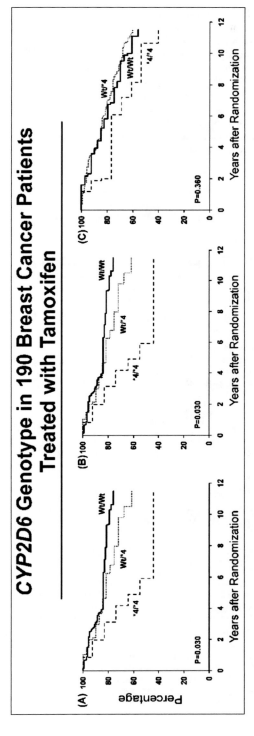

Figure 5. Kaplan-Meier curves for 190 women with breast cancer who were treated with tamoxifen and were genotyped for *CYP2D6*4*. Wt = wild type. (A) Relapse-free time, (B) disease-free survival and (C) overall survival for patients with the *CYP2D6* genotypes indicated (modified from Goetz MP, Rae JM, Suman VJ et al. J Clin Oncol 2005; 23(36):9312-9318.)

Aromatase Inhibitor Pharmacogenomics

The third generation aromatase inhibitors are much newer drugs than is tamoxifen.[36,37] Therefore, less is known with regard to the possible influence of inheritance on the pharmacokinetics or pharmacodynamics of letrozole, anastrozole and exemestane than is known with regard to tamoxifen. Although aromatase inhibitors, like tamoxifen, undergo biotransformation catalyzed by a variety of cytochromes P450,[36] there is currently no information with regard to the possibility that inherited variation in their metabolism or transport, i.e., their pharmacokinetics, might result in clinically relevant variation in their clinical effect. As in the case for tamoxifen, the question of greatest importance is whether inherited variation might influence outcomes relevant to the treatment of breast cancer (e.g., disease-free survival) and that type of study would require years to complete. In addition, these drugs are very potent and are used to treat postmenopausal women who already have very low circulating estrogen levels. Therefore, although there are data which indicate that individual differences in drug effect (inhibition of estrogen biosynthesis) occurs, no comprehensive studies of the effect of inheritance on the ability of third generation aromatase inhibitors to alter hormone levels have been published. However, as a step toward studies of the possible effects of inheritance on aromatase inhibitor "pharmacodynamics", resequencing of the

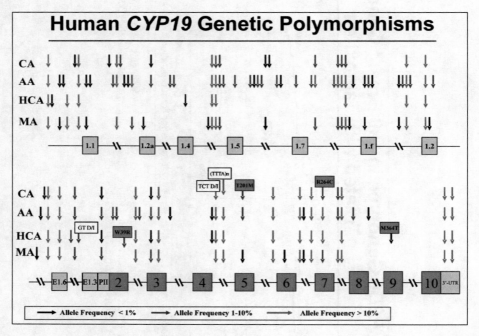

Figure 6. Human *CYP19* genetic polymorphisms. The figure shows a schematic representation of the *CYP19* gene structure, with arrows indicating the locations of polymorphisms in 60 DNA samples each from African-American (AA), Caucasian-American (CA), Han Chinese-American (HCA) and Mexican-American (MA) subjects. Orange rectangles represent the open reading frame and light blue rectangles represent untranslated regions. Red arrows represent minor allele frequencies (MAFs) greater than 10%; dark blue arrows frequencies from 1 to 10% and black arrows polymorphisms with MAFs of less than 1%. "I/D" indicates an insertion/deletion event. The GT and TTC I/D polymorphisms and the variable number of tandem repeat (TTTA)n polymorphism, as well as amino acids changes resulting from nonsynonymous cSNPs, are also indicated (modified from Ma CX, Adjei AA, Salavaggione OE et al. Cancer Res 2005; 65(23):11071-11082.)

gene encoding the target for these drugs, CYP19, aromatase, has been performed.[38] Specifically, *CYP19* was resequenced using 60 DNA samples (120 alleles) each from African-American, Caucasian-American, Han Chinese-American and Mexican-American subjects (Fig. 6). A total of 88 genetic polymorphisms, including four nonsynonymous coding single nucleotide polymorphisms (SNPs) that altered the encoded amino acid sequence, were identified.[38]

These *CYP19* gene resequencing studies were intended as a first step toward a determination of whether genetic variation in the target for these drugs might influence response to treatment with aromatase inhibitors. There is already a precedent for thinking that that type of effect can occur. That precedent involves the oral anticoagulant warfarin, a widely prescribed but potentially dangerous drug with a narrow therapeutic index, i.e., the difference between the therapeutic and toxic dose is small. Inherited variation in the gene encoding the target for warfarin and other coumarin-based anticoagulants, vitamin K oxidoreductase C1 (*VKORC1*), has been shown to have a striking effect on the dose of this drug required to achieve a target INR (the international normalized ratio, the universally used measure of the anticoagulant effect of this class of drugs).[39] Up to now, genetic polymorphisms in the aromatase gene, *CYP19*, have been genotyped predominantly to test their possible association with risk for diseases such as breast cancer, but they have not been studied systematically for a possible association with variation in response to treatment with aromatase inhibitors. The example provided by pharmacogenomic studies of tamoxifen and warfarin, among others, will undoubtedly serve as a "roadmap" for similar studies designed to test the hypothesis that individual variation in the sequence or structure of genes encoding proteins involved in the metabolism or transport of aromatase inhibitors—or in the gene encoding the target for these drugs—might contribute to variation in aromatase inhibitor response. The drug response phenotypes that might display individual variation include not only measures of drug efficacy, but also adverse drug reactions, in the case of aromatase inhibitors osteoporosis or musculoskeletal symptoms.[36,37]

Conclusions and Future Directions

Tamoxifen provides a striking example of the potential clinical relevance of pharmacogenomics. Although significant questions remain to be addressed with regard to tamoxifen pharmacogenomics and although the clinical application of genotyping for *CYP2D6* prior to the initiation of tamoxifen therapy remains controversial, there is a growing consensus, supported by a US FDA review panel, that genotyping might contribute to therapeutic decisions with regard to the adjuvant therapy of breast cancer. There is also a clear consensus that the treatment of patients on tamoxifen with drugs that are inhibitors of CYP2D6 should be discouraged.[25]

Tamoxifen is one of only four drugs for which the FDA has held public hearings with regard to the possible inclusion of pharmacogenomic information in labeling (see http://www.fda.gov). The first hearings involved thiopurine drugs such as 6-mercaptopurine and genetic variation in the thiopurine S-methyltransferase (*TPMT*) gene. *TPMT* polymorphisms are associated with life-threatening myelosuppression after exposure to "standard" doses of these drugs.[40] The second hearings involved another cytotoxic antineoplastic agent, irinotecan. The active metabolite of this anticancer drug is metabolized by glucuronidation catalyzed by UGT1A1 and the *UGT1A1 *28* variant allele that is associated with Gilbert's syndrome results in decreased irinotecan metabolism and increased toxicity, particularly diarrhea and myelosuppression.[41] The third example selected for public hearings was warfarin and genetic variation in both the warfarin-metabolizing enzyme CYP2C9 and the drug target, VKORC1. In the case of warfarin, the focus was on preventing both drug toxicity, hemorrhage and lack of the desired therapeutic effect. The fact that the FDA included tamoxifen among this highly select group of drugs is telling. It is also important to note that three of these four examples of the potential clinical relevance of pharmacogenomics involve drugs used in the treatment of cancer and all three involve polymorphisms in germline DNA. It is necessary to emphasize that fact because a bias exists in some quarters that the only genetic variation of importance in the treatment of cancer is variation involving somatic DNA in the tumor. Obviously, the tumor genome is important but, as demonstrated by this list, so is germline DNA, at least with regard to variation in drug response. It should also be emphasized that tamoxifen is the only member of this group for which the focus was squarely on genetic variation in efficacy rather than risk for toxicity, although pharmacogenomics might also provide insight into the possible contribution of inheritance to risk for the occurrence of serious tamoxifen side effects including thromboembolism or risk for endometrial cancer. Finally, the fact that the warfarin example involves two genes, *CYP2C9* on the pharmacokinetic (PK) side and *VKORC1* involving pharmacodynamics (PD), is a hint of possible future directions for pharmacogenomic studies of drugs used to treat breast cancer.

Pharmacogenomics, as a discipline, is rapidly moving beyond studies of single genes like *CYP2D6* to focus on entire pathways, pathways that include both PK and PD, as well as to genome-wide association studies. When genome-wide association studies have been applied to complex phenotypes such as risk for diseases like diabetes[42-44] and breast cancer,[45] multiple genes that could not have been anticipated are found to be associated with individual variation in disease risk. A similar approach is currently being applied to drug response phenotypes and is certain to be applied to complex therapeutic situations such as the endocrine therapy of breast cancer. Within that context, the "story" of tamoxifen and CYP2D6 represents only a first step toward truly individualized endocrine therapy of this important neoplastic disease.

Acknowledgements

Supported in part by National Institutes of Health (NIH) grants R01 GM28157, R01 GM35720, R24 GM078233 "The Metabolomics Research Network", U01 GM61388 "The Pharmacogenetics Research Network", P50CA116201 "The Mayo Clinic Breast Cancer SPORE" and a PhRMA Foundation Center of Excellence in Clinical Pharmacology Award. We thank Luanne Wussow for her assistance with the preparation of this chapter.

References

1. Weinshilboum RM, Wang L. Pharmacogenetics and pharmacogenomics: development, science and translation. Annu Rev Genomics Hum Genet 2006; 7:223-245.
2. Hayes DF. Why endocrine therapy? In: Miller WR, Ingle JN, eds. Endocrine Therapy in Breast Cancer. New York: Marcel Dekker, Inc; 2002:3-14.
3. Weinshilboum RM. The therapeutic revolution. Clin Pharmacol Ther 1987; 42:481-484.
4. Venter JC, Adams MD, Myers EW et al. The sequence of the human genome. Science 2001; 291:1304-1351 [Erratum, Science 2001; 1292:1838].
5. Lander ES, Linton LM, Birren B et al. Initial sequencing and analysis of the human genome. Nature 2001; 409:860-921 [Errata, Nature 2001; 2411:2720, 2412:2565].
6. Weinshilboum R. Inheritance and drug response. New Engl J Med 2003; 348:529-537.
7. Stearns V, Johnson MD, Rae JM et al. Active tamoxifen metabolite plasma concentrations after coadministration of tamoxifen and the selective serotonin reuptake inhibitor paroxetine. J Natl Cancer Inst 2003; 85(23):1758-1764.
8. Loprinzi CL, Kugler JW, Sloan JA et al. Venlafaxine in management of hot flashes in survivors of breast cancer: a randomised controlled trial. Lancet 2000; 356(9257):2059-2063.
9. Loprinzi CL, Sloan JA, Perez EA et al. Phase III evaluation of fluoxetine for treatment of hot flashes. J Clin Oncol 2002; 20(6):1578-1583.
10. Stearns V, Beebe KL, Iyengar M et al. Paroxetine controlled release in the treatment of menopausal hot flashes: a randomized controlled trial. JAMA 2003; 289(21):2827-2834.
11. Johnson MD, Zuo H, Lee KH et al. Pharmacological characterization of 4-hydroxy-N-desmethyl tamoxifen, a novel active metabolite of tamoxifen. Breast Cancer Res Treat 2004; 85(2):151-159.
12. Lim YC, Desta Z, Flockhart DA et al. Endoxifen (4-hydroxy-N-desmethyl-tamoxifen) has anti-estrogenic effects in breast cancer cells with potency similar to 4-hydroxy-tamoxifen. Cancer Chemother Pharmacol 2005; 55(5):471-478.
13. Lim YC, Li L, Desta Z et al. Endoxifen, a secondary metabolite of tamoxifen and 4-OH-tamoxifen induce similar changes in global gene expression patterns in MCF-7 breast cancer cells. J Pharmacol Exp Ther 2006; 318(2):503-512.
14. Goetz MP, Rae JM, Suman VJ et al. Pharmacogenetics of tamoxifen biotransformation is associated with clinical outcomes of efficacy and hot flashes. J Clin Oncol 2005; 23(36):9312-9318.
15. Bonanni B, Macis D, Maisonneuve P et al. Polymorphism in the CYP2D6 tamoxifen-metabolizing gene influences clinical effect but not hot flashes: data from the Italian Tamoxifen Trial. J Clin Oncol 2006; 24(22):3708-3709.
16. Goetz MP, Knox SK, Suman VJ et al. The impact of cytochrome P450 2D6 metabolism in women receiving adjuvant tamoxifen. Breast Cancer Res Treat 2007; 101(1):113-121.

17. Hoda D, Perez DG, Loprinzi CL. Hot flashes in breast cancer survivors. Breast J 2003; 9(5):431-438.
18. Coezy E, Borgna JL, Rochefort H. Tamoxifen and metabolites in MCF7 cells: correlation between binding to estrogen receptor and inhibition of cell growth. Cancer Res 1982; 42(1):317-323.
19. Jordan VC. Metabolites of tamoxifen in animals and man: identification, pharmacology and significance. Breast Cancer Res Treat 1982; 2(2):123-138.
20. Rodriguez-Antona C, Ingelman-Sundberg M. Cytochrome P450 pharmacogenetics and cancer. Oncogene 2006; 25(11):1679-1691.
21. Bertilsson L, Lou YQ, Du YL et al. Pronounced differences between native Chinese and Swedish populations in the polymorphic hydroxylations of debrisoquin and S-mephenytoin. Clin Pharmacol Ther 1992; 51:388-397 [Erratum, Clin Pharmacol Ther 1994; 1955:1648].
22. Jin Y, Desta Z, Stearns V et al. CYP2D6 genotype, antidepressant use and tamoxifen metabolism during adjuvant breast cancer treatment. J Natl Cancer Inst 2005; 97(1):30-39.
23. Borges S, Desta Z, Li L et al. Quantitative effect of CYP2D6 genotype and inhibitors on tamoxifen metabolism: implication for optimization of breast cancer treatment. Clin Pharmacol Ther 2006; 80(1):61-74.
24. Garber K. Tamoxifen pharmacogenetics moves closer to reality. J Natl Cancer Inst 2005; 97(6):412-413.
25. Young D. Genetics examined in tamoxifen's effectivness. Am J Health Syst Pharm 2006; 63(23):2286, 2296.
26. Van Poznak CH, Hayes DF. Aromatase inhibitors for the treatment of breast cancer: is tamoxifen of historical interest only? J Natl Cancer Inst 2006; 98(18):1261-1263.
27. Takimoto CH. Can tamoxifen therapy be optimized for patients with breast cancer on the basis of CYP2D6 activity assessments? Nat Clin Pract Oncol 2007; 4(3):152-153.
28. Choi JY, Nowell SA, Blanco JG et al. The role of genetic variability in drug metabolism pathways in breast cancer prognosis. Pharmacogenomics 2006; 7(4):613-624.
29. Marsh S, McLeod HL. Pharmacogenetics and oncology treatment for breast cancer. Expert Opin Pharmacother 2007; 8(2):119-127.
30. Beverage JN, Sissung TM, Sion AM et al. CYP2D6 polymorphisms and the impact on tamoxifen therapy. J Pharm Sci 2007; 96(9):2224-2231.
31. Wegman P, Vainikka L, Stål O et al. Genotype of metabolic enzymes and the benefit of tamoxifen in postmenopausal breast cancer patients. Breast Cancer Res 2005; 7(3):R284-R290.
32. Wegman P, Elingarami S, Carstensen J et al. Genetic variants of CYP3A5, CYP2D6, SULT1A1, UGT2B15 and tamoxifen response in postmenopausal patients with breast cancer. Breast Cancer Res 2007; 9(1):R7.
33. Nowell SA, Ahn J, Rae JM et al. Association of genetic variation in tamoxifen-metabolizing enzymes with overall survival and recurrence of disease in breast cancer patients. Breast Cancer Res Treat 2005; 91(3):249-258.
34. Schroth W, Antoniadou L, Fritz P et al. Breast cancer treatment outcome with adjuvant tamoxifen in relation to patient CYP2D6 and CYP2C19 genotypes. J Clin Oncol 2007; in press.
35. Hartman AR, Helft P. The ethics of CYP2D6 testing for patients considering tamoxifen. Breast Cancer Res 2007; 9(2):103.
36. Smith IE, Dowsett M. Aromatase inhibitors in breast cancer. N Engl J Med 2003; 348(24):2431-2442.
37. Swain SM. Aromatase inhibitors—a triumph of translational oncology. N Engl J Med 2005; 353(26):2807-2809.
38. Ma CX, Adjei AA, Salavaggione OE et al. Human aromatase: gene resequencing and functional genomics. Cancer Res 2005; 65(23):11071-11082.
39. Rieder MJ, Reiner AP, Gage BF et al. Effect of VKORC1 haplotypes on transcriptional regulation and warfarin dose. N Engl J Med 2005; 352(22):2285-2293.
40. Wang L, Weinshilboum RM. Thiopurine S-methyltransferase (TPMT) pharmacogenetics: insights, challenges and future directions. Oncogene Rev 2006; 25(11):1629-1938.
41. Innocenti F, Ratain MJ. "Irinogenetics" and UGT1A: from genotypes to haplotypes. Clin Pharmacol Ther 2004; 75(6):495-500.
42. Zeggini E, Weedon MN, Lindgren CM et al. Replication of genome-wide association signals in UK samples reveals risk loci for type 2 diabetes. Science 2007; 316(5829):1336-1341.
43. Scott LJ, Mohlke KL, Bonnycastle LL et al. A genome-wide association study of type 2 diabetes in Finns detects multiple susceptibility variants. Science 2007; 316(5829):1341-1345.
44. Diabetes Genetics Initiative of Broad Institute of Harvard and MIT, Lund University, Novartis Institutes of BioMedical Research et al. Genome-wide association analysis identifies loci for type 2 diabetes and triglyceride levels. Science 2007; 316(5829):1331-1336.
45. Easton DF, Pooley KA, Dunning AM et al. Genome-wide association study identifies novel breast cancer susceptibility loci. Nature 2007; 447(7148):1087-1093.
46. Desta Z, Ward BA, Soukhova NV et al. Comprehensive evaluation of tamoxifen sequential biotransformation by the human cytochrome P450 system in vitro: prominent roles for CYP3A and CYP2D6. J Pharmacol Exp Ther 2004; 310(3):1062-1075.

CHAPTER 15

Prevention of Breast Cancer Using SERMs

Trevor J. Powles*

Abstract

The development of breast cancer is dependant in part on oestrogen. Suppression of ovarian function or use of anti-oestrogens will reduce the incidence of breast cancer. Many trials have now been done involving tens of thousands of healthy women evaluating the use of selective oestrogen receptor modulators to reduce the risk of breast cancer in healthy women. Tamoxifen will reduce the early incidence of breast cancer in pre and postmenopausal women by about 40% but causes vasomotor symptoms, thromboembolism and gynaecological toxicity including polyps, endometrial atypia and rarely cancer. In long follow up trials the risk reduction for breast cancer extends beyond the treatment period out to at least 15 years appearing to get larger with time indicating a true long term prevention effect. The toxicity of tamoxifen is for the most part confined to the treatment period. Raloxifene also has similar breast cancer risk reduction activity to tamoxifen but has less toxicity with no evidence of an increased risk of endometrial atypia or cancer. Tamoxifen is licensed for breast cancer risk reduction in the USA and raloxifene has also recently been approved by the FDA for such use.

Introduction

Of all of the common cancers, breast cancer has provided one of the best opportunities for prevention because of the important involvement of oestrogen in its development. Early ovarian failure can substantially reduce the incidence of breast cancer,[1] but this is associated with the many associated problems of an early menopause. Another approach is to use a selective oestrogen receptor modulator (SERM) such as tamoxifen or raloxifene. Tamoxifen, used as adjuvant treatment in women with operable breast cancer has been clearly shown to reduce the incidence of second breast cancers[2] and tamoxifen has been shown to prevent oestrogen dependant tumours in rats.[3] Clinical trials of tamoxifen started in 1986 and raloxifene in 1994 followed by trials of other SERMs such as arzoxifene and lasoxifene. Nearly 100,000 healthy women have now been randomized into these trials. The results have been variable.

Tamoxifen Trials

The NSABP1 Trial

This trial included healthy pre and postmenopausal women with a risk of breast cancer of >1.65% over 5 years based on the Gail model,[4] randomized to tamoxifen 20 mg per day or placebo. Hormone replacement therapy (HRT) was not allowed for entry and women who started HRT were withdrawn from the trial and their data censored at that time. After a median follow up of 54 months a very significant 49% (p = 0.00001) reduction in the incidence of in invasive

*Trevor J. Powles—Parkside Oncology Clinic London, UK.
PA: Hilary Dummer Email: hilary.dummer@parkside-hospital.co.uk

Innovative Endocrinology of Cancer, edited by Lev M. Berstein and Richard J. Santen.
©2008 Landes Bioscience and Springer Science+Business Media.

breast carcinoma was reported, this reduction only occurring for oestrogen receptor (ER) positive cancers.[5] On the basis of this result the trial was unblinded in 1998 and participants on placebo offered tamoxifen. Analysis of further follow up showed a 43% reduction although this result may have been compromised by the unblinding.[6]

The IBIS1 Trial

This trial recruited healthy women at increased risk of breast cancer usually because of a family history. Participants were randomized to tamoxifen 20 mg per day or placebo but allowed HRT during the trial. After a median follow up of 50 months, there was a risk reduction of 32% but for invasive cancers this was not significant.[7] A recent update of this trial now shows a 27% reduction (p = 0.004) in all breast cancers. There was no benefit for oestrogen receptor negative (ER –ve) cancers but for ER +ve invasive cancers there was a 34% reduction which extended out to at least 10 years indicating a spillover benefit after the medication period.[8] This benefit was not apparent for women who used HRT during the trial.

The Italian Trial

The Italian National trial recruited women who were not at special risk of breast cancer but who had had a hysterectomy and also for the most part bilateral ovariectomy. Participants were randomized to tamoxifen 20 mg per day or placebo for 5 years. Use of HRT was allowed. The initial report after a median follow up of 81.2 mo showed no risk reduction with tamoxifen.[9] The trial remained blinded and after an average follow up of over 11 years, the incidence of all invasive and ER +ve invasive cancers was similar for the two treatment groups. There was a reduction for women who had not had ovariectomy and for those who received HRT indicating that loss of ovarian function before entry into the trial compromised the risk reduction effect of tamoxifen unless the women received HRT.

The Royal Marsden Trial

The Royal Marsden trial started in 1986 recruiting healthy women with a strong family history of breast cancer to tamoxifen 20 mg per day or placebo for 8 years. The participants in the Royal Marsden trial were generally younger and at higher risk than the other tamoxifen prevention trials. Most were premenopausal at entry most of whom became postmenopausal during the trial follow up period. HRT was allowed. The trial was originally a pilot trial to evaluate the feasibility of using tamoxifen in a placebo controlled trial in healthy high risk women. Satisfactory accrual, compliance and toxicity allowed the trial to develop into a single centre trial which accrued 2,500 women.[10] The first efficacy analysis of this trial after 70 events in 1998 showed no reduction in breast cancer incidence.[11]

The trial has remained blinded and now has 20 years (median over 13 years) of follow up and over 200 breast cancers have occurred. Recent analysis shows now a significant 39% reduction in ER +ve cancers (HR = 0.61, 95% CI 0.43-0.86 P = 0.005). This risk reduction was not significant during the 8 year treatment period (Tamoxifen n = 30; Placebo n = 39; HR = 0.77 CI 0.48-1.23 p = 0.3) but highly significant in the post treatment period (Tamoxifen n = 23; Placebo n = 47; HR = 0.48 CI 0.29-0.79 p = 0.004). There was no evidence of any interaction between HRT use during the trial and the observed post treatment risk reduction with tamoxifen.

Risk reduction during treatment reported from the NSABP-P1 trial after an average period of about 4 years on treatment is likely to be treatment of occult primary cancers some of which may be curable with tamoxifen. In the Marsden trial we saw no on treatment effect which may be related to the high risk characteristics of the population of participants in the Marsden trial. The risk reduction confined to the post treatment period, with this long duration of follow up and with the effect appearing to increase with longer follow up would seem to indicate a true prevention effect.

Status of Tamoxifen for Prevention

In 1998, the FDA approved the use of tamoxifen for risk reduction of breast cancer in women at a risk of greater than 1.65% over 5 years on the Gail score based principally on the data from the NSABP-P1 trial. Following this, tamoxifen use for breast cancer risk reduction in healthy high risk women has been poor in the USA probably in part because of toxicity and in part because of conflicting results from the 4 trials. A meta-analysis of all four trials in 2003 showed that tamoxifen caused about a 40% reduction in early breast cancer risk, together with a significant reduction in osteoporotic fractures and serum cholesterol. This meta-analysis confirmed that tamoxifen caused significant toxicity including an increased risk of thromboembolism, vasomotor symptoms and gynaecological problems including vaginal discharge, uterine fibroids, endometrial atypia, polyps and cancer and the overall need for hysterectomy.[12]

These data were not sufficiently compelling to encourage the licensing of tamoxifen for breast cancer risk reduction in healthy women in Europe.

Raloxifene Trials

The MORE Trial

The results from the tamoxifen breast cancer prevention trials encouraged the evaluation in 1994 of another SERM, raloxifene as an antiosteoporotic agent in the Multiple Outcomes Relevant to Evista trial (MORE). Two doses of raloxifene versus placebo were evaluated in 7700 postmenopausal women with osteoporosis. The results after about 3 years follow up indicated a significant reduction in the risk of vertebral fractures (RR 0.7; 95% CI 0.5-0.8 for 60 mg/day raloxifene, RR 0.5; 95% CI 0.4-0.7 for 120 mg/day raloxifene) but not in the risk of non vertebral fractures (RR 0.9; 95% CI 0.8-1.1).[13] A secondary outcome in the trial was breast cancer incidence which was reduced by 72% at 4 years.[14] Because this was not a primary outcome in the trial, it was not considered acceptable as support for the licensing of the drug for breast cancer risk reduction in healthy women. An extension of the MORE trial was therefore proposed with breast cancer as the primary outcome.

The CORE Trial

The extension of the MORE trial, the Continuing Outcomes Relevant to Evista trial (CORE), with breast cancer as a primary outcome continued raloxifene 60 mg/day or placebo in 4400 of the original participants according to their original randomization. The results indicated a 66% breast cancer risk reduction after 8 years of follow up.[15] Overall toxicity was low with some evidence of an increase in the risk of thromboembolism but no evidence of any increase in gynaecological toxicity including endometrial polyps, atypia or carcinoma.

The RUTH Trial

Another placebo controlled raloxifene trial in non cancer volunteers, the Raloxifene Use for the Heart trial (RUTH) has been reported. This trial randomized 10101 postmenopausal women at high risk of cardiac events to raloxifene 60 mg/day or placebo. The results indicated a significant reduction in the incidence of invasive breast cancer (HR 0.56 95% CI 0.38-0.83) and clinical vertebral fractures (HR 0.65 95% CI 0.47-0.89) but no effect on the incidence of heart events. The toxicity profile was similar to the MORE and CORE trials. There was no difference in overall risk of death or the risk of death from cardiovascular causes. There was no difference in the overall risk of stroke although there was a reported increased incidence of fatal stroke (59 vs 39; HR 1.44; 95% CI 1.06-1.95).[16] There was no effect of raloxifene on the incidence of stroke in the MORE trial and it is possible that this increase in the incidence of fatal stroke in the RUTH trial is a chance observation. There has been previous reports of increased risk of stroke with tamoxifen similar to the increased risk of stroke with HRT.

The NSABP P2 Trial

The NSABP P2 trial started in 1999, randomized a total of 19,747 post menopausal women with a moderately high risk of developing invasive breast cancer (Gail risk >1.65% at 5 years) to tamoxifen 20 mg/day or raloxifene 60 mg/day for 5 years. The overall mean Gail score for these women was 4.03% ± 2.17%.[17]

The results showed the same incidence of invasive breast cancer for tamoxifen and raloxifene (RR 1.02; 95% CI 0.82-1.28) indicating that both are equally effective at reducing breast cancer risk. However for non invasive breast cancer the incidence is higher for women on raloxifene than tamoxifen signifying a possible lesser risk reduction benefit for this condition. The toxicity data confirmed the previous reports of low uterine toxicity for raloxifene with a significant reduction in the incidence of endometrial hyperplasia, atypia and the requirement for hysterectomy. Endometrial cancer was less for raloxifene than tamoxifen (RR 0.62; 95% CI 0.35-1.08) confirming the previous indirect comparisons from placebo controlled trials showing no increase in endometrial cancer risk with raloxifene. Other toxicities were significantly less with raloxifene versus tamoxifen including thromboembolic events (HR 0.70; 95% CI 0.54-0.91) and cataracts. There was no difference in the incidence of ischaemic heart disease, stroke, osteoporotic fractures, other cancers or death.

Summary of SERM Breast Cancer Risk Reduction Trials

The toxicity of tamoxifen, particularly the gynaecological problems limited its clinical use for breast cancer risk reduction in healthy women. Raloxifene has significantly less thromboembolic and gynaecological toxicity and is as equally effective as tamoxifen at reducing the risk of invasive breast cancer and osteoporotic vertebral fractures. It is therefore an attractive alternative to tamoxifen as a risk reducing agent for invasive breast cancer and vertebral fractures in postmenopausal women.

For prevention agents such as SERMs for use in healthy women, the toxicity profile must be very low, multiple benefits are needed and women at high risk for more than one benefit may be needed in order to achieve a balance of overall benefit. Raloxifene has two clinical benefits for healthy women by reducing the risks of breast cancer and osteoporotic fractures which may be of special benefit for women at high risk of breast cancer for example because of a strong family history who also are at high risk of vertebral fractures, because of previous fractures, family history or low BMD. An algorithm of risk and clinical characteristics needs to be developed so that the benefits with use of SERMs for breast cancer risk reduction can be maximised. More clinical research is needed to better identify those women at special risk of developing endocrine sensitive invasive breast cancers and women at high risk of developing vertebral fractures.

Conclusion

The results of the clinical trials of SERMs in healthy women to prevent breast cancer are encouraging. The meta-analysis of the tamoxifen trials has shown a 40% risk reduction over the first few year whilst still on treatment and the longer blinded follow up of the IBIS and the Royal Marsden trials has shown a post treatment risk reduction which appears to be getting larger with longer follow up. Furthermore the IBIS trial shows that most of the toxicity occurs while on treatment indicating that the therapeutic benefit is likely to substantially improve with longer follow up. Other therapeutic benefits from SERM therapy, particularly reduction in osteoporotic fractures may add to the therapeutic benefit. It is possible that a relatively short intervention with a SERM may give a long lasting, possibly a lifetime of breast cancer risk reduction.

References

1. Pike M, Krailo M. Hormonal risk factors, breast tissue age and the age-incidence of breast cancer. Nature 1983; 303:767-770.
2. Cuzick J, Baum M. Tamoxifen and contralateral breast cancer (Letter). Lancet 1985; ii:282.
3. Jordan V. Effect of tamoxifen (ICI 46,474) on initiation and growth of DMBA-induced rat mammary carcinomata. Eur J Cancer 1976; 12:419-425.

4. Gail M, Brinton L, Byar D et al. Projecting individualised probabilities of developing breast cancer for white females who are examined annually. J Natl Cancer Inst 1989; 81:1879-86.

5. Fisher B, Bryant J, Wolmark N et al. Effect of preoperative chemotherapy on the outcome of women with operable breast cancer. J Clin Oncol 1998; 16(8):2672-85.

6. Fisher B, Costantino J, Wickerham D et al. Tamoxifen for the prevention of breast cancer: current status of the National Surgical Adjuvant Breast and Bowel Project P-1 study. J Natl Cancer Inst 2005; 97(22):1652-62.

7. Cuzick J, Forbes J, Edwards R et al. First results from the International Breast Cancer Intervention Study (IBIS-I): a randomised prevention trial. Lancet 2002; 360:817-24.

8. Cuzick J, Forbes J, Sestak I et al. Long-term results of tamoxifen prophylaxis for breast cancer—96 month follow-up of the randomised IBIS-I study. J Natl Cancer Inst 2007; 99:272-282.

9. Veronesi U, Maisonneuve P, Costa A et al. Prevention of breast cancer with tamoxifen: preliminary findings from the Italian randomised trial among hysterectomised women. Lancet 1998; 352:93-97.

10. Powles T, Hardy J, Ashley S et al. A pilot trial to evaluate the acute toxicity and feasibility of tamoxifen for prevention of breast cancer. Br J Cancer 1989; 60:126-131.

11. Powles T, Eeles R, Ashley S et al. Interim analysis of the incidence of breast cancer in the Royal Marsden Hospital tamoxifen randomised chemoprevention trial. Lancet 1998; 352:98-101.

12. Cuzick J, Powles T, Veronesi U et al. Overview of the main outcomes in the breast cancer prevention trials. Lancet 2003; 361:296-300.

13. Ettinger B, Black D, Mitlak B et al. Reduction of vertebral fracture risk in postmenopausal women with osteoporosis treated with raloxifene: results from a 3-year randomized clinical trial. Multiple Outcomes of Raloxifene Evaluation (MORE) Investigators. JAMA 1999; 282(7):637-645.

14. Cummings S, Eckert S, Krueger K et al. The effect of raloxifene on risk of breast cancer in postmenopausal women. Results from the MORE randomized trial. JAMA 1999; 281:2189-2197.

15. Martino S, Cauley J, Barrett-Connor E et al. Continuing outcomes relevant to Evista: Breast cancer incidence in postmenopausal osteoporotic women in a randomized trial of raloxifene. J Natl Cancer Inst 2004; 96(23):1751-1761.

16. Barrett-Connor E, Mosca L, Collins P. Effects of raloxifene on cardiovascular events and breast cancer in postmenopausal women. N Engl J Med 2006; 355:125-137.

17. Vogel V, Costantino J, Wickerham D et al. Effects of tamoxifen vs raloxifene on the risk of developing invasive breast cancer and other disease outcomes—The NSABP study of tamoxifen and raloxifene (STAR) P-2 trial. JAMA 2006; 295:2727-2741.

GENERAL CONCLUSION

Now we have come to the conclusion of this book.

What kind of thoughts were brought on by finishing this book? Was it a sigh of relief or on the contrary, some sense of scientific satisfaction?

Believing in the latter, we think about future pathways along which tumor endocrinology will achieve improvement and perfection. Some of these tracks are shared with principles and further goals of general oncology and endocrinology—and others are more specific to the endocrinology of cancer. The more we understand the causes of hormone-associated cancers and mechanisms of tumor developments under the action of steroidal and peptide hormones, the greater the chance that earlier and more efficient diagnostics and targeted treatment of these carcinomas (both based on high-tech achievements including nanotechnological approaches) will occur. Comprehensive and comparative analysis of the evolutionary aspect of the problem will start a new era in the progress of this discipline. Last but not least, 'An ounce of prevention is worth a pound of cure'—a phrase attributed to Benjamin Franklin—is considered in medicine without exception as a real truth. Consequently we await commentary on advancements in the prevention of endocrine-related cancer and how these methods will be elaborated in the future.

In closing, we have high hopes for the new developments and new innovations in endocrinology of cancer.

Lev M. Berstein and Richard J. Santen

Innovative Endocrinology of Cancer, edited by Lev M. Berstein and Richard J. Santen.
©2008 Landes Bioscience and Springer Science+Business Media.

INDEX